Emergency War Surgery

THIRD UNITED STATES REVISION

2004

"All the circumstances of war surgery thus do violence to civilian concepts of traumatic surgery. The equality of organizational and professional management is the first basic difference. The second is the time lag introduced by the military necessity of evacuation. The third is the necessity for constant movement of the wounded man, and the fourth — treatment by a number of different surgeons at different places instead of by a single surgeon in one place — is inherent in the third. These are all undesirable factors, and on the surface they seem to militate against good surgical care. Indeed, when the over-all circumstances of warfare are added to them, they appear to make more ideal surgical treatment impossible. Yet this was not true in the war we have just finished fighting, nor need it ever be true. Short cuts and measures of expediency are frequently necessary in military surgery, but compromises with surgical adequacy are not."

—Michael E. DeBakey, MD
Presented at Massachusetts General Hospital
Boston, October 1946

Published by Books Express Publishing
Copyright © Books Express, 2011
ISBN 978-1-780391-84-7

Books Express publications are available from all good retail and online booksellers. For publishing proposals and direct ordering please contact us at: info@books-express.com

THE THIRD UNITED STATES REVISION

of

EMERGENCY WAR SURGERY

IS DEDICATED TO THE

COMBAT PHYSICIAN

Contents

Editorial & Production

Borden Institute
Walter Reed Army Medical Center
Washington, DC

Andy C. Szul
Developmental/Production Editor

Lorraine B. Davis
Production Editor

Bruce G. Maston
Illustrator/Layout Editor

Douglas Wise
Layout Editor

Linette R. Sparacino
Production Editor

Jessica Shull
Illustrator

Editors

Contributors

Keith Albertson, COL, MC, US Army
Rocco A. Armonda, LTC, MC, US Army
Kenneth S. Azarow, LTC, MC, US Army
Gary Benedetti, LTC, MC, FS, US Air Force
Ronald F. Bellamy, COL, US Army (Ret.)
William Beninati, LTC, MC, US Air Force
Matthew Brengman, MAJ, MC, US Army
David G. Burris, COL, MC, US Army
Frank Butler, CAPT, US Navy
Mark D. Calkins, MAJ, MC, US Army
Leopoldo C. Cancio, LTC, MC, US Army
David B. Carmacke, MAJ, MC, FS, US Air Force
Maren Chan, CPT, US Army
David J. Cohen, COL, MC, US Army
Jan A. Combs, MAJ, MC, US Army
Paul R. Cordts, COL, MC, US Army
Nicholas J. Cusolito, MAJ, NC, US Air Force
Paul J. Dougherty, LTC, MC, US Army
David C. Elliot, COL, MC, US Army
Martin L. Fackler, COL, MC, US Army (Ret.)
John J. Faillace, MAJ, MC, US Army
Gerald L. Farber, LTC, MC, US Army
Joseph B. FitzHarris, COL, MC, US Army
Stephen F. Flaherty, LTC, MC, US Army
Roman A. Hayda, LTC, MC, US Army
John B. Holcomb, COL, MC, US Army
Stephen P. Hetz, COL, MC, US Army
Jeffrey Hrutkay, COL, MC, US Army
Donald H. Jenkins, LTC, MC, US Air Force
James Jezior, LTC, MC, US Army
Christoph Kaufmann, COL, MC, US Army (Ret.)
Kimberly L. Kesling, LTC, MC, US Army
Thomas E. Knuth, COL, MC, US Army
Wilma I. Larsen, LTC, MC, US Army
George S. Lavenson, Jr., COL, MC, US Army (Ret.)
James J. Leech, COL, MC, US Army
Dave Ed. Lounsbury, COL, MC, US Army

Craig Manifold, MAJ, MC, US Air Force
Patrick Melder, MAJ, MC, US Army
Alan L. Moloff, COL, MC, US Army
Allen F. Morey, LTC, MC, US Army
Deborah Mueller, MAJ, MC, US Air Force
Peter Muskat, COL, MC, US Air Force
Mary F. Parker, LTC, MC, US Army
George Peoples, LTC, MC, US Army
Karen M. Phillips, LTC, MC, US Army
Ronald J. Place, LTC, MC, US Army
Paul Reynolds, COL, MC, US Army
Lawrence H. Roberts, CPT, MC, US Navy
David Salas, Msgt, US Air Force (Ret.)
Scott R. Steele, CPT, MC, US Army
Allen B. Thach, COL, MC, US Army Reserve
Johnny S. Tilman, COL, MC, US Army
John M. Uhorchak, COL, MC, US Army
Steven Venticinque, MAJ, MC, US Air Force
Ian Wedmore, LTC, MC, US Army

Acknowledgments

Sections of this Handbook underwent review and comment by COL Michael Deaton (for the Surgeon General's Integrated Process Team on detainee medical care), LTC Glenn Wortmann, LTC Chester Buckenmaier, LTC Peter Rhee, COL (USAF) William Dickerson, and MAJ Clayton D. Simon.

Mr. Roy D. Flowers and Mr. Ronald E. Wallace deserve thanks.

The interest, efforts, and selfless service of Dr. Matthew Brengman (formerly MAJ, MC), COL Stephen Hetz, and Dr. Paul Dougherty (formerly LTC, MC) superseded their written contributions, were above and beyond the call, and deserve especial recognition.

Dave Ed. Lounsbury, MD, FACP
Colonel, MC, US Army
Director, Borden Institute

Foreword

It is an honor for me to acknowledge the time, efforts, and experience collected in this third revision of *Emergency War Surgery*. Once again a team of volunteers representing the Military Health System and numerous clinical specialties has committed itself to delimiting state-of-the-art principles and practices of forward trauma surgery.

War surgery, and treatment of combat casualties at far forward locations and frequently under austere conditions, continue to save lives. Military medical personnel provide outstanding health support to those serving in harm's way. As the face of war continues to evolve, so must the practice of medicine, to support those who so selflessly fight the global war on terrorism. Today, American military men and women face a new terrain of mobile urban terrorism and conflict. Despite advances in personal and force protection provided to our forces, they remain vulnerable to blast wounds, burns, and multiple penetrating injuries not usually encountered in the traditional civilian setting. This publication expertly addresses the appropriate medical management of these and other battle and nonbattle injuries.

The editors of this edition are to be congratulated for drawing on the experiences of numerous colleagues recently returned from tours of duty in Southwest Asia in order to provide as current a handbook as possible.

I wish to publicly extend my gratitude, and that of the American people, to the courageous men and women who serve in the medical departments of our Armed Services. I commend your dedicated service and acknowledge your sacrifices, and those of your families, to provide the best health care attainable to those who protect our nation by their military service. I, and all Americans, are indebted to your service.

William Winkenwerder, Jr., MD
Assistant Secretary of Defense
for Health Affairs

Preface

It is time for another revision of the *Emergency War Surgery* (*EWS*) handbook! In addition to the fundamental advances in the management of victims of trauma since the 1988 edition, the format of the earlier versions was distinctly "user unfriendly."

This edition contains new material that updates the management of war wounds and is filled with over 150 specially drawn illustrations. Equally important is the use of an outline, bulleted format that is so much more concise than the verbosity of the previous editions. Additionally, emphasis in this edition is on the all-important "Emergency" in *Emergency War Surgery*—surgery performed at levels II and III —that constitutes the raison d'être for military surgery. Our intent is that if given a choice of bringing a **single** book on a rapid or prolonged deployment, today's military surgeon would choose this edition over any other trauma book.

The last revision of the *Emergency War Surgery* handbook was published in 1988. Since then, world events have profoundly affected how the US Armed Forces fight and how their medical services provide combat casualty care. The threat of a massive conventional war with the Soviet Union has been replaced by a new enemy: those who espouse global terrorism.

There are ongoing conflicts against terrorists in both Iraq and Afghanistan, under conditions that differ radically from Operations Desert Shield/Storm of 1990–1991. In Iraq there is continuous urban warfare against fanatics who hide amongst the civilian population, while in Afghanistan isolated and sporadic but fierce small unit actions take place in mountainous terrain. Both tactical scenarios are quite different from what occurred in Vietnam and Operation Desert Storm, and in what was expected for a European war against the Soviet Union upon which the 1988 edition was predicated.

Military surgeons must assume a leadership role in combat casualty care especially when faced by such changing conditions of practice. The physicians must know what to expect, and how to configure and prepare the team in an austere and rapidly changing tactical environment with available and necessary equipment. They must know how to take care of an unfamiliar battlefield wound or injury and manage mass casualties. Finally, they must understand the next echelon of care, including any available capabilities, and how to safely evacuate their patient to the higher level. This handbook provides much of the information needed to answer these questions.

One of the most dramatic ways in which military surgery differs from civilian trauma management is the staged provision of care; emergency surgery is carried out at one locale, while definitive and reconstructive surgeries take place at different sites. This traditional aspect of military surgery has found new meaning in the increasing use of damage control surgery for the most critically wounded. Here, the initial operation is designed only to prevent further blood loss and contamination after which resuscitation and completion of surgery takes place, sometimes at larger, more capable medical treatment facilities remote from the battlefield. The US Air Force's fielding of Critical Care Air Transport Teams (CCATT) has revolutionized casualty care by transporting such stabilized patients to higher levels of care during active resuscitation. Efforts to standardize equipment across services are in place, with the use of smaller, lightweight diagnostic and therapeutic devices. Joint interdependence in the treatment and evacuation of the wounded is now the cornerstone of combat casualty care.

As a result of such advances, the Army has been able to restructure field medical facilities essentially making them small and mobile "building blocks."

Despite the changes in the conditions of practice, a military surgeon is far more likely to be deployed today than at any other time in our nation's history since World War II. In the 1988 version of this handbook, BG Thomas E. Bowen quoted Plato about the likelihood of future conflict: "Only the dead have seen the end of war!" As military surgeons, will we be capable and prepared to render the level of combat casualty care befitting the sons and daughters of America? This revision of the *Emergency War Surgery* handbook provides the information needed to save the country's and military's most precious resource: our soldiers, sailors, airmen, and marines.

Kevin C. Kiley, MD
Lieutenant General, Medical Corps, US Army
The Surgeon General

Prologue

Although called the *Third United States Revision*, this issue of *Emergency War Surgery* represents an entirely new Handbook. Format, intent, and much of the content are new. None of the chapters of the Second Revision has been preserved verbatim. All material has been rewritten by new authors. Flowing prose has been largely replaced by a bulleted manual style in order to optimize the use of this Handbook as a rapid reference. Illustrations are featured much more prominently than in the earlier edition. Lastly, this text is widely available (perhaps even more so than the printed version) electronically on the World Wide Web and as a CD-ROM; a format neither available nor imaginable when the second Revision was released in 1988.

In 2000, the Surgeon General of the US Army called on the Medical Department to revise *Emergency War Surgery*, published in 1988 as the *Second United States Revision* and *Emergency War Surgery NATO Handbook*. Responsibility for this revision was given to the Senior Clinical Consultant in the Directorate of Combat and Doctrine Development. He then collaborated with the Surgeon General's Consultant (General Surgery) to develop a plan. These two called upon consultants from all the Services and established an Editorial Board of volunteers committed to a complete overhaul of the previous Handbook. Through a series of on-line and personal meetings coordinated by the Senior Clinical Consultant, format and content were established. All of the chapters were drafted and underwent review and edit by the assembled Board at Fort Sam Houston, Texas.

Following terrorist attacks of 11 September 2001 on the United States, US military forces were mobilized and deployed to Afghanistan in 2001 and Iraq in 2003. The process in place to complete this now essential Handbook was necessarily disrupted by reassignments and deployments of the very people who had volunteered to produce it. In lieu of a completed text, Borden Institute hastily published and distributed (on-line and CD) the unedited draft manuscripts then available as *Emergency War Surgery Handbook, 2003 Draft Version*. This issue saw wide use in Southwest Asia in 2003.

In winter 2003 – 2004 Borden Institute took up the task of completing a final version of the Handbook. With numerous surgeons returning from yearlong tours at Combat Support Hospitals and Forward Surgical Teams in Iraq and Afghanistan, the decision was made to seek timely comment on the draft manuscript. Several surgeons with fresh field experience volunteered their subspecialty review. Substantial updates and changes were made to many chapters including: Anesthesia, Shock and Resuscitation, Infections, Damage Control Surgery, Face & Neck Injuries, Extremity Fractures, Abdominal Injuries, Burn Injuries, and Head Injuries.

At the same time material drawn from a Department of Defense Task Force on detainee medical care (July 2004) was adapted for the Care of Enemy Prisoners of War / Internees chapter of this Handbook. The chapter on Triage was expanded to include consideration of combat stress casualties.

The result of this two-stage process is this Handbook. Its intent, and the single-minded determination of the contributors, is the retention of lessons learned from recent, as well as past, battlefield surgery. War surgery in the 21st Century is not a jury-rigged art of accommodation and compromises. Although it can include these, it is a science, grounded on fundamentals of trauma surgery, which recognizes as well the overriding unique principles of harsh and austere environments, mass casualty, blast and penetrating injury, multiple trauma, triage, staged resuscitation, damage control surgery, time, and aeromedical evacuation. The adage that these principles have to be relearned by every generation of military surgeon is probably less true than in the past. *Emergency War Surgery* is a safeguard to assure this.

Mais, plus ça change, plus c'est la meme chose. (The more things change, the more they seem to remain the same.) Remarkable as the enormous changes in surgical diagnostics and therapeutics have been in the 16 years since the last edition of the Handbook, as noteworthy – and humbling – are what have *not* changed. Wound ballistics are the same and often injuries are due to the same projectiles used 35 years ago in Vietnam. The ghastly penetrating wounds, blast trauma, and burns produced by present day conventional and improvised weapons are essentially unchanged from those produced in the last half of the 20th Century. The automatic rifle, rocket-propelled grenade, mortar, and improvised explosive are widely available, easy to obtain, simple to use, ferociously lethal, and not confined to the arsenals of disciplined soldiers. Bearers of these arms today include suicidal fanatics, women, and children.

It is equally discouraging that although losses due to disease have plummeted, salvage rates from severe battlefield trauma sustained in conflict (ongoing as this Handbook goes to press) are similar to previous wars despite improvements in armor, surgery, critical care and evacuation. The died of wounds (% DOW) rate during the American campaign in northwestern Europe of 1944 – 1945 (approximately 3%) was markedly better than that of the American Civil War (14%) nearly a century earlier. But enormous advances in medicine and surgery have not been reflected in substantial improvement in lives saved in forward combat surgical facilities since then (in World War II and Vietnam the rates were 3.5% and 3.4% respectively).

Penetrating wounds of the head and chest are as lethal today as they were in biblical times. Extremity fractures are still best stabilized with external fixators, albeit a newer model. Human blood components, with a short demanding shelf life, have not yet been replaced despite longstanding forecasts of synthetic products. Whole blood continues to be collected and transfused in forward medical units as it was in the Second

World War. Bacteriologic capability to identify wound and cavity contaminants is still unavailable in forward facilities. Meanwhile, antibiotic resistance of numerous pathogens, Gram negative and Gram positive, is a growing problem no longer confined to level IV referral hospitals in the rear.

Though one can hope that major strides in these and other areas of trauma resuscitation will be reflected in a future edition, our more fervent hope is for mankind's dream of peace and the exercise of his better Angels, … whereby this Handbook becomes altogether unnecessary.

> Dave Ed. Lounsbury, MD
> Colonel, Medical Corps
>
> October, 2004
> Washington, DC

Chapter 1

Weapons Effects
and Parachute Injuries

Just as with any medical topic, surgeons must understand the pathophysiology of war wounds in order to best care for the patient.

Treat the wound, not the weapon.

Epidemiology of Injuries
- Weapons of conventional war can be divided into explosive munitions and small arms.
  - o Explosive munitions: artillery, grenades, mortars, bombs, and hand grenades.
  - o Small arms: pistols, rifles, and machine guns.
- Two major prospective epidemiological studies were conducted during the 20th century looking at the cause of injury as well as outcome.
  - o During the Bougainville campaign of World War II, a medical team was sent prospectively to gather data on the injured, including the cause of injury. This campaign involved primarily infantry soldiers and was conducted on the South Pacific island of Bougainville during 1944.
  - o US Army and Marine casualties from the Vietnam War collected by the Wound Data and Munitions Effectiveness Team (WDMET) in Vietnam.

US Casualties, Bougainville Campaign (WW II) and Vietnam

Weapon	Bougainville %	Vietnam %
Bullet	33.3	30
Mortar	38.8	19
Artillery	10.9	3
Grenade	12.5	11
Land mine/booby trap	1.9	17
RPG (rocket propelled grenade)	—	12
Miscellaneous	2.6	—

The most common pattern of injury seen on a conventional battlefield is the patient with multiple small fragment wounds of the extremity.

Anatomical Distribution of Penetrating Wounds (%)

Conflict	Head and Neck	Thorax	Abdomen	Limbs	Other
World War I	17	4	2	70	7
World War II	4	8	4	75	9
Korean War	17	7	7	67	2
Vietnam War	14	7	5	74	—
Northern Ireland	20	15	15	50	—
Falkland Islands	16	15	10	59	—
Gulf War (UK) **	6	12	11	71	(32)*
Gulf War (US)	11	8	7	56	18+
Afghanistan (US)	16	12	11	61	—
Chechnya (Russia)	24	9	4	63	—
Somalia	20	8	5	65	2
Average	**15**	**9.5**	**7.4**	**64.6**	**3.5**

*Buttock and back wounds and multiple fragment injuries, not included
+ Multiple wounds
** 80% caused by fragments; range of hits 1–45, mean of 9

Mechanism of Injury
● For missile injuries, there are two areas of projectile-tissue interaction, permanent cavity and temporary cavity (Fig. 1-1).

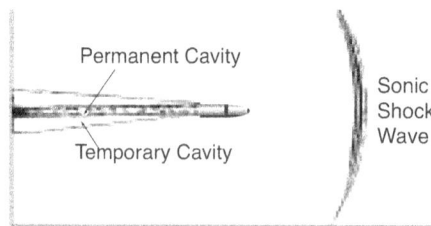

Permanent Cavity

Temporary Cavity

Sonic Shock Wave

Fig. 1-1. Projectile–tissue interaction, showing components of tissue injury.

o **Permanent** cavity. Localized area of cell necrosis, proportional to the size of the projectile as it passes through.

o **Temporary** cavity. Transient lateral displacement of tissue, which occurs after passage of the projectile. **Elastic tissue**, such as skeletal muscle, blood vessels and skin, may be pushed aside after passage of the projectile, but then rebound. **Inelastic tissue**, such as bone or liver, may fracture in this area.

- The **shock (or sonic) wave** (commonly mistaken for the temporary cavity), though measurable, has **not** been shown to cause damage in tissue.

Explosive munitions have three mechanisms of injury (Fig. 1-2):

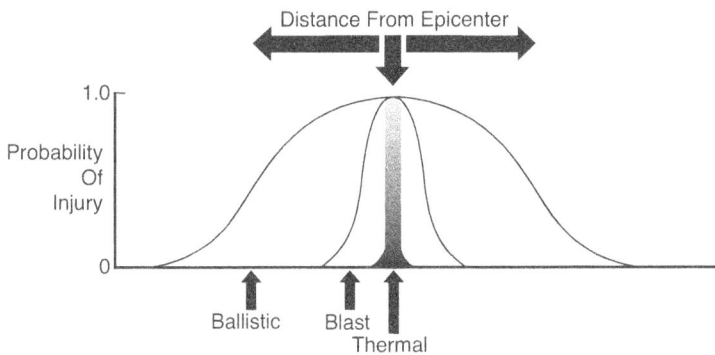

Fig. 1-2. The probability of sustaining a given trauma is related to the distance from the epicenter of the detonation.

- Ballistic.
  o Fragments from explosive munitions cause ballistic injuries.
  o Fragments are most commonly produced by mortars, artillery, and grenades.
  o Fragments produced by these weapons vary in size, shape, composition, and initial velocity. They may vary from a few milligrams to several grams in weight.
  o Modern explosive devices are designed to spread more uniform fragments in a regular pattern over a given area.

1.3

o Fragments from exploding munitions are smaller and irregularly shaped when compared to bullets from small arms.

o Although initial fragment velocities of 5,900 ft/s (1,800 m/s) have been reported for some of these devices, the wounds observed in survivors indicate that striking velocities were less than 1,900 ft/s (600 m/s). Unlike small arms, explosive munitions cause multiple wounds.

- Blast (see Fig. 1-2).
  o The blast effects take place relatively close to the exploding munition relative to the ballistic injury.
  o Blast overpressure waves, or sonic shock waves, are clinically important when a patient is close to the exploding munition, such as a land mine.
  o The ears are most often affected by the overpressure, followed by lungs and the gastrointestinal (GI) tract hollow organs. GI injuries may present 24 hours later.
  o Injury from blast overpressure is a pressure and time dependent function. By increasing the pressure or its duration, the severity of injury will also increase.
  o Thermobaric devices work by increasing the duration of a blast wave to maximize this mechanism of injury. The device initially explodes and puts a volatile substance into the air (fuel vapor). A second explosion then ignites the aerosolized material producing an explosion of long duration. The effects from this weapon are magnified when detonated in an enclosed space such as a bunker.
  o Air displaced on the site after the explosion creates a blast wind that can throw victims against solid objects, causing blunt trauma.

- Thermal.
  o Thermal effects occur as the product of combustion when the device explodes. Patients wounded near exploding munitions may have burns in addition to open wounds, which may complicate the management of soft tissue injuries.

Common Misconceptions About Missile Wounds

Misconception	Reality
Increased velocity causes increased tissue damage.	Velocity is one factor in wounding. An increase in velocity does not per se increase the amount of tissue damage. The amount of tissue damage in the first 12 cm of a M-16A1 bullet wound profile has relatively little soft tissue disruption, similar to that of a .22 long rifle bullet, which has less than half the velocity.
Projectiles yaw in flight, which can create irregular wounds.	Unless a projectile hits an intermediate target, the amount of yaw in flight is insignificant.
Exit wounds are always greater than entrance wounds.	This is untrue and has no bearing on surgical care.
Full metal-jacketed bullets do not fragment, except in unusual circumstances.	The M-193 bullet of the M-16A1 rifle reliably fragments at the level of the cannulure after traversing about 12 cm of tissue in soft tissue only.
All projectile tracts must be fully explored, due to the effects of the temporary cavity.	Elastic soft tissue (skeletal muscle, blood vessels, and nerves) generally heals uneventfully and does not require excision, provided the blood supply remains intact. Temporary cavity effects are analogous to blunt trauma.

Antipersonnel Landmines
- There are three types of conventional antipersonnel landmines available throughout the world: static, bounding, and horizontal spray.
  - o **Static** landmines are small, planted landmines (100–200 g of explosive) that are detonated when stepped on, resulting in two major areas of injury (Fig. 1-3).

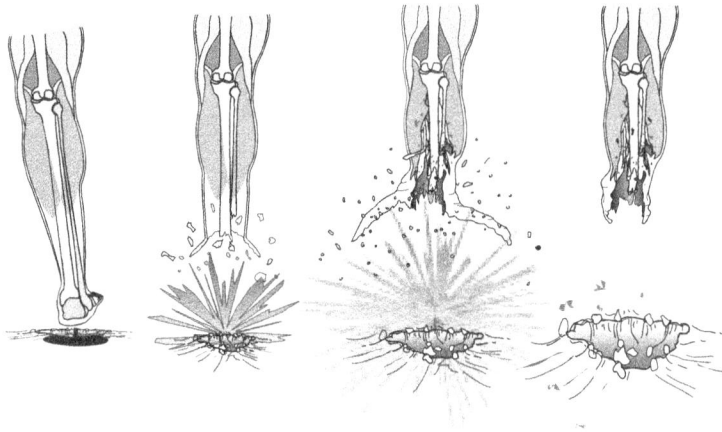

Fig. 1-3. Mechanisms of injuries caused by antipersonnel land mines.

  - ◆ Partial or complete traumatic amputation, most commonly at the midfoot or distal tibia.
  - ◆ More proximally, debris and other tissue is driven up along fascial planes with tissue stripped from the bone.
  - ◆ Factors influencing the degree of injury include size and shape of the limb, point of contact with the foot, amount of debris overlying the mine, and the type of footwear.
  - o **Bounding** mines propel a small explosive device to about 1–2 m of height and then explode, causing multiple small fragment wounds to those standing nearby. These landmine casualties have the highest reported mortality.

o **Horizontal spray** mines propel fragments in one direction. This land mine can be command-detonated or detonated by tripwire. The US Claymore mine fires about 700 steel spheres of ¾ g each over a 60° arc. Horizontal spray mines produce multiple small-fragment wounds to those nearby.

- An unconventional weapon (improvised explosive device, or IED) is a fourth type of antipersonnel landmine. Either another piece of ordnance is used, such as a grenade or a mortar shell, or the device is completely fabricated out of locally available materials.

Small Arms
- Pistols, rifles, and machine guns.
- Trends for small arms since World War II include rifles that have increased magazine capacity, lighter bullets, and increased muzzle velocity.
- Below are some examples of the characteristics of commonly encountered firearms seen throughout the world. The illustrations are of the entire path of missiles fired consistently at 5–10 m in range into ordnance gelatin tissue-simulant blocks. Variations of range, intermediate targets such as body armor, and body tissue will alter the wound seen.
  o The AK-47 rifle is one of the most common weapons seen throughout the world. For this particular bullet (full metal jacketed or ball) there is a 25 cm path of relatively minimal tissue disruption before the projectile begins to yaw. This explains why relatively minimal tissue disruption may be seen with some wounds (Fig. 1-4).

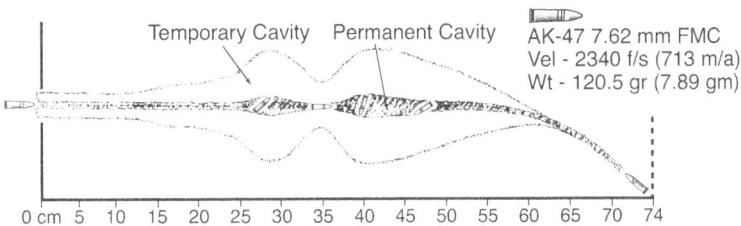

Temporary Cavity   Permanent Cavity   AK-47 7.62 mm FMC
Vel - 2340 f/s (713 m/a)
Wt - 120.5 gr (7.89 gm)

0 cm 5   10   15   20   25   30   35   40   45   50   55   60   65   70 74

Fig. 1-4. Idealized path of tissue disruption caused by an AK-47 projectile, (10% gelatin as a simulation).

1.7

o The AK-74 rifle was an attempt to create a smaller caliber assault rifle. The standard bullet does not deform in the tissue simulant but does yaw relatively early (at about 7 cm of penetration).

o The M-16A1 rifle fires a 55-grain full metal-jacketed bullet (M-193) at approximately 950 m/s. The average point forward distance in tissue is about 12 cm, after which it yaws to about 90°, flattens, and then breaks at the cannalure (a groove placed around the mid section of the bullet). The slightly heavier M-855 bullet used with the M-16A2 rifle, shows a similar pattern to the M-193 bullet (Fig. 1-5).

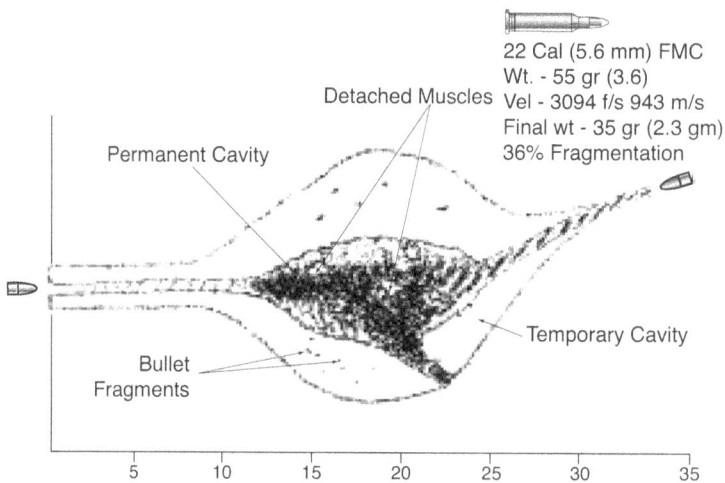

22 Cal (5.6 mm) FMC
Wt. - 55 gr (3.6)
Vel - 3094 f/s 943 m/s
Final wt - 35 gr (2.3 gm)
36% Fragmentation

Detached Muscles

Permanent Cavity

Temporary Cavity

Bullet Fragments

Fig. 1-5. Idealized path of tissue disruption caused by an M-193 bullet fired from the M-16A1 rifle (10% gelatin as a simulation).

o The 7.62 mm NATO rifle cartridge is still used in sniper rifles and machine guns. After about 16 cm of penetration, this bullet yaws through 90° and then travels base forward. A large temporary cavity is formed and occurs at the point of maximum yaw (Fig. 1-6).

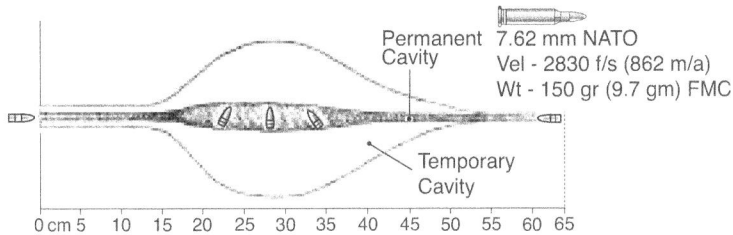

Fig. 1-6. Idealized path of tissue disruption caused by the 7.62 mm projectile, (10% gelatin as a simulation).

Armored Vehicle Crew Casualties
- Since the first large scale use of tanks during WWI, injuries to those associated with armored vehicles in battle have been a distinct subset of combat casualties.
- Tanks, infantry fighting vehicles, armored personnel carriers, armored support vehicles, and "light armored vehicles."
  - o Light armored vehicles tend to use wheels rather than tracks for moving and have lighter armor. The main advantage for these vehicles is to allow for greater mobility.

Compared to infantry, injuries to those inside or around armored vehicles are characterized by:
- **Decreased overall frequency.**
- **Increased severity of injury and mortality (up to 50%).**
- **Increased incidence of burns and traumatic amputations.**

- There are three main types of antiarmor weapons on the battlefield today.
  - o **Shaped charge** (Fig. 1-7a).
    - ♦ The shaped charge or high explosive antitank (HEAT) round consists of explosives packed around a reverse cone of metal called a melt sheet or a liner. This is the principle behind the warhead of the RPG.

a

b

Explosive Melt Sheet   Nose Cone

Fuse

Armor

Target Material

Jet

Gas and Fragments of
Exploding Charge   Melt Sheet

Spall Material

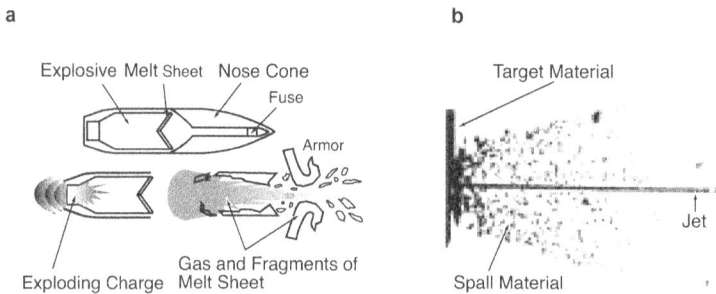

Fig. 1-7. (a) Disruptive mechanisms of the shaped-charge warhead, **(b)** diagram taken from photograph of an actual detonation of shaped-charged warhead against armor plate caused by antitank land mines.

- ◆ Shaped charges range in diameter from the 85 mm RPG-7 to the 6-in diameter tube launched, optically tracked, wire guided (TOW) missile.
- ◆ If the armor is defeated by the shaped charge, there are two areas of behind-armor debris.
  - ◊ First, there is the jet of the shaped charge itself. This may cause catastrophic wounds to soldiers who are hit, or it may ignite fuel, ammunition, or hydraulic fluid.
  - ◊ There is a second type of debris, called spall, which is material knocked off from the inside face of the armored plate. This produces a spray of small, irregularly shaped fragments inside of the compartment (Fig. 1-7b).
- o **Kinetic energy round.**
  - ◆ The kinetic energy (KE) round is a large, aerodynamically shaped piece of hard metal (such as depleted uranium or tungsten) shaped like a dart. Fragments of depleted uranium should be treated during initial wound surgery as any retained metal foreign body should. There is a hypothetical risk, over years, that casualties with retained depleted uranium fragments may develop heavy metal poisoning. This concern by itself does not justify extensive operations to remove such fragments during initial wound surgery. The metal is usually encased in a carrier or sabot that falls away from the projectile after it leaves the barrel.

♦ Injuries to those inside a vehicle are due to the direct effects of the penetrator or from fragments knocked off the inside face of the armored plate. The range of fragment masses may be from a few milligrams to over a kilogram.

o **Antitank landmines**.

♦ Blast mines are those with a large explosive filler of 4–5 kg. Injuries are often from blunt trauma due to crewmembers being thrown around inside the vehicle after it detonates the mine.

♦ Closed fractures of the upper and lower extremities and spine are common (Fig. 1-8).

♦ A modification of the shaped charge is the Miznay-Schardin antitank mine that creates a projectile or large metal slug to cause damage to the vehicle. This is less likely than a conventionally shaped charge to be broken up by intermediate targets.

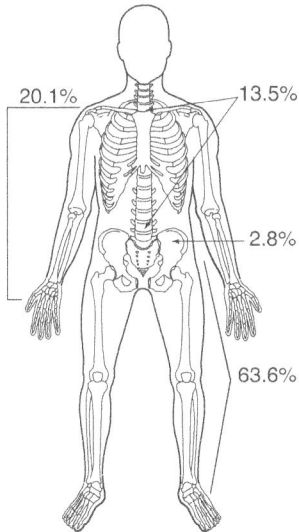

Fig. 1-8. Distribution of fracture sites sustained within an armored vehicle that had detonated a land mine (Soviet data from Afghanistan, early 1980s).

Mechanisms of Injury (Fig. 1-9)
- **Ballistic** injuries take place as the result of defeated armor as described above.

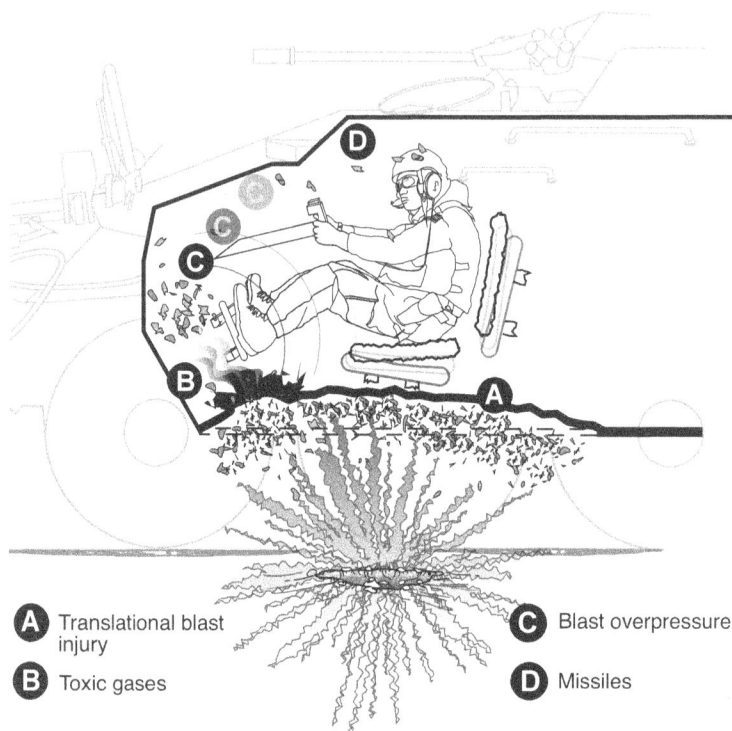

A Translational blast injury

B Toxic gases

C Blast overpressure

D Missiles

Fig. 1-9. Injuries sustained as a result of defeated armor, (**a**) translational blast injury, (**b**) toxic gases, (**c**) blast overpressure, (**d**) penetrating missile wounds.

- **Thermal**. Burns occur because of ignited fuel, ammunition, hydraulic fluid, or as the direct result of the antiarmor device.
  - Two large studies, one from British WWII tank crewmen and one from Israeli casualties in Lebanon, showed that about 1/3 of living wounded casualties have burns.

o The severity of burns range from a mild 1ˢᵗ degree burn to full thickness burns requiring skin coverage. Most burns are superficial burns to exposed skin, most often of the face, neck, forearms, and hands. These are often combined with multiple fragment wounds.

- **Blast overpressure** occurs from the explosion occurring inside a confined space. One study from WWII showed 31% of armored crewmen casualties had ear injury due to blast overpressure, including ruptured tympanic membranes.
- **Toxic Fumes** are secondary to phosgene-like combustion byproducts in Teflon coated interiors of armored vehicles (antispall liners).
    o HCL is produced at the mucous membrane.
    o Treatment is supportive and may require IV steroids (1,000 mg methylprednisolone, single dose).
    o Surgical triage considerations. Emergent if pulmonary edema, expectant if hypotensive and cyanotic. Reevaluate nonemergent patients q 2 h.
- **Blunt Trauma** is due to acceleration mechanisms.

Unexploded Ordnance (UXO)
- UXOs are embedded in the casualty without exploding.
    o Rockets, grenades, mortar rounds.
    o UXO must travel a distance (50–70 m) without arming.
    o Fuses are triggered by different stimuli (impact, electromagnetic, laser).
- **Notify explosive ordnance disposal immediately!**
- ³¹⁄₃₁ victims lived after removal (from recent review).
- The casualty should be triaged as **nonemergent**, placed far from others, and **operated on last**.
- Preplan for how to handle both transport and operation.
    o Transport.
        ♦ If by helicopter, ground the casualty to the aircraft (there is a large electrostatic charge from rotors).
    o Move into **safe area**.
        ♦ Revetment, parking lot, or back of building.
    o **Operate in safe area, not in main OR area.**
- Operative management.
    o Precautions for surgeon and staff.

- ◆ Sandbag operative area, use flak vests and eye protection.
  - o Avoid triggering stimuli.
    - ◆ Electromagnetic (no defibulator, monitors, Bovie cauterizer, blood warmers, or ultrasound or CT machines).
    - ◆ Metal to metal.
    - ◆ Plain radiography is safe. It helps identify the type of ammunition.
  - o Anesthesia.
    - ◆ Regional/spinal/local preferred.
    - ◆ Keep **oxygen** out of OR.
    - ◆ Have anesthesiologist leave after induction.
  - o Operation: The surgeon should be alone with the patient.
    - ◆ Employ gentle technique.
    - ◆ Avoid excessive manipulation.
    - ◆ Consider amputation if other methods fail.
    - ◆ Remove en-block if possible.
- **The decision to remove a chemical/biological UXO is a command decision.**
- Immediately after removal, hand to explosive ordnance disposal (EOD) personnel for disposal.

Parachute Injuries
- Dependent on several factors: **Weather** (wind), **day/night, drop zone hazards/terrain,** low **drop altitude**, and **level of opposition** (enemy resistance) at the drop zone.
- Caused by improper aircraft exit, parachute malfunction, hazards (including enemy) on descent or in the landing zone, entanglements, or an improper parachute landing fall (PLF).
- Peacetime rate of injuries is 0.8%.
- Combat injury **rate** is historically higher (subject to above listed factors).
  - o As high as 30% overall.
  - o Majority of injuries are minor.
  - o 8% to 10% of total jumpers are rendered either combat ineffective or significantly limited.

Injury Site/Type	%	Injury Site/Type	%
Ankle	20	Sprain/Strains	37.7
Back	11.1	Contusions	30.1
Knee	10.7	Lacerations	14.7
Head/Neck	8.7	Closed Fractures	11.1
Leg	8.3	Concussions	2.0
Open Fractures	2.0	—	—

● Fractures result in a higher percentage of removal from combat.

Fractures of the calcaneus are associated with fractures of the axial skeleton (10%). Patients should be placed on spinal precautions until such injuries are ruled out.

Chapter 2

Levels of Medical Care

Military doctrine supports an integrated health services support system to triage, treat, evacuate, and return soldiers to duty in the most time efficient manner. It begins with the soldier on the battlefield and ends in hospitals located within the continental United States (CONUS). Care begins with first aid (self-aid/buddy aid, and combat lifesaver), rapidly progresses through emergency medical care (EMT) and advanced trauma management (ATM) to stabilizing surgery, and is followed by critical care transport to a level where more sophisticated treatment can be rendered.

There are **five levels of care (also known as "roles")**, previously referred to as echelons by NATO and ABCA (USA, Britain, Canada, Australia) countries. Levels should **not to be confused with American College of Surgeons use of the term in US trauma centers**. Different levels denote differences in capability, rather than the quality of care. Each level has the capability of the level forward of it and expands on that capability. Soldiers with minor injuries can be returned to duty after simple treatments at forward locations, all others are prepared for evacuation with medical care while en route to a higher level.

Level I
- Immediate first aid delivered at the scene.
  - First aid and immediate life-saving measures provided by self-aid, buddy aid, or a **combat lifesaver** (nonmedical team/squad member trained in enhanced first aid).
  - Care by the trauma specialist (91W) (**combat medic**), assigned to the medical platoon, trained as an Emergency Medical Technician-Basic (EMT-B). Some other primary

care providers, with various levels of training, include the Special Forces Medical Sergeant 18D, Special Operations Combat Medic 91W, SEAL Independent Duty Corpsman, Special Boat Corpsman, Pararescueman, and Special Operations Medical Technician.

o Initial treatment of nuclear, biological, and chemical casualties, treatment of toxic industrial material casualties, primary disease prevention, combat stress control measures, and nonbattle injury prevention.

- Level I medical treatment facility (MTF) (commonly referred to as the Battalion Aid Station [BAS]).
  o Provides triage, treatment, and evacuation.
  o Physician, Physician Assistant (PA), and medics.
  o Return to duty, or stabilize and evacuate to the next level.
  o Can be chem/bio protected.
  o No surgical or patient holding capability.
- US Marine Corps (USMC): Shock Trauma Platoon (STP).
  o Small forward unit supports the Marine Expeditionary Force (MEF).
  o Stabilization and collecting/clearing companies.
  o 1 physician.
  o No surgical capability.
  o Patient holding time limited to 3 hours.

Level II

- Increased medical capability and limited inpatient bed space.
- Includes basic primary care, optometry, combat operational stress control and mental health, dental, laboratory, surgical (when augmented) and X-ray capability.
- 100% mobile.
- Each service has a slightly different unit at this level.

- **Army.**
  o **Level II MTFs** operated by the treatment platoon of divisional/nondivisional medical companies/troops.
    ◆ Basic/emergency treatment is continued.
    ◆ Packed RBCs (Type 0, Rh positive and negative), limited X-ray, laboratory, and dental.
    ◆ 20–40 cots with 72-hour holding.

◆ Can be chem/bio protected.
◆ No surgical capability.

o **Forward Surgical Team (FST).**
  ◆ Continuous operations for up to 72 hours.
  ◆ Life-saving resuscitative surgery, including general, orthopedic, and limited neurosurgical procedures.
  ◆ 20-person team with 1 orthopedic and 3 general surgeons, 2 nurse anesthetists, critical care nurses and technicians.
  ◆ The supporting medical company must provide logistical support and security. (Doctrinally, the FST is collocated with a Medical Company.)
  ◆ ~1,000 sq ft surgical area.
  ◆ Can be chem/bio protected.
  ◆ Operational within 1 hour of arrival at the supported company.
  ◆ May be transported by ground, fixed wing, or helicopter; some fleet surgical teams (FSTs) are airborne deployable.
  ◆ 2 operating tables for a maximum of 10 cases per day and for a total of 30 operations within 72 hours.
  ◆ Post-op intensive care for up to 8 patients for up to 6 hours.
  ◆ X-ray, laboratory, and patient administrative support provided by the supporting medical company.
  ◆ Requires additional electricity, water, and fuel from the supporting medical company.
  ◆ The FST is not designed, staffed, or equipped for stand alone operations or conducting sick-call operations. Augmentation requirements are discussed in FM 4-02.25.

● **Air Force.**
  o **Mobile Field Surgical Team (MFST).**
    ◆ 5-person team (general surgeon, orthopedist, anesthetist, emergency medicine physician, and OR nurse/tech).
    ◆ 10 life/limb saving procedures in 24–48 hours from five backpacks (350 lb total gear).
    ◆ Designed to augment an aid station or flight line clinic.
    ◆ Not stand alone, requires water, shelter of opportunity, communications, among other things.

- ♦ Integral to remainder of Air Force (AF) Theater Hospital System.
  - o **Small Portable Expeditionary Aeromedical Rapid Response (SPEARR) team.**
    - ♦ 10-person team: 5-person MFST, 3-person CCATT (see Chapter 4, Aeromedical Evacuation) and a 2-person preventive medicine (PM) team (flight surgeon, public health officer).
    - ♦ Stand alone capable for 7 days, 600 sq ft tent.
    - ♦ 10 life/limb saving procedures in 24–48 hours.
    - ♦ Designed to provide surgical support, basic primary care, post-op critical care, and PM for early phase of deployment.
    - ♦ Highly mobile unit, with all equipment fitting in a one-pallet–sized trailer.
  - o **Expeditionary Medical Support (EMEDS) Basic.**
    - ♦ Medical and surgical support for an airbase, providing 24-hour sick call capability, resuscitative surgery, dental care, limited laboratory and X-ray capability.
    - ♦ 25 member staff includes SPEARR team.
    - ♦ 4 holding beds, 1 OR table, 3 climate controlled tents, and 3 pallets.
    - ♦ 10 life/limb saving procedures in 24–48 hours.
    - ♦ ~2,000 sq ft.
  - o **EMEDS + 10.**
    - ♦ Adds 6 beds to EMEDS Basic, for total of 10.
    - ♦ No additional surgical capability.
    - ♦ 56-person staff.
    - ♦ 6 tents, 14 pallets.
    - ♦ Can be chemically hardened.

- • Navy.
  - o **Casualty Receiving & Treatment Ships (CRTS)**. CRTSs are part of an Amphibious Ready Group (ARG) and usually comprise one landing helicopter assault or amphibious (LHA) Tarawa-class or landing helicopter deck (LHD) Wasp-class ship, which are Marine amphibious

assault helicopter carriers that function as casualty receiving platforms. An ARG includes up to 6 ships with surgical capability only on the CRTS.

- ♦ 45 beds, 4 ORs, 15 ICU beds.
- ♦ 300 additional medical care beds are available.
- ♦ Fleet Surgical Teams (FSTs): 4 surgeons and support staff.
- ♦ Usually 2 general surgeons and 2 orthopedic surgeons. OMFS (oral maxillofacial surgery) support available through the dental department.
- ♦ Laboratory, X-ray.
- ♦ Excellent casualty flow capability (large helicopter flight deck and landing craft units [LCU] well deck).
- ♦ Mass casualty (MASCAL) capability with triage area for 50 casualties.
- ♦ Doctrinally, holding capability is limited to 3 days.

- **Aircraft Carrier (CVN) Battle Group.**
  - o 1 OR, 40–60 beds, 3 ICU beds.
  - o 1 surgeon, 5 other medical officers.
  - o Up to 9 ships, but usually only the CVN has physicians.
- **USMC.**
  - o **Surgical Company**.
    - ♦ Provides surgical care for a MEF (Marine Expeditionary Force).
    - ♦ 3 ORs, 60-bed capability.
    - ♦ Patient holding time up to 72 hours.
    - ♦ Stabilizing surgical procedures.
  - o **Forward Resuscitative Surgical System (FRSS)**.
    - ♦ Rapid assembly, highly mobile.
    - ♦ Resuscitative surgery for 18 patients within 48 hours without resupply.
    - ♦ 1 OR, 2 surgeons.
    - ♦ No holding capability.
    - ♦ No intrinsic evacuation capability.
    - ♦ Chem/bio protected.
    - ♦ Stand alone capable.

Level III

Represents the highest level of medical care available within the combat zone with the bulk of inpatient beds. Most deployable hospitals are modular, allowing the commander to tailor the medical response to expected or actual demand.

- **Army.**
    - o Two different Corps-level Combat Support Hospital (CSH) designs.
        - ♦ Medical Force 2000 (MF2K) CSH.
        - ♦ Medical Reengineering Initiative (MRI) CSH will replace the MF2K.
    - o **Combat Support Hospital.**
        - ♦ **MF2K CSH.**
            - ◊ Resuscitation, initial surgery, post-op care, and either return to duty or stabilize for further evacuation.
            - ◊ Up to 296 patients, typically divided into 8 ICUs (96 ICU beds), and 7 Intermediate Care Wards (ICWs) (140 beds), 1 neuropsychiatric (NP) ward (20 beds), and 2 minimal care wards (40 beds).
            - ◊ 175 officers, 429 enlisted; specialty attachments may increase numbers.
            - ◊ Up to 8 OR tables for a maximum of 144 operating hours per day.
            - ◊ General, orthopedic, urologic, neurosurgical, dental and oromaxillofacial surgery.
            - ◊ Blood bank, laboratory, X-ray/computer tomography (CT); nutrition, physical therapy and NP capabilities.
            - ◊ Dependent on a number of Corps support elements for personnel, finance, mortuary, legal, laundry, security, and enemy prisoners of war (EPW) management, support.
            - ◊ Transportation support required for both incoming and outgoing patient evacuation, and to transport the hospital.
            - ◊ Transported via semitrailer, railcar, air cargo, or ship.
            - ◊ Fully deployed CSH (including motor pool, billeting, heliport, and other life support activities) covers 30.3 acres.

◊ Divided into modules, deployed as a single unit or separately as the mission dictates. The main modules are the Hospital Unit-Base (HUB) and the Hospital Unit-Surgical (HUS).

- HUB is the infrastructure of the CSH.
  □ Up to 236 patients, divided into 36 ICU, 140 intermediate, 40 minimal, and 20 NP beds.
  □ Two operating modules with specialty surgical care capability.
  □ HQ, administrative, personnel, chaplain, laboratory, pharmacy, X-ray, and blood bank services.
  □ Part of the HUB can be chem/bio protected (FM 4-02.7).
- HUS capabilities.
  □ 60 ICU patients, 2 OR modules, X-ray.
  □ Dependent on the HUB for all logistical support.
  □ Can be deployed forward, separate from the HUB, for brief periods as the mission dictates.

- **MRI CSH (Corps).**
  o Provides hospitalization and outpatient services for all classes of patients in the theater, either returned to duty or stabilized for further evacuation.
  o Headquarters/headquarters detachment: 15 officers and 44 enlisted.
  o Up to 248 patients, typically divided into an 84-bed hospital company and a 164-bed hospital company, with split base operations capability.
    ♦ **84-bed hospital company.**
      ◊ 24 ICU beds.
      ◊ Up to 2 OR tables, maximum of 36 operating hours per day.
      ◊ 3 ICWs (total 60 beds, including NP patients).
      ◊ 56 officers and 112 enlisted personnel.
        - Some patient care areas can be chem/bio protected.
    ♦ **164-bed hospital company.**

◊ 24 ICU beds.
◊ Up to 4 OR tables, maximum of 60 operating hours per day.
◊ 7 ICWs (total 140 beds, including NP patients).
◊ 84 officers and 169 enlisted personnel.
▪ Some patient care areas can be chem/bio protected.
♦ **Applicable to 84-, 164-, and 248-bed (see CSH [Echelon of Care, EAC] below) hospital companies.**
◊ General, orthopedic, urologic, thoracic, OB/GYN, neurosurgical, dental and oromaxillofacial surgery.
◊ Blood bank, laboratory, X-ray, nutrition, and physical therapy.
◊ Dependent on EAC support elements for personnel, finance, mortuary, legal, laundry services, security and EPW support.
◊ Parts can be chem/bio protected.
◊ Transportation support required for both incoming and outgoing patient evacuation, and to transport the hospital.
◊ Transported by semi-trailer, railcar, air cargo, or ship.
◊ Fully deployed, covers 5.7 acres.
◊ Minimal care wards are provided by an attached minimum care detachment.
● **Air Force.**
o **EMEDS +25.**
♦ 25-bed version of EMEDS Basic.
♦ 84 personnel, 2 OR tables, 9 x 600 sq ft tents, and 20 pallets.
♦ 20 operations in 48 hours.
♦ Can be chemically hardened.
♦ Additional specialty modules can be added, including vascular/cardiothoracic, neurosurgery, OB/GYN, ear, nose and throat (ENT), ophthalmology teams; each comes with own personnel and equipment.
● **Navy.**
o **Fleet Hospital.**
♦ 500-bed hospitals, 80 ICU beds, and 6 ORs.
♦ 1,000 personnel.
♦ Stand alone; full ancillary services.

- 8–10 days to be operational.
- Large footprint — 28 acres, 450 isolation (ISO) shelters.
- No limit on holding capability.
- o **Hospital Ships (TAH) — USNS Mercy and USNS Comfort**.
  - 1,000 beds, 100-bed ICU capability, and 12 ORs.
  - 1,000 staff, over 50 physicians.
  - Extensive laboratory and X-ray capabilities.
  - Patient holding is doctrinally limited to 5 days.

Level IV

- Definitive medical and surgical care outside the combat zone, yet within the communication zone/EAC of the theater of operations (TO).
- Patients requiring more intensive rehabilitation or special needs.
- Traditionally includes the MF2K Field Hospital (FH) and General Hospital (GH).
- In some situations, the MF2K CSH or a fixed hospital may act as a Level IV facility (eg, Landstuhl Army Regional Medical Center, Germany).
  - o **Field Hospital.**
    - Semipermanent hospital that provides primarily convalescent care.
    - At least 2 OR tables for 24 OR hours per day.
    - General, orthopedics, OB/GYN, urologic, oral surgery, and dental services.
    - Up to 504 patients, with 2 ICUs (24 patients), 7 ICWs (140 patients), 1 NP ward (20 patients), 2 minimum care wards (40 patients), and 7 patient support sections (280 patients).
  - o **General Hospital.**
    - Usually a permanent or semipermanent facility.
    - At least 8 OR tables for 144 OR hours per day.
    - General, orthopedic, gynecologic, urologic, and oral surgery.
    - Dental and optometry services.
    - Outpatient specialty and primary care services.
    - Up to 476 patients, with 8 ICUs (96 patients), 16 ICWs (320 patients), 1 NP ward (20 patients), and 2 minimum care wards (40 patients).

> **The MRI CSH Echelon Above Corps (EAC) will replace the FH and GH.**

- **CSH (EAC).**
  - Headquarters/headquarters detachment: 17 officers and 33 enlisted.
  - Cannot operate in a split-based mode like the CSH (Corps).
  - 248-bed hospital company.
    - 4 ICUs (total 48 ICU beds), and 10 ICWs (total 200 beds, including NP patients). A specialty clinic section that can treat NP patients. Minimal care wards are provided by attached minimum care detachments.
    - 140 officers, 244 enlisted personnel.
    - Up to 6 OR tables for 96 operating hours per day.
    - Fully deployed (including motor pool, troop billeting, heliport, and other life support activities), covers 9.3 acres.
    - See other general characteristics under MRI CSH (Corps).

Level V

This level of care is provided in the CONUS. Hospitals in the CONUS sustaining base will provide the ultimate treatment capability for patients generated within the theater. Department of Defense (DoD) hospitals (military hospitals for the tri-services) and Department of Veterans Affairs (DVA) hospitals will be specifically designated to provide the soldier with maximum return to function through a combination of medical, surgical, rehabilitative, and convalescent care. Under the National Disaster Medical System, patients overflowing DoD and DVA hospitals will be cared for in designated civilian hospitals.

Chapter 3

Triage

Introduction

Modern combat casualty evacuation has become so immediate and efficient that it can result in a mass casualty situation at military treatment facilities (MTFs) within the military medical care system. Consequently, a method of dealing with the conflicting factors of severity of injury, the tactical situation, the mission, and the resources available for treatment and evacuation is essential. **Triage is an attempt to impose order during chaos and make an initially overwhelming situation manageable.**

> **Triage is the dynamic process of sorting casualties to identify the priority of treatment and evacuation of the wounded, given the limitations of the current situation, the mission, and available resources (time, equipment, supplies, personnel, and evacuation capabilities).**

Triage occurs at every level of care, starting with buddy and medic care, extending through the OR, the ICU, and the evacuation system.

> **The ultimate goals of combat medicine are the return of the greatest possible number of soldiers to combat and the preservation of life, limb, and eyesight in those who must be evacuated.**

The decision to withhold care from a wounded soldier who in another less overwhelming situation might be salvaged, is difficult for any surgeon or medic. Decisions of this nature are infrequent, even in mass casualty situations. Nonetheless, this is the essence of military triage.

Triage Categories

It is anticipated that triage will be performed at many levels, ranging from the battlefield to the battalion aid station to the field hospital. Traditional categories of triage are **Immediate, Delayed, Minimal, and Expectant**. This classification scheme is useful for mass casualties involving both surgical and medical patients. An additional category of **Urgent** has been used to describe surgical patients who need an operation but can wait a few hours.

- **Immediate**: This group includes those soldiers requiring life-saving surgery. The surgical procedures in this category should not be time consuming and should concern only those patients with high chances of survival (eg, respiratory obstruction, unstable casualties with chest or abdominal injuries, or emergency amputation).
- **Delayed**: This group includes those wounded who are badly in need of time-consuming surgery, but whose general condition permits delay in surgical treatment without unduly endangering life. Sustaining treatment will be required (eg, stabilizing IV fluids, splinting, administration of antibiotics, catheterization, gastric decompression, and relief of pain). (The types of injuries include large muscle wounds, fractures of major bones, intra-abdominal and/or thoracic wounds, and burns less than 50% of total body surface area (TBSA).
- **Minimal**: These casualties have relatively minor injuries (eg, minor lacerations, abrasions, fractures of small bones, and minor burns) and can effectively care for themselves or can be helped by nonmedical personnel.
- **Expectant**: Casualties in this category have wounds that are so extensive that even if they were the sole casualty and had the benefit of optimal medical resource application, their survival would be unlikely. The expectant casualty should not be abandoned, but should be separated from the view of other casualties. Expectant casualties are unresponsive patients with penetrating head wounds, high spinal cord injuries, mutilating explosive wounds involving multiple anatomical sites and organs, second and third degree burns in excess of 60% TBSA, profound shock with multiple injuries, and agonal respiration. Using a minimal but competent staff, provide comfort measures for these casualties.

Alternative Triage Categories

In practice, however, the division of patients into these four categories is not useful for a surgical unit. The casualties should be divided into emergent, nonemergent, and expectant. These divisions are useful in dividing casualties into those requiring further surgical triage (emergent), and those that are less injured, still require care, but have little chance of dying (nonemergent). It is anticipated that 10%–20% of casualties presenting to a surgical unit will be in the emergent category, requiring urgent surgery. The vast majority of wounded will not require intensive decision-making, intervention, and care.

- **Emergent**: Although this category has been historically subdivided into **Immediate** (unstable and requiring attention within 15 minutes) and **Urgent** (temporarily stable but requiring care within a few hours), except in the most overwhelming circumstances, such division is rarely of practical significance. This group of wounded will require attention within minutes to several hours of arriving at the point of care to avoid death or major disability.
  - o Types of wounds include:
    - ♦ Airway obstruction/compromise (actual or potential).
    - ♦ Uncontrolled bleeding.
    - ♦ Shock.
      - ◊ Systolic BP < 90 mm Hg.
      - ◊ Decreased mental status without head injury.
    - ♦ Unstable penetrating or blunt injuries of the trunk, neck, head, and pelvis.
    - ♦ Threatened loss of limb or eyesight.
    - ♦ Multiple long-bone fractures.
- **Nonemergent**: This category was historically divided between **Delayed** (would require intervention, however, could stand significant delay) and **Minimal**. This is the group of patients that, although injured and may require surgery, does not require the attention of the emergent group and lacks significant potential for loss of life, limb, or eyesight. Examples include:
  - o Walking wounded.
  - o Single long-bone fractures.
  - o Closed fractures.
  - o Soft tissue injuries without significant bleeding.
  - o Facial fractures without airway compromise.

- **Expectant**: This group of wounded, **given the situation and resource constraints**, would be considered unsalvageable. Examples may include:
  o Any casualty arriving without vital signs or signs of life, regardless of mechanism of injury.
  o Transcranial gunshot wound (GSW).
  o Open pelvic injuries with uncontrolled bleeding; in shock, with decreased mental status.
  o Massive burns.
- **Special categories**: Patients who do not easily fit into the above categories and casualties who pose a risk to other casualties, the medics, and the treatment facility, may require special consideration:
  o **Wounded contaminated in a biological and/or a chemical battlefield environment.** The threat posed by these patients mandates decontamination prior to entering the treatment facility. Appropriately protected medical personnel may treat emergent casualties prior to decontamination.
  o **Retained, unexploded ordnance:** These patients should be segregated immediately. See Chapter 1, Weapons Effects and Parachute Injuries, which describes the special handling of these wounded.
  o **Enemy Prisoners of War (EPWs)/Internees:** Although treated the same as friendly casualties, it is essential that the threat of "suicide bombers" and "human booby traps" be prevented by carefully screening all EPWs prior to moving into patient areas, including the triage area. See Chapter 34, Care of Enemy Prisoners of War/Internees.
- **Combat stress:** Rapid identification and immediate segregation of stress casualties from injured patients will improve the odds of a rapid recovery. With expeditious care these casualties can be returned to duty (80%). Do not use them as litter bearers as this may increase the trauma you seek to treat.
  o **Place patient in one of two groups.**
    ♦ **Light stress**: Immediate return to duty or return to unit or unit's noncombat support element with duty limitations and rest.

- **Heavy stress:** Send to combat stress control restoration center for up to 3 days reconstitution.
- Use **BICEPS** mnemonic where resources/tactical situations allow.
  ◊ **Brief**: Keep interventions to 3 days or less of rest, food, reconditioning.
  ◊ **Immediate**: Treat as soon as symptoms are recognized—do not delay.
  ◊ **Central:** Keep in one area for mutual support and identity as soldiers.
  ◊ **Expectant**: Reaffirm that we expect return to duty after brief rest; normalize the reaction and their duty to return to their unit.
  ◊ **Proximal**: Keep them as close as possible to their unit. This includes physical proximity and using the ties of loyalty to fellow unit members. Do this through any means available. **Do not evacuate away from the area of operations or the unit, if possible.**
  ◊ **Simple**: Do not engage in psychotherapy. Address the present stress response and situation only, using rest, limited catharsis, and brief support (physical and psychological).
  ◊ Or, refer: Must be referred to a facility that is better equipped or staffed for care.

If battlefield casualties do not have physical injuries, DO NOT send them out of the battle area, as this will worsen stress reactions, and possibly start evacuation syndromes!

Triage is a fluid process at all levels, with altered situations and resources requiring a change in category at any time and in any setting. In the extreme example, a casualty may be triaged from emergent to expectant during surgery, abruptly terminating the procedure ("on-the-table triage").

Resource Constraints

Including all of the factors that influence triage decision making would be encyclopedic and of little benefit. Rather, a framework for thinking about this process in a logical fashion is presented here.

- **External factors.** The surgeon/medic may have limited knowledge of and no control over external issues. Nonetheless, optimal casualty care requires at least an assessment of these factors.
  - o **Tactical situation and the mission.** The decision to commit scarce resources cannot be based on the current tactical/medical/logistical situation alone. One severely wounded, resource-consuming casualty may deplete available supplies, and thus prevent future, less seriously injured casualties from receiving optimal care. Liaison with the tactical force operating in your area is essential to making sound triage decisions. Operational security may make this kind of information difficult to obtain in a timely fashion. **Education of, and communication with, line commanders about the critical nature of this information is essential.**
  - o **Resupply**: Having a sense of how and when expended internal resources will be resupplied may prove critical to making the decision to treat or not treat the individual casualty.
  - o **Time.**
    - ♦ **Evacuation to the MTF.** The shorter this time interval, expect the complexity of triage decisions to increase, especially sorting the worst emergent patients from the expectant. Longer intervals will result in the opposite, with "autotriage" of the sicker patients from the emergent to the expectant/dead on the battlefield category.
    - ♦ **Time spent with the individual casualty.** In a mass casualty situation, time itself is a resource that must be carefully triaged/husbanded. All patients receive an evaluation, but only some receive operative intervention. Time on the OR table is usually the choke point. Apply the concepts of damage control to minimize the time casualties spend in surgery. On-table triage to expectant may be necessary due to deteriorating casualty physiologic response and/or the pattern of injury (aorta-vena cava GSW, dual

      exsanguination sites, extensive pancreatic-duodenal injury, and so forth).

     ◆ **Evacuation out.** Casualties must move expeditiously to the next echelon of care (EOC), otherwise valuable local resources will be consumed in maintaining patients, thereby preventing additional patients from receiving care.

- **Internal factors.** These issues are known to the surgeon/nurse/medic and should be factored into triage decisions.
  - o **Medical supplies.** These supplies include equipment, drugs, oxygen, dressings, sutures, sterilization capability, blood, etc. **Immediate** liaison with the logistics system in the MTF and the theater of operation is essential to ensure the availability and timely resupply of these items, to include "surge" capabilities and local resource availability.
  - o **Space/Capability.** This category includes the number of OR tables and ICU beds: the holding capacity and ward capacity; and the available diagnostic equipment—ultrasound (US), X-ray, computed tomography (CT)—and laboratory tests. For example, if your MTF has the only CT scanner in theater, plan for an increased number of head-injured patients.
  - o **Personnel.** This includes knowing the professional capability (type and experience of individual physician/nurse/medic), and the emotional stability, sleep status, and so forth, of your hospital personnel. This perishable resource must be preserved; for example, 24 hours of continuous operation may exhaust your only OR crew, and may necessitate diversion of casualties to another facility.
  - o **Stress.** Soldiers, including medical personnel, are affected by the consequences of war; individual and unit capability is degraded during sustained operations. The personal impact of military triage on the medical team cannot be overemphasized. It is extremely emotional, and measures should be undertaken to minimize these effects. This is best provided by trained staff. Cohesive groups may tolerate stress better and assist each other in dealing with traumatic events when allowed to

process the event in a group format according to their
own traditions.

Triage Decision Making

The complexity of decision making in triage varies greatly, often
depending on the level of training and experience of the triage
officer, as well as the location where the triage decision is being
made. At the front line, the medic must make a decision about
whether or not to evacuate patients from the battlefield and how
fast. The following decision tree is an example of a triage tool
that may be used in the field as an initial decision-making aid.

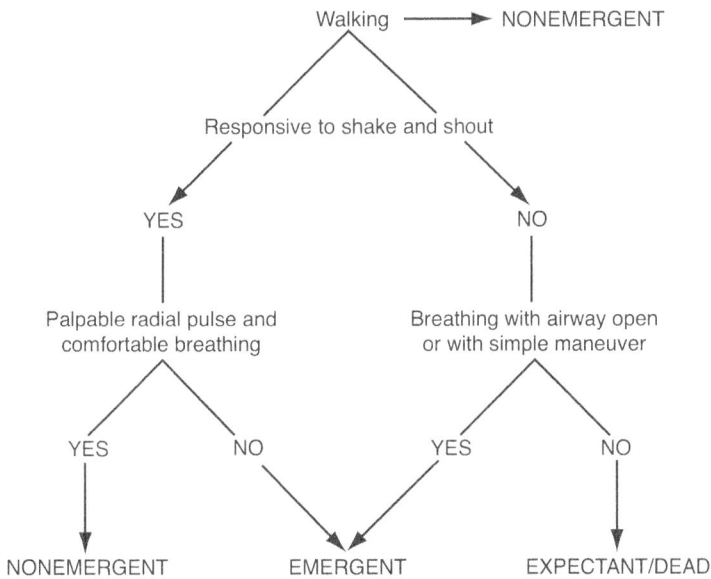

Walking ⟶ NONEMERGENT

Responsive to shake and shout

YES   NO

Palpable radial pulse and   Breathing with airway open
comfortable breathing   or with simple maneuver

YES   NO   YES   NO

NONEMERGENT   EMERGENT   EXPECTANT/DEAD

In the emergent treatment area, the surgeon must make decisions
about whether surgery is needed, the timing of the surgery, and
the priority of multiple surgical patients. Regardless of the type
of triage decision needed, the following information is of critical
importance in reaching that decision:

● **Initial vital signs.** Pulse (rate and quality), mentation,
difficulty breathing (eg, a casualty with normal mentation

and radial pulse quality is nonemergent). Respiratory rate alone is not predictive of the appropriate triage category.

- **Pattern of injury.** A historical perspective aids the triage decision maker in understanding the distribution of wounds encountered on the modern battlefield and the likely mortality associated with those wounds. **The majority of combat wounded will suffer nonfatal extremity injuries.** In general, these will be triaged as nonemergent.

- **Response to initial intervention.** Does the shock state improve, remain unchanged, or worsen with initial resuscitative efforts? A patient who fails to respond rapidly to initial fluid resuscitation should be triaged ahead of a patient with a good response to minimal fluid replacement; alternatively, this nonresponder in a mass casualty situation may need to be placed in the expectant category.

- The following data from the Vietnam War indicate the numerical distribution of diagnoses that were seen in the low-intensity light-infantry combat that characterized that war. Casualties from armored combat can be expected to have a higher prevalence of burns and multiple injuries. Of 100 injuried in combat:

  o **30%—Minor or superficial wounds** (minor burns, abrasions, intraocular foreign body, ruptured tympanic membrane/deafness).

  o **16%—Open comminuted fractures of a long bone.** Several patients with multiple fractures and injuries to named nerves and blood vessels.

  o **10%—Major soft tissue injury or burn** requiring general anesthesia for treatment. Several had an injury to major nerves.

  o **10%—Had laparotomies,** two of which were negative, and several involved extensive, complicated procedures.

  o **6%—Open comminuted fractures of hand, fingers, and feet.**

  o **5%**—Required closed thoracostomy and had soft tissue wounds.

  o **4%—Major multiple trauma.**

  o **3%—Major amputations** (above the knee [AK], below the knee [BK], below the elbow [BE], above the elbow [AE]). In three out of four cases, the surgical procedure simply required completion of the amputation.

o **3%—Craniotomies.** Two were for fragments and one for a depressed skull fracture.

o **3%—Vascular repair** (one half was to repair a femoral artery, and the other half involved named nerves or fractures).

o **3%—Major eye injuries,** one involving enucleation.

o **2%—Minor amputations** (toes, fingers, hand, foot).

o **2%—Maxillofacial reconstructions** (one half were mandibular injuries, and most of the rest were maxillary).

o **1%—Formal thoracotomy.**

o **1%—Neck exploration.**

o **1%—"Miscellaneous."**

Data from more recent American combat operations in Iraq (OIF) and Afghanistan (OEF), 2003–2004, indicating the spectrum of injury type (Table 3-1), mechanism (Table 3-2), and anatomical location (Table 3-3) are found below.

Table 3-1. Type of Injury.[*]

Type of Injury	Frequency	Percent
Penetrating	645	35.7%
Blast	425	23.5%
Blunt	410	22.7%
Unknown	84	4.6%
Crush	63	3.5%
Mechanical	49	2.7%
Thermal	48	2.7%
Undetermined	21	1.2%
Other	16	0.9%
Chemical agent	10	0.6%
Bites/Stings	8	0.4%
Degloving	8	0.4%
Electrical	7	0.4%
Heat Injury	7	0.4%
Inhalation	3	0.2%
Multiple Penetration System	3	0.2%
Total	1807	100%

[*] A casualty may have more than one type of injury. These numbers are based on 1530 Level III casualties.

Table 3-2. Mechanism of Injury.*

Mechanism of Injury	Frequency	Percent
IED	310	18.4%
MVA	207	12.3%
Gun Shot Wound (GSW)	188	11.1%
Grenade (includes RPG)	170	10.1%
Shrapnel/Fragment	141	8.3%
Unknown	119	7.0%
Machinery or Equipment	95	5.6%
Fall or Jump from height	90	5.3%
Mortar	84	5.0%
Burn	53	3.1%
Aggravated Range of Motion	31	1.8%
Landmine	29	1.7%
Other	27	1.6%
Knife or other sharp object	21	1.2%
Helicopter Crash	19	1.1%
Blunt object (eg, rock or bottle)	17	1.0%
Pedestrian	16	0.9%
Free Falling Objects	14	0.8%
Bomb	12	0.7%
None	12	0.7%
UXO	10	0.6%
Environmental	9	0.5%
Exertion/overexertion	5	0.3%
Flying debris	5	0.3%
Building Collapse	2	0.1%
Hot Object/Substance	2	0.1%
Altercation, fight	1	0.1%
Total	**1689**	**100%**

* A casualty may have more than one mechanism of injury. These numbers are based on 1530 Level III casualties.

Setup, Staffing, and Operation of Triage System
- Initial Triage Area.

  All casualties should flow through a **single triage area** and undergo rapid evaluation by the **initial triage officer**. Casualties will then be directed to separate treatment areas (emergent, nonemergent, and expectant), each with its own triage/team leader. The expectant will have a medical attendant, ensuring optimal pain control. The dead should

Table 3-3. Anatomical Location of Injury.[*]

Anatomical Location	Frequency	Percent
Multiple Sites	761	49.7%
Lower Extremity	248	16.2%
Upper Extremity	223	14.6%
Head/Face	174	11.4%
Thorax/Back	48	3.1%
Neck	20	1.3%
None	20	1.3%
Abdomen	16	1.0%
Unknown	9	0.6%
Buttock	6	0.4%
N/A	3	0.2%
Genitalia	1	0.1%
Soft Tissue	1	0.1%
Total	**1530**	**100%**

[*] Casualties with more than one injury location are included in 'Multiple Sites'. These numbers are based on 1530 Level III casualties.

be sent to the morgue and must remain separate from all other casualties, especially the expectant. Unidirectional flow of patients is important to prevent clogging the system. Reverse patient flow in any treatment area is highly discouraged.

> **No significant treatment should occur in the triage area. Casualties should be rapidly sent to the appropriate treatment area for care.**

- o Qualities of an ideal initial triage area should include
  - ♦ **Proximity** to the receiving area for casualties—LZ, ground evacuation, decontamination area.
  - ♦ **One-way flow** both into and out of the triage area through separate routes to **easily identified, marked** (signs, colors, chemical lights, etc.) treatment areas.
  - ♦ **Well-lit, covered, climate-controlled** (if possible) area with sufficient space for easy access, evaluation, and transport of casualties in and out.
  - ♦ Dedicated **casualty recorders** to identify, tag, and record initial triage/disposition.

◊ Using an indelible marker to place numbers on the casualty's forehead is an easy, fast way to track patients. Any method that is reproducible and simple will suffice.

◊ If resources allow, casualty tracking may include stationing administrative personnel at every entry/exit.

♦ Sufficient **litter bearers** (controlled by an NCO) to ensure continuous casualty flow.

o Initial triage office.

♦ Ideally, a surgeon experienced in dealing with combat trauma should be used in this capacity. Unfortunately, using a surgeon outside of the OR is a luxury that most small forward surgical units cannot afford.

♦ It is essential that another person with clinical experience be trained to assume this function. Using mass casualty exercises or limited mass casualty situations is one way to train/identify the right person to fill this role in the absence of a surgeon.

• Emergent treatment area.

o Setup.

♦ Close proximity to initial triage area with direct access.

♦ Administrative personnel stationed at entry and exit doors to record patient flow. Ideally, a display board or a computer should be used to record patient identity, location, and disposition.

♦ Series of resuscitation bays (number depends on available resources/personnel).

◊ Allow sufficient room for 3-person team to work.

◊ Easy access in and out of bay.

◊ Availability of equipment needed for ATLS style resuscitation (Fig. 3-1 a,b).

o Staffing.

♦ Team leader: a surgeon serves as the surgical triage officer.

◊ Responsible for determining priority for operative interventions.

◊ Needs to identify patients that require early evacuation.

◊ If a surgeon is unavailable, may be a physician who maintains close communication with the operating surgeons.

♦ Administrative person. Responsible for recording flow of patients through unit.

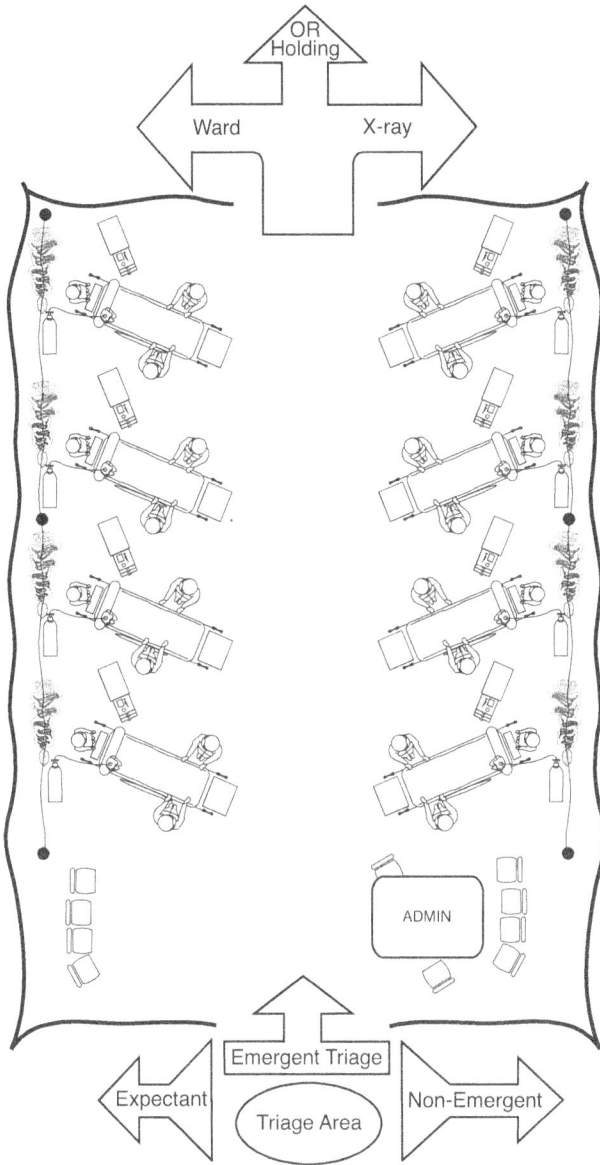

Fig. 3-1a. Triage.

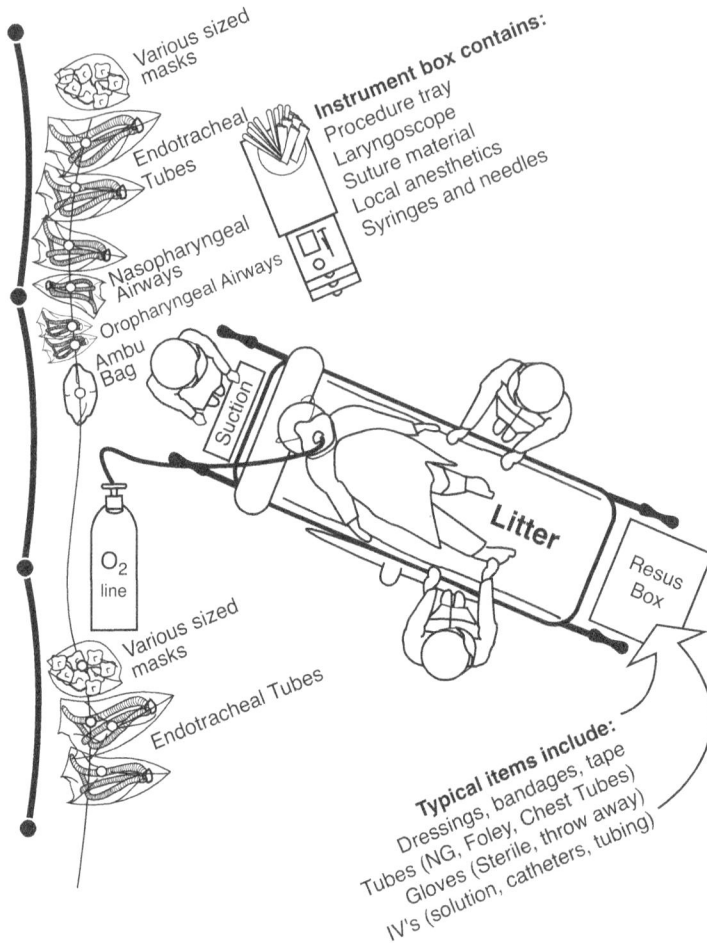

Fig. 3-1b. Resuscitation Station.

♦ Resuscitation team. A physician, nurse, and medical
  technician, ideally.
  ◊ Each individual treatment team will coordinate
    movement of its patient via the team leader.
o Operation.
  ♦ Manpower team delivers patient.

◆ Team Leader retriages patient and assigns resuscitation team to patient.
◆ Resuscitation team treats patient and determines required disposition (surgery, ICU, ward, air evacuation).
◆ Resuscitation team communicates to Team Leader the recommended disposition.
◆ Team Leader coordinates movement of patient to next stop.
◆ Administrative person records disposition.

● Nonemergent treatment area.
An empty ward, a cleared out supply area, or other similar space can be utilized. Appropriate medical and surgical supplies should be stockpiled and easily identifiable. A team consisting of a physician and several nurses and medical technicians can form the nucleus of the treatment team. Lacerations can be sutured, closed fractures splinted, IVs placed, and radiographs taken. The team leader should be alert to changing vital signs, mental status changes, and any failure to respond to appropriate treatment measures. Any evidence of deterioration should prompt a retriage decision and a possible transfer to the emergent treatment area.

● Expectant area.
Ideally, expectant casualties should be kept in an area away from all other treatment areas. The team leader can be anyone capable of giving parenteral pain medications. The patient should be kept comfortable. **After all other patients have been treated, a retriage of these patients should be done and treatment instituted if appropriate.**

Additional Triage Operation Tips
● Diversion of casualties to another facility should be considered. These options (sister service, local national assistance, or local NATO assets) should be established prior to the mass casualty event.
● As the casualties finally clear the OR suites, the pace will slow for the surgeons. ICU and ward care will supplant operative procedures. Casualties initially undertriaged (~10%) will be discovered and will require care. The recovery room and ICUs will become crowded, nursing

shifts will have to be extended, and fatigue will rapidly become a hospital-wide factor.

- Numerous authors have stated that after the first 24 hours of a mass casualty ordeal, the activities of the care providers must be decreased by 50%, allowing for recovery and rest for the participants, and a new rotation must be established to sustain a modified but continuous effort. Once the press is over, personnel must be encouraged to rest rather than to socialize. Rest must be enforced because the entire scenario may recur at any time.
- Prior to an actual mass casualty situation, all deployable units should exercise a variety of triage scenarios to ensure smooth patient flow and identification. "Driving" litters without running into things can be difficult unless practiced! These scenarios should evaluate personnel, supplies, and equipment.

Conclusion

Small, highly mobile units, either Special Operations or conventional forces, are currently performing military operations around the globe. These units are usually supported by highly mobile, small footprint surgical elements that have limited diagnostic, operative, holding, and resupply capability. Evacuation may entail an extremely long transport from point of wounding to the forward surgery team, then another long transport directly to a Level IV/V. Air superiority may be in question, especially the use of helicopters for initial patient evacuation. In these situations the tactical, logistic, and physiologic integration of triage concepts becomes of paramount importance and needs to be considered and extensively discussed prior to arrival of the first casualty.

Chapter 4

Aeromedical Evacuation

Introduction

Evacuation of injured personnel using aircraft, fixed or rotary wing, has revolutionized the rapid transport of casualties from areas where there is either inadequate or no care available to medical treatment facilities (MTFs) where essential and/or definitive care can be rendered. While an aircraft can decrease transport time, the aeromedical environment creates unique stresses on the injured patient. The following are terms that describe evacuation of patients using aircraft.

- Casualty evacuation (CASEVAC): The movement of a casualty from the point of injury to medical treatment by nonmedical personnel. Casualties transported under these circumstances do not receive en route medical care; if the casualty's medical condition deteriorates during transport, an adverse impact on the casualty's prognosis and long-term disability may result. Traditionally, this situation involves a helicopter mission returning from the battlefield.

- Medical evacuation (MEDEVAC): The timely, efficient movement and en route care provided by medical personnel to the wounded being evacuated from the battlefield to MTFs, using medically equipped vehicles or aircraft. Examples include civilian aeromedical helicopter services and Army air ambulances. This term also covers the transfer of patients from the battlefield to an MTF or from one MTF to another by medical personnel, such as from a ship to shore.

- Aeromedical evacuation (AE): Providing USAF fixed-wing **intra**theater (Tactical Evacuation [TACEVAC]: from the combat zone to points outside the combat zone, and between points within the communications zone) and **inter**theater (Strategic Evacuation [STRATEVAC]: from out of the theater of operations to a main support area) movement of sick or injured personnel, with enroute care provided by AE crewmembers and critical care air transport teams (CCATTs), to locations offering appropriate levels of medical care.

● Enroute care: Maintenance of treatment initiated prior to evacuation and sustainment of the patient's medical condition during evacuation.

Medical Considerations for Patients Entering the Medical Evacuation System

Medical Considerations/Requirements
- Medical evacuation request includes requirement for surgical equipment and/or providers.
- Patient is sufficiently stabilized for the anticipated mode and duration of travel.
- Patient's airway and breathing is adequate for movement.
- Patient's IV lines, drainage devices, and tubes are fully secured and patent.
- Patient at high risk for barotrauma should be considered for prophylactic chest tube placement before prolonged aeromedical evacuation.
- Heimlich valves on chest tubes are functioning.
- Foley catheters and nasogastric (NG) tubes are placed and allowed to drain.
- Patient is securely covered with both a woolen and aluminized blanket for air transport, cold environment, or postoperative hypothermia.
- 3 litter straps are used to secure the patient to the litter.
- Personal effects and all medical records accompany the patient.

● The evacuation of a patient is initiated by the surgeon according to established procedures. The support patient administration personnel normally provide the administrative details and coordination required to accomplish the evacuation. Due to differences in the type of evacuation assets used and their effect on the patient's medical condition (such as flying in the pressurized cabin of an aircraft), patients entering the USAF AE system must also be validated for evacuation by the supporting flight surgeon.

- For patients evacuated from Level II MTFs or forward surgical teams (FST), the brigade surgeon (or designee) determines the evacuation precedence for all patients requiring evacuation from that facility. This is done in consultation with the forward surgical team's chief surgeon and/or senior nurse. When a patient is readied for evacuation from the forward surgical team by USAF assets, the supporting patient movement requirements center (PMRC) should be established at the earliest possible time. This allows the PMRC sufficient time to coordinate airlift and patient movement items requirements.

Implications of Aviation Environment
- General Considerations Prior to Transport.
  - o Due to altitude effects, limited mobility, decreased staffing enroute, and unpredictable evacuation times, the referring physician should tailor vital signs (VS) monitoring requirements, and frequency of wound and neurovascular checks.
  - o Some therapies that might not be used in a fixed MTF are appropriate for AE.
    - ♦ For example, patients with significant medical or surgical conditions should have Foley catheters, NG tubes, provisions for IV pain medications, extended duration IV antibiotics.
  - o Consider liberal use of fasciotomies/escharotomies.
  - o Consider securing airway with prophylactic endotracheal (ETT) tube.
  - o Wounds dressed for delayed primary closure. Unless directed otherwise, AE crew should not routinely re-dress wounds. If a patient develops fever or sepsis enroute, wounds must be inspected.
  - o Casts must be bivalved. If the cast is over a surgical wound site, "window" the cast to allow for tissue expansion and emergency access. Document neurovascular checks prior to and frequently during flight.

- Decreased Barometric Pressure.
  - o The diameter of a gas bubble in liquid doubles at 5,000 ft above sea level, doubles again at 8,000 ft, and doubles again at 18,000 ft. Cabin pressures in most military aircraft are maintained at altitudes between 8,000 and 10,000 feet. If an aircraft has the capability, the cabin altitude can be maintained at lower levels, with increased flight time and fuel.
- Consider a Cabin Altitude Restriction (CAR) for the following:
  - o Penetrating eye injuries with intraocular air.
  - o Free air in any body cavity.
  - o Severe pulmonary disease.
  - o Decompression sickness and arterial gas embolism require CAR at origination field altitude. Destination altitude should not be higher than origination altitude. Transport on 100% oxygen (by aviator's mask if available).
- Pneumothorax: Chest tube required, even for small, asymptomatic lesions. A Heimlich valve or collection system must be in place prior to patient transfer to the flight line.
- Air Splints: Should not be used if alternate devices are available. Because air expands at altitude, air splints require close observation and adjustments during flight.
- Ostomy Patients: Vent collection bags to avoid excess gas dislodging the bag from the stoma wafer. Use a straight pin to put two holes in the bag above the wafer ring.
- Decreased Partial Pressure of Oxygen: Ambient partial pressure of oxygen decreases with increasing altitude. At sea level, a healthy person has an oxygen saturation of 98%–100%. At a cabin altitude of 8,000 ft, this drops to 90%, which corrects to 98%–100% with 2 L/min of oxygen.
- Neurosurgical Patients: Hypoxia may worsen neurological injury. Adjust ventilator settings to meet increased oxygen demands at altitude.
- Gravitational Stress: Traumatic brain injury patients can experience transient marked increases in intracranial pressure during takeoff or landing. Patient positioning onboard the aircraft helps minimize this risk (head forward on takeoff, head rearward on landing).

- Thermal Stress: Plan for cabin temperature changes from 15°C (59°F) to 25°C (77°F) on winter missions, and from 20°C (68°F) to 35°C (95°F) on summer missions.
- Noise: Exposure to noise can produce problems with communication and patient evaluation (auscultation is impossible — use noninvasive blood pressure [NIBP] and an arterial line). Provide hearing protection. Audible medical equipment alarms are useless.
  - Decreased Humidity: Airplanes have very low cabin humidity at altitude. Evaporative losses will increase; therefore, patients will require additional fluids, especially those with large burns, and those at risk for mucous plugging.
- Patient movement in nuclear, biological and chemical (NBC) environments.
  - Nuclear and chemical casualties must be externally decontaminated, and time allowed for off-gassing of residual chemical agent.
  - Movement of biological casualties varies by the nature of the agent, its mechanism of transmission, and the period of communicability during the course of illness.
  - Any NBC AE movement may be delayed due to the following:
    - Aircraft decontamination time.
    - Availability of noncontaminated aircrew.
    - Cohorting of similarly exposed patients.
    - Quarantinable diseases (eg, plague and smallpox) require special approval (command and diplomatic) before AE.

Medical Evacuation Precedences
- Depending on the Service and the type of evacuation assets used, the timeframes for affecting evacuation differ. Refer to Table 4-1.

Table 4-1. Evacuation Precedences.

Movement Precedence	Army, Navy, Marine (MEDEVAC)	Air Force (AE)	Description
Urgent	Within 2 h.	ASAP	Immediate AE to save life, limb, or eyesight.
Priority	Within 4 h.	Within 24 h.	Prompt medical care not available locally. Medical condition could deteriorate and patient cannot wait for routine AE.
Routine	Within 24 h.	Within 72 h or next available mission.	Condition is not expected to deteriorate significantly while awaiting flight.

● **Concept of Operations. The USAF AE system.**
  o Command and control (C2) of casualty movement by air transport.
  o AE personnel and equipment for inflight supportive patient care and flight line support operations.
  o Organic communication network for medical facilities and airlift C2 agencies.
    ◆ Aeromedical Evacuation Liaison Team (AELT): 4–6 person communication team, usually collocated with an MTF, to coordinate requests with the AE system.
  o Facilities and personnel at airheads for the administrative processing, staging, and limited medical care of casualties entering or transiting the AE system. Patients are normally held only for 2–6 hours prior to evacuation.
    ◆ USAF units provide aeromedical staging support through incrementally sized elements ranging in size/ capability from forward deployed special operations forces (SOF) to 100-bed facilities.
● Reporting a Patient for AE. Originating physician consults with local FS to determine the en route care plan and timing of evacuation.

> Due to the complexity of the AE system, physicians must identity points of contact (POCs) (local Flight Surgeons [FSs], AELT, aeromedical staging elements, PMRC); verify and test lines of communication; and rehearse patient evacuation drills and procedures, **before** the actual need arises.

- Patient Stability. Patients validated for transport by AE must be stabilized as well as possible (secure airway, controlled hemorrhage, treated shock, and immobilized fractures).
  - o Communicate the condition, AE category (ambulatory or litter), and movement precedence (Table 4-1) of the patient to the PMRC, as communications assets allow. See PMRC contact information below.

PMRC	Commercial telephone number	Military telephone number
Global-Scott AFB, IL	1-800-303-9301 or 1-800-874-8966	DSN 779-4200 or 8184
EUCOM Theater-Ramstein Air Force Base, Germany	011-49-6371-47-2264 or 2235	DSN 314-480-2264 or 2235
PACOM Theater-Yakota Air Force Base, Japan	011-81-3117-55-4700	DSN 315-225-4700 or 7660

  - o To ensure optimum care, communicate with the accepting physician, and provide diagnosis, care rendered, and subsequent medical care plan (next 24–48 h).
  - o Ensure the patient has adequate quantities of supplies and medications for duration of transfer (at least 72 h).
- **Local Flight Surgeon Responsibilities.**
  - o Authority for determining whether patients are physiologically ready for air transport.
  - o Resource for AE system information, communication, and coordination.

AE Process

Activity	Location at Which the Activity Occurs
Request for AE mission (see end of chapter for format).	Originating physician.
Validation for Aeromedical Evacuation.	PMRC (establishes AE requirement).
Clearance to move by air.	MTF (referring physician and local FS).

- Request versus Requirement. AE **requests** and patient movement **requirements** are different. Physicians at originating MTFs submit requests for movement, timing, destination, suggested support therapies, and so forth. Only the validating Flight Surgeon (usually located at PMRC; not the local FS) and the PMRC can validate those requests, which then become AE requirements.
- Validation versus Clearance for USAF AE.
  - o Aeromedical evacuation **clearance** is a medical care event; **validation** is a logistical event.
  - o **Clearance** is a decision between the referring physician and the local FS, addressing
    - ◆ Description of the medical condition of the patient.
    - ◆ Probability that patient can survive transit through an aviation environment?
    - ◆ What the patient needs to make the trip safely.
    - ◆ Enroute medical capability requirements.
- Key Steps for USAF AE Patient Request.
  - o Contact local FS and AE liaison for clearance consultation.
  - o Determine the patient's AE category, based on diagnosis and ability to self-help in an emergency during flight.
  - o Determine need for CCATT (see below). The CCATT adds an additional level of support to the AE system for movement of stabilized patients who require a higher level of medical therapy or have the potential to experience significant deterioration during movement. The CCATT physician is the clinical authority and, with the other team members, is responsible for documenting and providing

care. CCATT members may be called on to consult and/
or assist in the care of other patients.

o A four-person burn transport team can augment a CCATT
team as required for inhalation injury and/or severe burns.

o Determine if special requirements exist for transport; eg,
CAR, and splinting.

o Determine patient movement items (PMI) required (eg,
ventilators, pulse oximeters, among others).

o Determine the patient's movement precedence.

o Submit request.

Critical Care Air Transport Teams

Intensivist physician.
- Capable of providing short term life-support, including advanced airway management, ventilator management, and limited invasive (nonoperative) procedures.
- Trained in critical care medicine, anesthesiology, or emergency medicine.

Critical care or emergency medicine nurse.
- Experienced in managing patients requiring mechanical ventilation, invasive monitoring, and hemodynamic support.

Cardiopulmonary technician.
- Experienced in management of patients requiring mechanical ventilation, and invasive monitoring.
- Experienced in troubleshooting ventilatory support and monitoring systems.

Chapter 5

Airway/Breathing

Introduction

Skillful, rapid, assessment and management of airway and ventilation are critical to preventing morbidity and mortality. Airway compromise can occur rapidly or slowly and may recur. Frequent reassessment is necessary. Preventable causes of death from airway problems in trauma include the following:

- Failure to recognize the need for an airway.
- Inability to establish an airway.
- Failure to recognize the incorrect placement of an airway.
- Displacement of a previously established airway.
- Failure to recognize the need for ventilation.
- Aspiration of the gastric contents.

Initial airway management at any level, but especially outside of medical treatment facilities (MTFs).

Immediate goal: Move tongue, pharyngeal soft tissues, and secretions out of airway. **Until a formal airway is established, place patients in the lateral or prone position (rescue position).**

- Chin-lift and head tilt: Place fingers under the tip of the mandible to lift the chin outward from face.
- Two-Handed Jaw Thrust: Place both hands behind the angles of the mandible and displace forward. This method can be used on the patient with cervical injury.
- Oropharyngeal airway:
  - Insert oral airway upright if a tongue depressor is used (preferred method).
  - Keep the airway inverted past the tongue then rotate 180°.
  - Too small an airway will not alleviate the obstruction. Too long an airway may fold the epiglottis caudally, worsening the obstruction.
  - Estimate airway size by distance from corner of mouth to ear lobe.
  - Oral airways are not used in conscious patients.

- Nasopharyngeal airway.
  - o Pass lubricated nasal airway gently through one nostril.
  - o Not used in suspected facial or basal skull injuries.
  - o Is tolerated by conscious patients.
- Field expedient.
  - o Pull tongue forward and safety pin or suture it to corner of mouth.
- Cricothyrotomy.

Ventilation

- Ventilate patient with bag valve mask (BVM).
  - o **Bring the face into the mask rather than pushing the mask onto the face.**
  - o The chin-lift and head tilt are also employed during mask ventilation unless they are contraindicated due to cervical spine precautions.

> **Assess air movement during mask ventilation by observing rise and fall of the chest, auscultation, absence of a mask leak, compliant feel of self-inflating bag, and stable oxygen saturation.**

  - o If air movement is not achieved, use **two-person mask ventilation** (Fig. 5-1).
    - ♦ One person lifts the jaw aggressively at the angles of the mandible; the other holds the mask and ventilates.
    - ♦ If air movement is still not present, obtain a definitive airway.

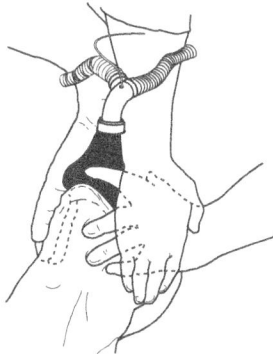

Fig. 5-1. Two-person mask ventilation.

o Unsuccessful and aggressive attempts at ventilation may result in inflation of the stomach, placing the patient at increased risk for vomiting and aspiration.

Positive pressure ventilation can convert a simple pneumothorax into a tension pneumothorax. Perform frequent assessment and have equipment available for needle chest decompression.

Orotracheal Intubation

Rapid Sequence Intubation (RSI)—7 steps.
1. Preoxygenate with 100% oxygen by mask.
2. Consider fentanyl—titrate to maintain adequate blood pressure and effect (2.0–2.5 µg/kg).
3. Cricoid Pressure—Selleck maneuver until endotracheal tube (ETT) placement is confirmed and balloon is inflated.
4. Induction Agent: etomidate 0.1–0.4 mg/kg IV push.
5. Muscle Relaxant: succinylcholine 1.0–1.5 mg/kg IV push.
6. Laryngoscopy and orotracheal intubation.
7. Verify tube placement.

- Direct laryngoscopy technique.
  o Ensure optimal "sniffing" position is achieved unless contraindicated by cervical spine injury.
  o Open the mouth by scissoring the right thumb and middle finger.
  o Hold the laryngoscope in the left hand and insert the blade along the right side of the mouth, slightly displacing the tongue to the left.
    ♦ **Macintosh** (curved) blade: Advance the tip of the blade into the space between the base of the tongue and the epiglottis (valecula). Apply force at a 30°–45° angle, lifting the entire laryngoscope/blade, without rocking it backward (Fig. 5-2).
    ♦ **Miller** (straight) blade: Advance the tip of the blade into the posterior oropharynx, picking up the epiglottis and tongue base anteriorly and laterally, and apply a force vector like that of the Macintosh blade. Avoid rocking the laryngoscope backward (Fig. 5-3).

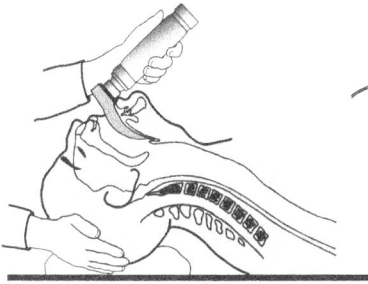

Fig. 5-2. Use of curved blade laryngoscope.

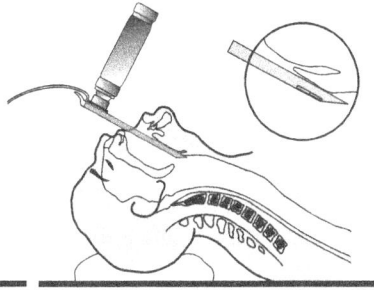

Fig. 5-3. Use of straight blade laryngoscope.

- o Visualize the vocal cords.
- o Consider the "BURP" maneuver when the laryngoscopic view is poor (Fig. 5-4).
  - ◆ "Backward-Upward-Rightward-Pressure" of the larynx, also referred to as external laryngeal manipulation.
  - ◆ Place the fingers of an assistant onto the larynx with your right hand and manipulate the glottic opening into the field of view.
  - ◆ Assistant then holds the position for intubation.

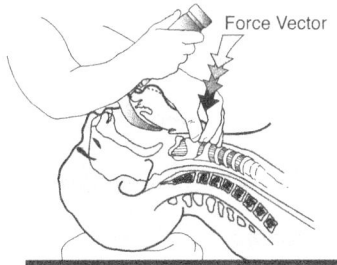

Force Vector

Fig. 5-4. BURP maneuver.

Eschmann stylet or Gum Elastic Bougie (GEB) (Fig. 5-5).
  - ◆ Blindly guide the tip of the stylet beneath the epiglottis, then anteriorly through the vocal cords.
  - ◆ Advance the bougie deeply. Placement into the trachea results in the sensation of tracheal ring "clicks", and turning of the stylet as it passes airway bifurcations.

♦ The patient may cough as the stylet passes through the airway.
♦ When passed into the trachea, the stylet will stop at a terminal bronchus. If placed into the esophagus, it will pass indefinitely into the stomach without any tactile feedback.
♦ The ETT is guided over the stylet into the airway, and tracheal intubation is confirmed.

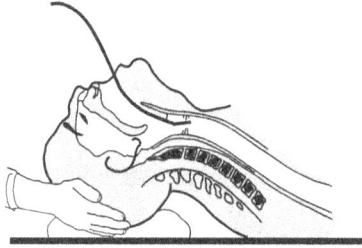

Fig. 5-5. Eschmann stylet in place.

o Advance the ETT between the vocal cords, withdraw stylet, and advance the ETT to 20–21 cm at the teeth for adult females, 22–23 cm for adult males. Deeper placement may result in right mainstem intubation.
o Confirm placement of the ETT in the trachea.
o Auscultate over the axilla to ensure breath sounds are equal.

Avoid making more than 3 attempts at direct laryngoscopy. Excessive attempts may result in airway trauma and swelling, potentially turning a "cannot intubate" urgency into a "cannot intubate-cannot ventilate" emergency.

Difficult Airway
After three unsuccessful attempts at direct laryngoscopy, abandon the technique and try alternatives.
● Alternative intubation techniques.
  o Tactile intubation.
    ♦ Requires no instruments.
    ♦ No light use—good in light control situations.
    ♦ Slide hand closest to patient over tongue to hold it down.

- ♦ Lift epiglottis with first two fingers.
- ♦ Slide ETT along the "v" between the two fingers into the airway.
  - o Lighted stylet or "light wand" intubation.
    - ♦ Flexible wand, lighted at the tip, is placed through the ETT.
    - ♦ Wand is advanced by tactile guidance into the trachea.
    - ♦ Position in trachea is verified by transillumination.
    - ♦ The ETT is advanced over the wand.
  - o Flexible fiberoptic oral or nasal intubation.
  - o Retrograde wire intubation.
  - o Rigid fiberoptic intubation (Bullard laryngoscope).
  - o Alternative Airways.
    - ♦ May NOT be definitive airways.
    - ♦ Allow for oxygenation and ventilation when standard airways cannot be placed.
    - ♦ "Fastrach" model laryngeal mask airway (LMA).
    - ♦ Esophageal-tracheal combitube (ETC).
- Perform a surgical airway.
- Wake the patient up and attempt an awake technique if possible.

Surgical Cricothyrotomy
- Identify cricothyroid membrane (between cricoid ring and thyroid cartilage [Fig. 5-6a]).
- Prep skin widely.
- Grasp and hold trachea until airway is completely in place.
- Make a **vertical SKIN** incision down to the cricothyroid membrane (a No. 10 or 11 blade).
- Bluntly dissect the tissues to expose the membrane.
- Make a **horizontal MEMBRANE** incision (Fig. 5-6b).
- Open the membrane with forceps or the scalpel handle.
- Insert a small, cuffed ETT, 6.0–7.0 inner diameter (ID), to just above the balloon (Fig. 5-6c).
- Confirm tracheal intubation.
- Suture the ETT in place, and secure it with ties that pass around the neck.

a

b

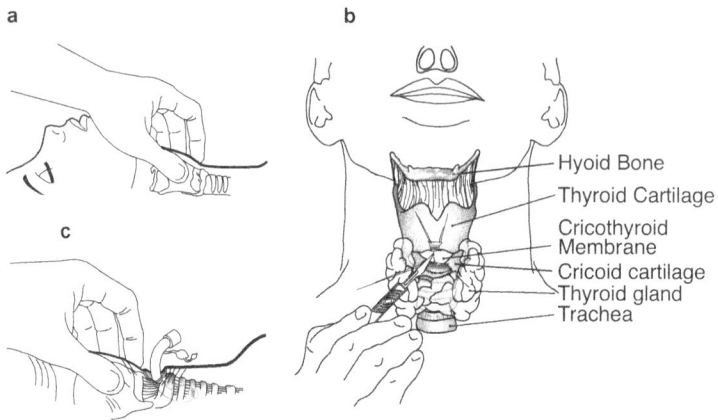

Hyoid Bone
Thyroid Cartilage
Cricothyroid Membrane
Cricoid cartilage
Thyroid gland
Trachea

c

Fig. 5-6 a,b,c. Steps of surgical cricothyrotomy.

Laryngeal Mask Airway

> **Do NOT use in penetrating upper airway trauma or central airway obstruction (foreign body).**

- Insert blindly without a laryngoscope. LMA rests over the laryngeal inlet (Fig. 5-7).

a   b   c

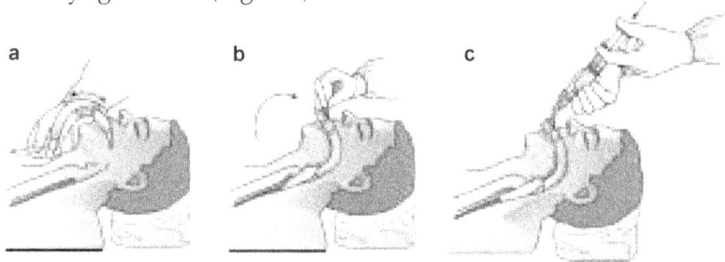

Fig. 5-7 a,b,c. Fastrach laryngeal mask airway placement. Illustration courtesy of LMA North America, Inc.

- May be used alone or as a conduit to advance an ETT.
- Compared to an ETT, the LMA supports less airway pressures, and offers less aspiration protection.

- Check LMA cuff, then deflate it until the down side (inner) surface is smooth and flat; lubricate the pharyngeal (upper) side of LMA.
- The sniffing position works best, but LMA may be inserted in different patient positions.
  - o Insert LMA (3–4 for women, 4–5 for men) with upper (pharyngeal) side **gliding along the hard palate, down and around into the posterior pharynx**—this allows proper direction and reduces the chance of cuff folding.
  - o Do **NOT** push the LMA directly back into the mouth— this folds the cuff and prohibits proper placement.
  - o Inflate cuff with 20–30 cc of air via syringe—slight upward movement of LMA tubing is seen.
  - o Secure the LMA.

Blind nasal-tracheal intubation

Contraindications: Coagulopathy, midface trauma, basilar skull fracture, and suspected elevated intracranial pressure.

- Nasal-trachael intubation is better tolerated than orotracheal techniques and requires less sedation and no paralysis.
- Prepare the nasopharynx and larynx (as conditions allow).
  - o Spray vasoconstrictor into the nostril that appears largest and most patent.
  - o Insert a nasal trumpet soaked in lidocaine gel and leave in place for a brief period.
  - o Apply Cetacaine spray to oropharynx.
  - o Administer a transtracheal injection of 4 cc lidocaine via cricothyroid membrane.
- Insert an ETT (~ 7.0 ID for adults) slowly into the nostril, perpendicular to the face.
- Advance the ETT slowly past the nasal turbinates and around the curve of the posterior nasopharynx.
- **Do not use excessive force!**
- The ETT is advanced as breath sounds of increasing volume are heard at the distal end of the tube.
- The ETT is advanced beyond the vocal cords into the trachea. If the tube fails to advance into the trachea, several maneuvers can be employed.

o Tilt the head.
o Apply external, downward pressure to the larynx.
o Inflate the ETT balloon to help center the tube, then deflate and advance it once it is engaged in the glottic opening.

Chapter 6

Hemorrhage Control

"The hemorrhage that takes place when a main artery is divided is usually so rapid and so copious that the wounded man dies before help can reach him." – COL H.M. Gray, 1919

Stop the Bleeding!
- Hemorrhage is the leading cause of preventable death on the battlefield.
  - o 90% of combat fatalities occur forward of medical care.
  - o Half of these casualties bleed to death, $1/5$ from extremity trauma (10%–15% of all deaths).
  - o Although bleeding is a main cause of death, the vast majority of wounds do not have life-threatening bleeding.

Under Fire

Get the patient out of the line of fire — prevent further injury.
Control obvious external bleeding once out from under fire.
If you must remain under fire, stop external bleeding with use of a tourniquet.
Do not endanger the casualty or yourself with unnecessary treatment.
Stay engaged in the firefight if necessary.

Keep Your Head Down

Sites of Hemorrhage
- External.
  - o Extremity injury (most common cause of massive external blood loss in combat), scalp, and torso wounds.
  - o Usually associated with an open fracture or amputation.

Direct Pressure Is Central to Treatment

- Internal.
  - ◆ Chest, abdomen, pelvis, and closed extremity fractures.

♦ High mortality if the casualty is not expeditiously transported and salvage surgical procedures performed.
♦ Controlled (hypotensive) resuscitation may be necessary.

Internal Torso Bleeding Requires Surgical Control

Treatment—First Responder

- External hemorrhage from extremity wounds.
  - o **Direct pressure** at site of injury is the most effective and preferred method of hemorrhage control.
    - ♦ If direct pressure fails to stop the hemorrhage, it signifies deep, massive, or arterial injury, and will require surgery or advanced hemostatic agents.
    - ♦ Hold pressure for at least 5 minutes before looking to see if it is effective.
    - ♦ Impaled foreign bodies should not be removed because profuse bleeding may occur.

Pitfall: A Bandage Does Not Equal Direct Pressure!

A bandage may wick blood from the wound without stopping the bleeding.

A bandage hides ongoing bleeding.

Hemostatic bandages currently being developed may stop bleeding.

- ♦ **Elevation** of the extremity will decrease most bleeding—this is an under-appreciated technique.
- ♦ **Point compression of the proximal artery.**

Pitfalls of Blind Clamping

Blind clamping into the wound is more likely to cause additional injury than to control bleeding.

Risk–Benefit Decision: Judgment that other measures are not successful should be exercised before applying clamps in a wound. Field wound exploration is not recommended.

◊ May help slow bleeding while attempting to gain better control at the wound site.
◊ May require compression at the pressure point for up to 20 minutes to provide hemostasis.
◊ Table 6-1 shows the recognized pressure points.

Table 6-1. Recognized pressure points.

Bleeding Site	Hand	Forearm	Lower Arm	Leg	Thigh
Artery	Radial/Ulnar	Brachial	Axillary	Popliteal	Femoral
Pressure Point	Wrist	Inner upper arm	Axilla	Behind knee	Below groin crease

---

Tourniquet May Be First Choice in Combat

♦ A **tourniquet** should be applied if previous techniques fail.
◊ Use a tourniquet early, rather than allow ongoing blood loss. Substitutes for issued tourniquet include belt, torn cloth, gauze, and rope, among others.
◊ Rapid method to secure hemorrhage control.
◊ Does not require constant attention; allows first responder to care for others — extends resources.
◊ Tourniquets should not be removed until the hemorrhage can be reliably controlled by advanced hemostatic agents or until arrival at surgery.
◊ Tourniquet placement on the forearm or leg may not compress the vessels, which lie between the double long bones. Tourniquets on the upper extremity should be placed on the upper arm and if bleeding from the lower extremity is not controlled by a tourniquet on the leg, it should be moved to the thigh where the vessel may be more easily compressed.

Pitfalls of Tourniquet

Application for more than 2 hours may increase limb loss.

Risk–benefit decision: Don't avoid a tourniquet in order to save a limb, and then lose a life! Use of tourniquet does not always lead to limb loss.

- ◆ **Clamping vessels:** If there is continued bleeding and a damaged vessel can be readily identified, a hemostat may be used to clamp the vessel.
- ◆ **Limb splints** will decrease bleeding associated with fractures and soft tissue injury by aligning, stabilizing, and returning the limb to length.
- ◆ Military Anti-Shock Trousers (MAST) possible uses.
    - ◊ Controls hemorrhage from massively injured/ mangled lower extremities.
    - ◊ Provides temporary stabilization of pelvic fractures to decrease hemorrhage.
    - ◊ Splints fractures of lower extremities.

Pitfalls of MAST

Protracted MAST use leads to compartment syndrome and ischemic limbs.

Respiratory compromise occurs due to diaphragmatic elevation.

Increased torso bleeding.

Pressure changes within aircraft (caused by altitude changes) affect inflation pressure.

Requires close monitoring in aircraft.

- ◆ **Scalp bleeding:** can be significant due to the rich vasculature of the scalp.
    - ◊ Responds to direct pressure.
    - ◊ Compression dressings must be applied if you cannot provide ongoing direct pressure.
    - ◊ Difficult to apply and maintain direct pressure.

◊ Requires circumferential head application.
◊ Vertical mattress suture closure sometimes is necessary to control bleeding scalp edges.
◊ A readily identified bleeding vessel can be clamped, but the wound should generally not be explored.
◊ Avoid pushing fragments into brain when applying pressure, but control hemorrhage even at the expense of exposed brain.
◊ Protection of exposed brain with nonadherent gauze or plastic can minimize injury.

♦ **Internal bleeding.**
◊ Blood loss into the abdomen or chest cannot be controlled in the field and requires immediate evacuation for salvage or definitive surgery.
◊ Stabilization of pelvic fracture with MAST garment, or by wrapping the pelvis tightly with a wide strap (such as a folded sheet), may reduce pelvic bleeding.
◊ Open torso injuries. If direct pressure does not stop the hemorrhage, consider inserting a tamponade with a balloon (Foley) catheter into the wound, and then with balloon inflated pulling back to compress the bleeding site.

Dressings, bandages, hemostatic agents, and controlled hypotension. Dressings promote hemostasis, protect wounds from mechanical injury and contamination, immobilize tissues, and provide physical and psychological support to the patient.
● **Application of dressings and bandages.**
o Control all bleeding.
o Assess neurologic status and circulation of extremity before and after applying a dressing or bandage.
o Immobilize suspected fractures.
o Keep dressing as clean as possible.
o Dressings should cover the entire wound.
o Bandages should cover the entire dressing.
o Avoid skin-to-skin contact.
o Leave fingers and toes exposed.

o **Reinforcement.**
  ♦ If at all possible, **do not** remove the first dressing.
  ♦ If the dressing becomes thoroughly saturated, reevaluate the wound for a source of bleeding amenable to direct pressure, and consider advanced hemostatic agents or a proximal tourniquet. Blood loss into the dressing can be estimated from Table 6-2.

Table 6-2. Blood loss.

Size designation	Small	Medium	Large	ABD
Measurement (inch)	4 x 7	7.5 x 8	11.75 x 11.75	18 x 22
Saturation (mL)	300	750	1,000	2,500

o Coagulopathy. Blood loss, massive fluid resuscitation, and drop in body temperature may lead to inability to form clot.
  ♦ Keep patient warm (above 34°C).
  ♦ Use warm fluids.
  ♦ Use crystalloid fluids sparingly.
  ♦ Transfuse with fresh whole blood (less than 24 h old).

o Hemostatic agents: new products and bandages are available in several forms:
  ♦ Powders: placed in wound, then covered with a dressing.
  ♦ Dressings: impregnated with hemostatic agents.
  ♦ Injectables.
    ◊ Intravenous: augment clotting cascade of body.
    ◊ Intracavitary: through wounds to control internal bleeding.
  ♦ Two=component "glues".
  ♦ If an advanced hemostatic agent is used after a tourniquet has been placed, the tourniquet may be carefully removed after the agent has achieved hemostasis and the wound observed for hemorrhage. If hemorrhage recurs, return to the tourniquet.

Hemostatic Agents

Product	Source	Mechanism	Advantages	Disadvantages
Hem-Con	Shrimp shell poly-saccharide & vinegar	Sticks to blood forming plug	FDA approved, inexpensive	
Quik-Clot	Volcanic rock	Acts as a selective sponge for water/ dehydrates blood	FDA approved, inexpensive, easy to store, long shelf life	Thermal injury, requires removal from wound
Fibrin bandage	Fibrinogen/ thrombin	Activates clotting mechanism	Natural clotting mechanism reactions	Not FDA approved, allergic expensive

---

Two Field Hemostatic Agents

- Two agents are recommended by the US Tactical Combat Casualty Care Committee: 1) HemCon, 2) QuikClot.
- If standard measures such as elevation and pressure dressings do not control bleeding, it is recommended that tourniquet be used and that the first agent be HemCon. If this dressing fails, it should be removed and QuikClot used if the bleeding is life threatening.
- If the bleeding is external and not at a site where a tourniquet can be applied, HemCon and QuikClot can be used if conventional pressure dressings fail.
- Both products are to be used only on external sources of hemorrhage.
- HemCon dressing is a firm 4 x 4 inch dressing that is sterile and individually packaged. It works by adherence to the bleeding wound and has some vasoconstrictive properties. The blood and clot in the wound should be removed before application.

- QuikClot is a granular zeolite that absorbs fluid and causes hemostasis. It has handling properties similar to sand. When applied it can generate significant heat during the absorption process. Blood and clot should be wiped out of the wound prior to application.
- Remember, pressure must be applied for 3–5 minutes at the bleeding site, after application of a hemostatic dressing.

Field Hemostatic Dressings Considerations

Use should be delayed until after a trial of conventional dressings.

Do not use on minor injuries.

Use on internal wounds is not yet recommended.

Must apply pressure to the bleeding site after application.

Risk of inadequate contact of HemCon to the bleeding tissues in deep wounds.

Heat generation from QuikClot.

---

o **Controlled resuscitation** (hypotensive resuscitation).
   ◆ Resuscitation as a method of hemorrhage control. The needs of organ perfusion must be carefully balanced against the risk of increased bleeding as blood pressure rises. Excessive fluid resuscitation may increase bleeding and rebleeding. Prior to definitive hemorrhage control, a lower-than-normal blood pressure may be accepted. Small volumes of resuscitation fluid are still required in those casualties with decreased mentation due to hypotension (ie, decreased or absent radial pulse).

Chapter 7

Shock and Resuscitation

Introduction
The goal of fluid resuscitation is to maintain adequate perfusion. Fluid resuscitation of the wounded combatant remains a formidable challenge on the modern day battlefield. Routine resuscitation using 2 L of crystalloid through two large bore IVs is not appropriate in all situations and **the vast majority of the casualties do not need any IV resuscitation prior to arrival at a forward medical treatment facility** (MTF).

This chapter will briefly address shock, including recognition, classification, treatment, definition, and basic pathophysiology. Initial as well as sustained fluid resuscitation and a review of currently available fluids and potential future products will be described.

Recognition and Classification of Shock
Shock is a clinical condition marked by inadequate organ perfusion and tissue oxygenation, manifested by poor skin turgor, pallor, cool extremities, capillary refill greater than 2 seconds, anxiety/confusion/obtundation, tachycardia, weak or thready pulse, and hypotension. Lab findings include base deficit > 2, and lactic acidosis > 2.5 mmol/L.

- Hypovolemic shock: Diminished volume resulting in poor perfusion as a result of hemorrhage, diarrhea, dehydration, and burns (see Chapter 28, Burns). This is the most common type of shock seen in combat soldiers (see Table 7-1).

> **Hypotension is a late finding in shock, after 30%–40% lost blood volume. Earlier signs are tachycardia, decreased pulse pressure, and mental status changes. Tachycardia is often not reliable; however, and relative bradycardia is common.**

Table 7-1. Clinical Correlates in Hypovolemic Shock.

Blood Vol. Lost*	Heart Rate	Respiratory Rate	Blood Pressure	Central Nervous System
≤ 15%	Minimal tachycardia	No change	No change	No change
15%–30%	Tachycardia	Tachypnea	Decreased pulse pressure	Anxiety or combativeness
30%–40%	Marked tachycardia	Marked tachypnea	Systolic hypotension	Depressed mental status
> 40%	Marked tachycardia	Marked tachypnea	Severe systolic hypotension	Comatose

*Blood volume is approximately 7%, so a 70 kg patient has a blood volume of 4,900 mL.

- **Cardiogenic** shock: Pump failure from intrinsic cardiac failure or obstructive cardiac dysfunction from a tension pneumothorax, or cardiac tamponade with distended neck veins, or unilateral absence of breath sounds.
- **Distributive** shock: Poor perfusion due to loss of vascular tone; **neurogenic** shock: **bradycardia** with hypotension, seen with spinal cord injury.
  - o **Treat hemorrhagic shock first.**
  - o Volume resuscitation to maintain systolic BP > 90 mm Hg.
  - o Consider the addition of a vasopressor to address the loss in vascular tone—phenylephrine (50–300 µg/min) or dopamine (2–10 µg/kg/min).
- **Septic** shock: Fever, hypotension, and warm extremities from massive vasodilation, usually seen 5–7 days after initial trauma.

Treatment of Traumatic Shock—Control Bleeding!

The goal in the treatment of shock is to restore tissue perfusion and oxygen delivery (dependent on hemoglobin, cardiac output, and oxygenation).
- Secure the airway and administer O_2 for Sao_2 < 92%.
- Diagnose and treat tension pneumothorax.
- Control obvious bleeding and assess for occult hemorrhage.
- Assess circulation and establish IV access.

o Consider cardiac tamponade even if no distended neck veins.
- Administer IV fluids.
  o Hemorrhagic shock: Initially, any fluid available.
    ♦ LR: 1,000 mL expands intravascular volume by ~ 250 mL within 1 hour after injection.
    ♦ 6% hetastarch: 500 mL expands intravascular volume by ~ 800 mL in 1 hour, is functionally equivalent to 3 bags of LR, and is sustained for at least 8 hours.
    ♦ 7.5% hypertonic saline (HTS) results in the same physiologic response with $^1/_8$th the volume of LR or saline. Two infusions of 250 cc can be used. Although this recommendation has been made by the Institute of Medicine (Washington, DC) and two military consensus groups, 7.5% HTS is not commercially available. 3% and 5% HTS can be used instead and are formulary stock items.
  o Nonhemorrhagic shock: Crystalloid is the fluid of choice.
    ♦ Within 1 hour, resuscitate to a mean arterial pressure of > 60 mm Hg, a urine output of 0.5 cc/kg/h, and Sao_2 of > 92%.
- Based on response to fluids, casualties will fall into 3 groups:
  o **Responders**: Casualties with a sustained response to fluids probably have had significant blood loss but have stopped bleeding. However, they may still require definitive surgery.
  o **Transient** and **nonresponders** are continuing to bleed. They need immediate surgical intervention.
    ♦ Start blood transfusion as soon as possible.
    ♦ For nonresponders, fluids may be given to keep the patient alive, but one should not attempt to restore pressure to normal. Consideration should be taken into account of the futility of the resuscitation depending on the tactical scenario.
    ♦ Follow **controlled resuscitation** guidelines presented below.

Exsanguinating hemorrhage is the cause of most preventable deaths during war. Combat casualties in shock should be assumed to have hemorrhagic shock until proven otherwise.

- Vasopressors have no role in the initial treatment of hemorrhagic shock.
- Fluid choices.

The ideal fluid for resuscitation is still debated despite decades of research that began during WW I (see chart on next page).

Concept of Controlled (Hypotensive/Limited/Balanced) Resuscitation

- Raising the blood pressure with fluid resuscitation may dislodge established clots leading to more blood loss. Prior to establishing definitive hemorrhage control, use controlled resuscitation to **achieve and maintain** adequate perfusion as demonstrated by at least one of the following prioritized goals:
  - o Regains consciousness (follows commands).
  - o Palpable radial pulse.
  - o SBP ~90 mm Hg.
  - o MAP of ~60 mm Hg.

> **Controlled resuscitation is NOT a substitute for definitive surgical control. It is an attempt to keep a very sick patient alive until he can get to definitive treatment.**

- Endpoints of resuscitation.
  - o **Following definitive hemorrhage control**, more traditional endpoints of resuscitation include
    - ◆ Blood pressure: SBP > 120 mm Hg, MAP > 70 mm Hg.
    - ◆ Urine output: > 0.5 mL/kg/h (approximately 30 mL/h).
    - ◆ Correction of acidosis:
      - ◊ base deficit < 2.
      - ◊ serum lactate < 2.5 mmol/L.
    - ◆ Hypothermia: It is important to maintain normal body temperature. Fluids and patient care areas should be warmed. This is often not possible in the deployed environment. Patients frequently arrive at the facility already hypothermic. Keep patients covered when on litters, radiograph tables, and operating tables. External warmers (such as contained forced warm air devices, eg, Bair Hugger) should be employed in all patient care

Fluid/Initial Dose	Indication	Advantages	Cautions
Crystalloids Saline Ringer's Lactate	Hypovolemia, dehydration, hemorrhage, shock, burns	Easy to store Inexpensive Proven effectiveness Isotonic	Weight ratio – requires 3:1 for lost blood Dilution, edema, coagulopathy
Hypertonic saline (HTS) 3%–5% 7.5%* Hypertonic saline- colloid combinations* HTS dextran* HTS hetastarch*	Hemorrhagic shock: 4cc/kg or 250 cc bolus, may repeat once Burns—only one dose initially	Lighter weight Small volume = large effect Increased cardiac contractility Longer duration of effect than plain HTS?	>500cc – Risk of hypernatremia, seizures Do not use for dehydration from vomiting, diarrhea or sweating, or heat injuries Do not repeat without addition of other fluids Must replace depleted extravascular fluid

Colloids
Albumin
Artificial colloids
Dextran
6% hetastarch
(Hextend, Hespan)
10% Pentastarch*
Gelatin-based colloids*
	Hemorrhagic shock
	250–500 mL bolus
	Burns? Third day
		Longer duration
		1:1 replacement for blood
		Raises plasma oncotic pressure
		Recruits extravascular fluid
		Weight/cube better than crystalloids
			Overuse may lead to "leak" into tissue
			Binds immunoglobulins and Ca++
			Must replace depleted extravascular fluid
			Artificial colloids:
			  Coagulopathy, allergic reaction, osmotic
			  diuresis, interferes with crossmatching
			  Hetastarch: ↑ fibrinolysis, ↑ Amylase
			  Max dose: 20 mL/kg/d (about 1.5 L)

Oral rehydration fluids	Dehydration controlled hemorrhage Burns	Fluids of opportunity Nonsterile ingredients: 4 tsp sugar, 1 tsp salt, 1 L water	Austere option in abdominal wounds and unconscious patients, but use with caution
Blood	Hemorrhagic—Type O universal donor	Carries oxygen Autotransfusion Walking blood bank	Storage, type and cross-match Transfusion reactions, infection, immunogenic
Artificial blood Hemoglobin based Fluorocarbon based	Hemorrhage	Easy storage No type and cross matching	Experimental only, not yet available for use Fluorocarbons require supplemental O$_2$ Future option?

*Not FDA approved

areas from initial emergency area through operating room and ICU. Hypothermia is much easier to prevent than it is to treat. See further discussion of hypothermia in Chapter 12, Damage Control Surgery.

Transfusion Therapy
● Blood transfusion.

Blood should be added to the resuscitation of patients who have lost 30%–40% of their blood volume. Blood may also be necessary in patients who have not reached this threshold but have ongoing blood loss. Whole blood has a greater risk for immunologic reactions than packed cells.

Blood products fielded with forward medical units (FST, CSH) are predominantly group O packed red cells and FFP. Upon reaching a stabilization phase of operations, type-specific packed cells and platelets will be supplied through theater specific channels. Storage, shelf-life, and availability of these products are outlined in Table 7-2.

Table 7-2. Blood Products Available to the Theater.

Product	Unit of Issue	Storage	Shelf Life for Transfusion	Echelon Availability	Blood Group Availability			
					O+/-	A+/-	B+/-	AB+/-
Liquid PRBCs	~250mL	35d	35d	Second & third (MASH)	100%	—	—	—
				Third (CSH) & fourth	50%	40%	10%	—
Frozen/ deglyc- erolized RBCs	~250mL	10y	3d (postwash)	Third & fourth	100%	—	—	—
FFP	~250mL	1y	24h (postthaw)	Third & fourth	—	50%	25%	25%
Platelet concen- trate	~60mL	5d	5d	Third & fourth	50%	50%	—*	—*

* Will be provided by blood bank platoon and medical treatment facilities by in-theater blood collections.
CHS: combat support hospital; FFP: fresh frozen plasma; MASH: mobile army surgical hospital; PRBCs: packed red blood cells; RBCs: red blood cells
Adapted from US Department of the Army. *Planning for Health Service Support*. Washington, DC: Headquarters, DA; approved final draft January 1994. Field Manual 8-55: 8-6.

Familiarity with transfusion technique, patient-donor unit infusion connections, and walking blood bank connections, is essential and should be practiced routinely. Most serious transfusion reactions are the result of an error at the bedside, not an error in typing and cross-matching (ie, transfusing "the right unit to the wrong patient").

- **Transfusion reactions** may be difficult to recognize in severely or multiply injured casualties. Hemolytic (ABO mismatch) reactions present acutely (< 24 hours) with fever, chills, back pain, dyspnea, and renal failure. Delayed reactions may occur. Transfusion should be halted immediately in all cases, except minor allergic reactions (urticaria, fever, +/- mild bronchospasm), which are treated with diphenhydramine (25–50 mg IV or PO), H-2 blocker, methylprednisolone, +/- epinephrine.

Field Management of a Transfusion Reaction
- Stop the infusion of blood. Continue to infuse normal saline through the intravenous line.
- Examine the urine for hemoglobinuria. Examine plasma for hemoglobinemia.
- Maintain blood pressure and urinary output with saline. Consider administering mannitol or furosemide after volume repletion if the patient is oliguric.
- Reexamine the donor unit for seal integrity, evidence of hemolysis or infection, and recheck the transfusion log for clerical error.
- Annotate the field medical card with a description of the suspected reaction and the therapy provided. Transfer the unit suspected of causing the reaction to the next echelon of care with the casualty.

- **Clinical relevance of the Rh bloodgroup in female casualties**.
  Women, military and civilian, are becoming more frequent victims of conflict. Approximately 85% of the American population is Rh positive. Serious consequences to Rh incompatible blood are rare in men. Data predict that 10% of

group O blood transfusions will be of Rh positive units to Rh negative female recipients. An Rh negative woman transfused with Rh positive blood is very likely (approximately 80%) to produce anti-D (Rh positive) antibodies. This seroconversion can jeopardize a subsequent pregnancy when this Rh negative mother, now sensitized by Rh positive transfusion, conceives an Rh positive fetus. Chronic hemolytic disease of the newborn may result.

Under no circumstances should a life-saving transfusion be withheld because of Rh incompatibility; saving a life takes precedence over Rh immunization.

Prevention: When the supply of group O blood permits, group O Rh negative blood should be reserved for women.

- **Massive transfusions.**
    - o Definition.
        - ♦ >10 Units of PRBC's in <24 hours.
        - ♦ Whole body blood volume transfusion in a 24-hour period.
    - o Consequences of massive blood loss.
        - ♦ Shock.
        - ♦ Hypothermia.
        - ♦ Acidosis.
        - ♦ Decrease of coagulation factors.
        - ♦ Decrease of platelets.
    - o Consequences of massive blood transfusions.
        - ♦ Dilution of coagulation factors.
        - ♦ Dilution of platelets.
        - ♦ Acidosis.
        - ♦ Hypothermia.
        - ♦ Hypocalcaemia (citrate toxicity) associated with rapid transfusions.
    - o For every 10 units of PRBCs give:
        - ♦ 4 units of FFP.
        - ♦ 1 unit of platelets (6 pack of 1 aphresis unit).
        - ♦ Consider 1 dose of cryoprecipitate (10 single units of Cryo).
    - o What blood to use?

- ◆ Type specific if at all possible.
- ◆ O positive (preferred) in males and postreproductive females.
- ◆ O negative (if available) in females of reproductive age.
- ◆ If still using O after 8 units, stick with O, even if blood type is determined. Stick with O until the patient's forward and back typed appropriately.
- o Which FFP to use?
  - ◆ There is no such thing as emergency release FFP.
  - ◆ Type specific if at all possible.
  - ◆ AB when in doubt.
  - ◆ A as a second choice.
  - ◆ Unless you KNOW that the patient is Type O blood, **DO NOT use Type O FPP**.

- ● **Walking blood bank.**
When standard blood component therapy is unavailable, the use of fresh whole blood can be lifesaving. Because whole blood contains clotting factors, it is effective for treating dilutional coagulopathy associated with massive blood loss and fluid resuscitation.
  - o Equipment.
    - ◆ Blood recipient set (bag), indirect Tx Y-type (NSN 6515 01 128 1407).
    - ◆ Stopcock, IV therapy 3 way, with Luer lock (NSN 6515 00 864 8864).
  - o Cautions.
    - ◆ Field conditions increase the risk of bacterial contamination.
    - ◆ Definitive testing of blood for transfusion virus diseases is not available.
    - ◆ "Dog tag" blood typing wrong 2%–11% of the time.
    - ◆ Donor performance may be impaired by donation.
      - ◊ Good for small numbers of patients—large numbers lead to doubling of unit ineffectiveness.
      - ◊ Should not be the "default" answer for standard blood program planning.
      - ◊ Donate only once a month.
      - ◊ Avoid donation at high altitudes.

> **Even in an emergency, try to get regularly issued blood products.**

- ◊ Women—ideally on supplemental iron before/after donation.
- o Planning.
  - ◆ Predeployment.
    - ◊ Develop a current prescreened donor roster.
      - ▪ Blood type and Rh.
      - ▪ Nonreactive transfusion transmissible disease tests (if available).
  - ◆ Onsite.
    - ◊ Update prescreening donor roster.
      - ▪ Tent/cot location.
      - ▪ Duty location.
- **Emergency (no roster in place).**
  - o Establish blood types with local testing or previous donor history.
  - o Choose prior blood donors in preference to nondonors because they have been tested for the infectious diseases in the past.
  - o Rely on "dog tags" only as a last resort.
  - o Draw only type "O" universal donors in mass casualty situations to reduce the confusion of handling.
  - o Draw universal or type specific donors in case of single patient incidents. (Type O donors are 46% of the US population.)
- Procedure for walking blood bank.
  - o Clean donor's arm with povidone iodine for at least 1 minute.
  - o Draw the blood from an arm vein into an unexpired, intact commercial blood bag.
  - o The bag has a 600 ml capacity and contains 63 mL of CPD or CPDA-1 anticoagulant.
  - o Draw about 450 mL, a "pint," so that the bag is almost full.
  - o Draw tubes for typing, cross-matching, and transfusion transmissible disease testing (if available).

o Send tubes to a supporting laboratory (if available). Even after-the-fact testing is useful to provide reassurance of safety or explanations of untoward events.

o Label the bag clearly with blood type and donor identification information.

- Whole blood crossmatching.
  o The white tile method uses a drop of the donor blood mixed with the recipient serum on a white ceramic tile and is examined in 4 minutes.
  o If no agglutination occurs, the blood is suitable for transfusion into that recipient. A hand lens may be useful.

- Storage.
  o Keep at room temperature no longer than 24 hours.
  o Blood stored warm for more than 24 hours has a significant risk of bacterial growth and clotting factors will be lost. If the blood has been kept at room temperature for less than 8 hours, it can be kept in a refrigerator or on wet ice for up to 3 weeks.
  o Although RBCs remain viable, platelets may become inactive in whole blood stored cold (1°C–10°C) for greater than 24 hours, losing one of the main benefits of fresh whole blood.
  o Ensure that anesthetist/anesthesiologist and surgeon are aware that this is an emergency-drawn unit and tell them the history of the unit.
  o After 24 hours, destroy warm-stored, whole-blood units. (Stateside hospitals would do so after exceeding 10°C for 30 minutes.) They are no longer safe or fresh. You may save cold-stored units until a regular supply of tested blood is reestablished.
  o Keep a record of donors and patients transfused so they can be tested on return to stateside.
  o Keep a record of number of units transfused, donor names, and outcome.

- Autotransfusion.
  o Blood collected into sterile containers (eg, suction, chest tube, among others) may be returned to the patient through a blood filter.

o Blood from sterile cavities, such as the chest or abdomen without visceral injuries is preferred.

o Blood from contaminated abdominal wounds can be used at an increased risk of systemic infection.

o Blood may be filtered through sterile gauze as a field expedient method.

The Future

Because the definition of shock is inadequate oxygenation at the cellular level, the most ideal fluid would provide volume expansion and oxygen-carrying capacity. For this fluid to be useful in deployed settings it needs to be stable at a variety of temperatures and have a low-risk profile. Hemoglobin based oxygen carrying compounds (HBOCs) currently under investigation may be such fluids. There are HBOCs derived from either bovine or human sources that require no refrigeration, have a shelf life of up to 3 years, are disease free, and require no crossmatching.

Chapter 8

Vascular Access

Introduction
Vascular access is a critical early step in the management of trauma. Peripheral access should be attempted first; if unsuccessful, additional percutaneous central access locations include the subclavian vein, the internal and external jugular veins, and the common femoral veins. Cutdowns for the saphenous vein at ankle or femoral sites are alternative options.

- Basic Equipment.
  - o Tourniquet.
  - o 1%–2% Lidocaine.
  - o Sterile prep solution, drape, gloves, and 4 x 4 gauze pads.
  - o 3mL syringe with 25-gauge needle.
  - o Scalpel, hemostat, 11 blade scalpel and fine scissors.
  - o Vein introducer or "vein pick".
  - o IV catheter; IV tubing (modified with distal connector cut off), and 8 F NG tube, are field expedients.
  - o 3-0 or 4-0 silk ties to secure catheter in vein.
  - o 2-0 or 3-0 suture to secure catheter to skin.
  - o Central catheter kit (for central lines) or intraosseous device for intraosseous insertion.

Subclavian Vein Access or Internal Jugular Venipuncture
- Place the patient supine in Trendelenburg (15° head down).
- Prep and drape subclavian/jugular area. Sterile gloves should be worn.
  - o Subclavian line.
    - ♦ With an index finger placed at the sternal notch, the thumb is placed at the junction of the medial and middle third of the clavicle.
    - ♦ 1% lidocaine is infiltrated into the skin, subcutaneous tissue and periosteum of the clavicle.

- ♦ Introduce a large caliber needle with attached 5 mL syringe. Insert with the bevel of the needle up, directing the needle towards the contralateral clavicular head. Keep the needle horizontal to avoid a pneumothorax.
- ♦ While aspirating, slowly advance the needle underneath the clavicle.
- o Jugular vein line.
  - ♦ Turn the patient's head 45° toward the contralateral side to expose the neck.
  - ♦ Identify the apex of the anterior cervical triangle formed by the heads of the sternocleidomastoid muscle to locate the carotid artery.
  - ♦ Palpate the carotid artery and stay lateral with your venipuncture.
  - ♦ Introduce a large-bore needle on 10mL syringe at a 45° angle into the apex of the triangle, lateral to the carotid pulse.
  - ♦ Carotid Puncture: Immediately withdraw the needle and place pressure on site for a minimum of 5 minutes.
  - ♦ Advance the needle caudally, parallel to the sagittal plane and at a 30° posterior angle (eg, toward the ipsilateral nipple).
  - ♦ When free flow of venous blood appears, advance the needle an additional 4 mm (the length of the needle bevel), then remove the syringe and quickly cover the hub of the needle to prevent air embolism.
    - ◊ If air or arterial blood appears, stop immediately. Withdraw needle immediately and place pressure at the site for at least 5 minutes.
  - ♦ If no venous blood return after advancing 5 cm, slowly withdraw the needle while aspirating. If this fails, redirect the needle.
- o Subclavian vein or internal jugular vein catheter insertion.
  - ♦ Once the needle is in the vein, introduce the "J" wire through the needle (Seldinger technique). The wire should pass with minimal resistance. If wire does not pass easily, withdraw the entire apparatus and reattempt line placement.
  - ♦ Remove the needle.

◆ Enlarge the puncture site with a scalpel and dilator.
◆ Pass the catheter over the wire while holding the wire in place, to a depth of 18 cm on the left and 15 cm on the right for subclavian, and to a depth of 9 cm on the right and 12 cm on the left for jugular vein, then remove the wire.
◆ Aspirate from all ports, flush all ports, suture in place, apply antibiotic ointment, dress area, secure tubing, and label date of insertion.
◆ Chest radiograph to ensure line position and rule out pneumothorax.

Greater Saphenous Vein Cutdowns
● **Contraindications.**
  o Deep vein thrombosis (DVT) or severe ipsilateral lower extremity trauma.
● **Procedure.**
  o Expose, prep, and drape ankle or femoral site.
  o For ankle, administer local anesthetic proximal to the medial malleolus.
  o Make a superficial transverse incision through the skin over the entire width of the flat tibial edge (~3cm) in the area of the saphenous vein.
  o Using a curved hemostat, isolate the greater saphenous vein from the nerve and underlying bone.
  o Using the open hemostat as a platform, cut a 1–2 mm venotomy in the anterior surface of the vein with a number 11 blade (Fig. 8-1a).
  o Place the intravenous tubing (previously beveled) or angiocatheter at least 4 cm into the vein (may require use of a vein introducer) (Fig. 8-1b).
  o Secure the catheter with a proximal silk ligature, and tie off the distal vein.
  o Secure the catheter with a suture.
  o Apply a clean dressing.
  o Femoral procedure is essentially the same, with site being a handbreadth below the inguinal ligament, medial to the midline of the thigh. After skin incision, finger bluntly dissects through the fat to the fascia. Hook the finger and lift, and the vein comes up with it.

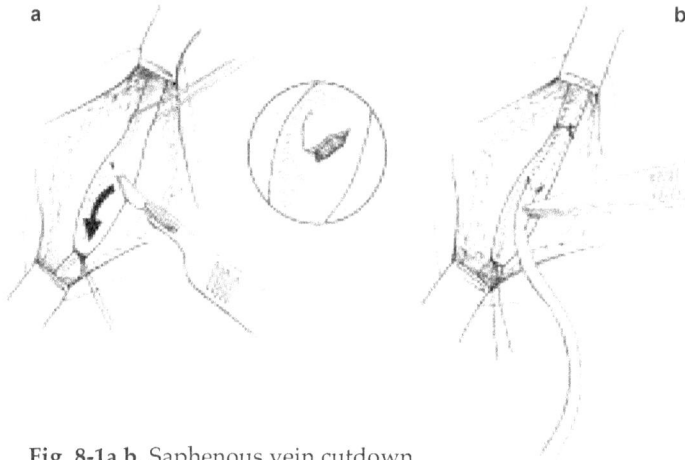

Fig. 8-1a,b. Saphenous vein cutdown.

- Cutdown can also be performed on the common femoral veins, the jugular veins, and on veins of the forearm.

IO Infusion
- **Contraindications.**
    - o Trauma or infection at insertion site.
    - o Recent IO device at the same site.
    - o Fracture of insertion bone.
    - o Recent sternotomy.
- **Devices/ Procedure.**
    - o F.A.S.T. 1, BIG, SurFast, Jamshidi Needle, VidaPort.
    - o Procedures vary based on model; all IV fluids acceptable except possibly hypertonic solutions.
    - o BIG, SurFast, and Jamshidi may be placed in proximal medial tibia, distal medial tibia, or the radius.
    - o F.A.S.T. 1 is designed for sternal placement, 1.5 cm below the sternal notch.
    - o Pediatric: Insert a bone-marrow aspiration needle or 14–19-gauge spinal needle, directing it caudally through the outer cortex. Common sites: tibia, distal femur.
    - o Aspirate to confirm placement.

Chapter 9

Anesthesia

Introduction
Battlefield anesthesia primarily describes a state of balanced anesthesia using **adequate amounts of anesthetic agents** to minimize cardiovascular instability, amnesia, analgesia, and a quiescent surgical field in a technologically austere environment. Adapting anesthetic techniques to battlefield conditions requires flexibility and a reliance on fundamental clinical skills. While modern monitors provide a wealth of data, the stethoscope may be the only tool available in an austere environment. Thus, the value of crisp heart sounds and clear breath sounds when caring for an injured service member should not be underestimated. In addition, close collaboration and communication with the surgeon is essential.

Airway
Many methods for securing a compromised airway exist, depending on the condition of the airway, the comorbid state of the patient, and the environment in which care is being rendered. When a definitive airway is required, it is generally best secured with direct laryngoscopy and an endotracheal tube (ETT), firmly secured in the trachea.

Indications for a Definitive Airway
- Apnea/airway obstruction/hypercarbia.
- Impending airway obstruction: facial fractures, retropharyngeal hematoma, and inhalation injury.
- Excessive work of breathing.
- Shock (bp $\leq$ 80 mm Hg systolic).
- Glasgow Coma Scale (GCS) $\leq$ 8. (See Appendix 2.)
- Persistent hypoxia ($Sao_2 < 90\%$).

Secondary Airway Compromise Can Result From
- Failure to recognize the need for an airway.
- Inability to establish an airway.
- **Failure to recognize an incorrectly placed airway.**
- Displacement of a previously established airway.
- Failure to recognize the need for ventilation.

Induction of General Anesthesia
The Anesthesia Provider Must Evaluate the Patient for
- Concurrent illness and current state of resuscitation.
- Airway — facial trauma, dentition, hyoid-to-mandibular symphysis length, extent of mouth opening.
- Cervical spine mobility (preexistent and trauma related).
- Additional difficult airway indicators.
  - o Immobilization.
  - o Children.
  - o Short neck/receding mandible.
  - o Prominent upper incisors.

Rapid Sequence Intubation Checklist
- Equipment.
  - o Laryngoscope, blades, and batteries (tested daily).
  - o Suction, O_2 setup.
  - o Endotracheal tubes and stylet.
  - o Alternative tubes (oro, nasopharyngeal, LMA [laryngeal mask airway]).
  - o IV access items.
  - o Monitors — pulse ox, ECG, BP, end-tidal CO_2.
  - o Positive pressure ventilation (Ambu bag or anesthesia machine).
- Drugs.
  - o Narcotics.
  - o Muscle relaxants.
  - o Anxiolytics and amnestics.
  - o Induction agents and sedatives.
  - o Inhalation agents.
- Narcotics.
  - o **Fentanyl**, 2.0–2.5 µg/kg IV bolus, then titrate to effect.

- o **Morphine**, 5–10 mg IV bolus to load, then 2 mg q5min to effect.
- o **Dilaudid** (Hydromorhone), 1–2 mg IV to load, then 0.5 mg q5min to effect.
- Muscle relaxants.
  - o Depolarizing.
    - ◆ **Succinylcholine**.
      - ◊ 1.0–1.5 mg/kg.
      - ◊ Onset 30–60 sec.
      - ◊ Duration 5–10 min.
      - ◊ Can cause bradycardia, fasciculations, elevated intragastric pressure, elevated ICP, elevated intra-cranial pressure, potassium release (especially in "chronic" burn or immobile patients).
      - ◊ Potent trigger of malignant hyperthermia (MH).

> **Succinylcholine should be NOT be used in patients with burns or crush injuries > 24 hours old or chronic neuromuscular disorders due to risk for hyperkalemia — rocuronium is the next best choice.**

  - o Nondepolarizing.
    - ◆ **Vecuronium**: induction dose of 0.1 mg/kg with an onset of 2–3 minutes and duration of action of 30–40 minutes.
    - ◆ **Rocuronium**: induction dose of 0.6 mg/kg with an onset of 1.5–2.5 minutes and duration of action of 35–50 minutes. At 1.2 mg/kg onset similar to succinyl-choline, but, unfortunately, a duration of action that can exceed 60–90 minutes.
    - ◆ **Pancuronium**: induction dose of 0.15 mg/kg with an onset of 3.5–6 minutes and duration of action of 70–120 minutes.
- Anxiolytics and amnestics.
  - o **Versed** (midazolam), 1–2 mg IV slowly (over 2 min).
  - o **Scopolamine**, 0.4 mg IV.
- Induction agents and sedatives (Table 9-1).

Table 9-1. Induction Agents and Sedatives.

Agent	Routine Dose[*]	Characteristics	Concerns
Ketamine	1.0–2.0 mg/kg IV	Dissociative anesthetic and amnestic. Sympathomimetic effects (useful in hypovolemia). Potent bronchodilator.	Varying degrees of purposeful skeletal movement despite intense analgesia and amnesia.
	4.0–8.0 mg/kg IM	Onset within 30–60 sec. Emergence delirium avoided with concomitant benzodiazepine use.	Increased salivation, consider an antisialagogue.
Barbiturates (eg, thiopental)	3–5 mg/kg	Onset within 30–60 seconds.	May cause profound hypotension in hypovolemic shock patients.
Propofol	1.5–2.5 mg/kg	Mixed in lipid, strict sterility must be ensured. Rapid onset and rapidly metabolized. Onset within 30–60 seconds.	Contraindicated in acute hypovolemic shock patients.
Etomidate	0.2–0.4 mg/kg	Onset within 30–60 seconds. Duration 3–10 min. Minimal cardiac effects. Minimal effects on peripheral and pulmonary circulation. Maintains cerebral perfusion.	May cause clonus.

* All induction agents can be used for induction of severely injured patients if reduced dosages are used (eg, $^{1}/_{2}$ of the lower recommended dose). However, the recommended choice for hypovolemic patients would be Ketamine > etomidate >> thiopental > propofol.

Rapid Sequence Intubation (RSI) 7 steps*

1. Preoxygenate with 100% oxygen by mask.
2. Consider fentanyl—titrate to maintain adequate blood pressure and effect (2.0–2.5 µg/kg).
3. Cricoid pressure—Selleck maneuver until endotracheal tube (ETT) placement is confirmed and balloon is inflated.
4. Induction agent: etomidate 0.1–0.4 mg/kg IV push.
5. Muscle relaxant: succinylcholine 1.0–1.5 mg/kg IV push.
6. Laryngoscopy and orotracheal intubation.
7. Verify tube placement.

*For children, see page 33.6.

- Endotracheal intubation.
  - o Orotracheal.
    - ◆ Direct laryngoscopy 60–90 seconds after administration of induction agents and neuromuscular blockade.
    - ◆ First attempt is the best chance for success, but have a backup plan:
      - ◊ Optimize positioning of patient and anesthesia provider.
      - ◊ Have adjuncts readily available (stylet, smaller diameter tubes, alternative laryngoscope blades, suction, laryngeal mask airway, lighted stylet).
  - o Nasotracheal should generally not be performed.
  - o Other considerations.
    - ◆ Maintain cricoid pressure until balloon inflated and tube position is confirmed.
    - ◆ Hypertension can be managed with short-acting medications such as beta blockers (labetalol, esmolol) or sodium nitroprusside.
    - ◆ May treat induction-related (transient) hypotension initially with small dose of ephedrine (5–10mg) or Neosynephrine (50 µg), but if hypotension persists after induction agents are metabolized, use fluids to treat the persistent hypovolemia. The anesthesiologist must convey this situation to the surgeon, as the need to control bleeding becomes urgent.

♦ A sensitive airway can be topically anesthetized with lidocaine 1.5 mg/kg 1–2 minutes before laryngoscopy.
- Verify ETT placement.
  - o Auscultate the lungs.
  - o Measure the end-tidal CO_2.
  - o Ensure that the Sao_2 remains high.
  - o Palpate cuff of ETT in sternal notch.
  - o Place the chemical CO_2 sensors in the airway circuit.

Verification of tube placement is VITAL. Any difficulty with oxygenation/ventilation following RSI should prompt evaluation for immediate reintubation.

The Difficult Airway (see Chapter 5, Airway and Breathing)
Initially provide airway management with jaw-thrust, facemask oxygenation, and assess the situation. Failed RSI may be due to inadequate time for induction agents to work; inadequate time for muscle relaxation to occur; anatomically difficult airway; or obstruction due to secretions, blood, trauma, or foreign material.
- Resume oxygenation; consider placing a temporary oral airway.
- Reposition patient and anesthesia provider.
- Call for help.
- Consider alternatives to RSI.
  - o Awake intubation.
  - o Laryngeal mask airway.
  - o Regional anesthesia or local anesthesia.
  - o Surgical airway.

Maintenance of General Anesthesia
General Anesthesia Is Maintained After Intubation With
- Oxygen. Titrate to maintain $Sao_2 > 92\%$.
- Ventilation.
  - o Tidal volume (TV) 10–15 cc/kg.
  - o Respiratory rate (RR) 6–10/min.
  - o PEEP (positive end-expiratory pressure) if desired at 5 cm H_2O, titrate as necessary.
- Minimal alveolar concentration (MAC).
  - o 0.3–0.5 MAC: awareness abolished although 50% of patients respond to verbal commands.

o 1 MAC: 50% of patients do not move to surgical stimulus.
o 1.2 MAC: 95% of patients do not move to surgical stimulus.
o Common inhalation agent MACs:
  ♦ Halothane: 0.75%.
  ♦ Sevoflurane: 1.8%.
  ♦ Isoflurane: 1.17%.
  ♦ Enflurane: 1.63%.
  ♦ Nitrous Oxide (N_2O) = 104%.
  ♦ Additive effects (eg, 60% N_2O mixed with 0.8% sevoflurane yields 1 MAC).
- Total intravenous anesthesia (TIVA).
  o Mix midazolam 5 mg, vecuronium 10 mg, ketamine 200 mg in 50 cc normal saline (NS) and infuse at 0.5 cc/kg/h (stop 10–15 minutes before end of surgery).
  o Mix 50–100 mg of ketamine with 500 mg of propofol (50 cc of 10% propofol) and administer at 50–100 µg/kg/min (21–42 mL/h for a 70 kg patient).
- Balanced anesthesia (titration of drugs and gases) combine:
  o 0.4 MAC.
  o Versed 1–2 mg/h.
  o Ketamine 2–4 mg/kg/h.

Conclusion of General Anesthesia
- If the patient is to **remain intubated**, anesthetics may be terminated but sedatives and muscle relaxants are maintained.
- If the patient is to be **extubated**, ventilation is decreased to allow the patient to spontaneously breathe.
  o Anesthetic agents are stopped 5 minutes before conclusion of surgery.
  o Glycopyrrolate (Robinul) (0.01–0.02 mg/kg IV over 3–5 minutes) to decrease parasympathetic stimulation and secretions. This can be administered at the same time or before neostigmine.
  o Muscle relaxation reversal with neostigmine (0.04–0.08 mg/kg IV over 3–5 minutes, can be mixed in same syringe as glycopyrrolate).
- Extubation criteria include reversal of muscle relaxation, spontaneous ventilation, response to commands, eye

opening, and head lifting for 5 seconds. **When in doubt, keep the patient intubated.**

- Amnestic therapy with midazolam and analgesic therapy with a narcotic is appropriate in small amounts so as not to eliminate the spontaneous respiratory drive.

Regional Anesthesia

Regional anesthesia (RA) is a "field friendly" anesthetic requiring minimal logistical support while providing quality anesthesia and analgesia on the battlefield. Advantages of RA on the modern battlefield are listed below.

- Excellent operating conditions.
- Profound perioperative analgesia.
- Stable hemodynamics.
- Limb specific anesthesia.
- Reduced need for other anesthetics.
- Improved postoperative alertness.
- Minimal side effects.
- Rapid recovery from anesthesia.
- Simple, easily transported equipment needed.

Recent conflicts have revealed that the majority of casualties will have superficial wounds or wounds of the extremities. RA is well suited for the management of these injuries either as an adjunct to general anesthesia or as the primary anesthetic. The use of basic RA blocks is encouraged when time and resources are available.

- Superficial cervical plexus block.
- Axillary brachial plexus block.
- IV regional anesthesia.
- Wrist block.
- Digital nerve block.
- Intercostobrachial nerve block.
- Saphenous nerve block.
- Ankle block.
- Spinal anesthesia.
- Lumbar epidural anesthesia.
- Combined spinal-epidural anesthesia.
- Femoral nerve block.

Prior training in basic block techniques is implied, and use of a nerve stimulator, when appropriate, is encouraged to enhance block success. More advanced blocks and continuous peripheral nerve blocks are typically not available until the patient arrives at a combat support hospital (CSH) or higher level health care facility where personnel trained in these techniques are available. A long-acting local anesthetic such as 0.5% ropivacaine is used for most single-injection peripheral nerve blocks. Peripheral nerve blocks can often be used to treat pain (without the respiratory depression of narcotics) while patients are waiting for surgery.

- **Neuraxial anesthesia.**
  - o Subarachnoid block (SAB).
  - o Epidural block.

When the patient's physical condition allows the use of spinal or epidural anesthesia those techniques are encouraged. The sympathectomy that results is often poorly tolerated in a trauma patient and this must be factored into any decision to use those techniques. Peripheral nerve blocks do not have this limitation.

- **Local anesthesia.**

When local anesthesia would suffice, such as in certain wound debridements and wound closures, it should be the technique of choice.

Field Anesthesia Equipment

There are two anesthesia apparatuses currently fielded in the forward surgical environment: (1) the draw-over vaporizer and (2) a conventional portable ventilator machine. A schematic of the draw-over system is shown in Figure 9-1.

- **Draw-over vaporizer.**
  - o Currently fielded model: Ohmeda Portable Anesthesia Complete (PAC).
  - o Demand type system (unlike the plenum systems in hospital-based ORs).
    - ♦ When the patient does not initiate a breath or the self-inflating bag is not squeezed, there is **no flow of gas**. No demand equals no flow.
  - o Temperature-compensated flow-over in-line vaporizer.

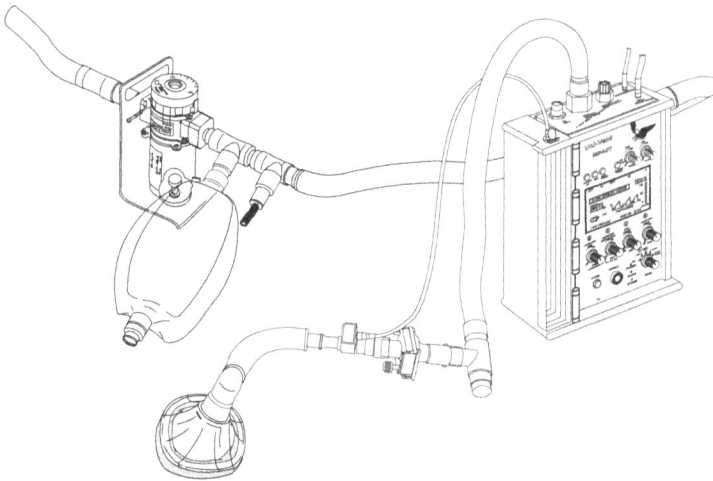

Fig. 9-1. Draw-over apparatus in combination with the ventilator.

o Optimal oxygen conservation requires a larger reservoir (oxygen economizer tube [OET]) than is described in the operator's manual — a 3.5 ft OET optimizes F_{IO_2}.
o May be used with spontaneous or controlled ventilations.
o Bolted-on performance chart outlines dial positions for some commonly used anesthetics (eg, halothane, isoflurane, enflurane, and ether). **Ether is highly flammable; use extreme care.**

Ohmeda UPAC Draw-Over Apparatus in Combination With the Impact Uni-Vent Eagle 754 Portable Ventilator:
• Currently, there is no mechanical ventilator specifically designed for use with the UPAC draw-over apparatus, but use with various portable ventilators has been studied in both the draw-over and push-over configuration.
o Adding the ventilator frees the anesthesia provider's hands while providing more uniform ventilation and more consistent concentrations of the inhalational anesthetic agent.

o The **draw-over** configuration places the ventilator distal to the vaporizer, entraining ambient air and vapor across the vaporizer in the same manner as the spontaneously breathing patient. Do not attach a compressed source of air to the Impact Uni-Vent Eagle 754 in this configuration because the Uni-Vent Eagle 754 will preferentially deliver the compressed gases and will not entrain air / anesthetic gases from the UPAC draw-over.

o The **push-over** configuration places the ventilator proximal to the vaporizer, effectively pushing entrained ambient air across the vaporizer and then to the patient.

● The Impact Uni-Vent Eagle 754 portable ventilator (Figure 9-1) is not part of the UPAC apparatus but is standard equipment for the US military. It has been used in combination with the Ohmeda UPAC Draw-Over Apparatus.

o The air-entrainment (side intake) port is used to create the draw-over / ventilator combination.

♦ The side intake port of the ventilator contains a nonreturn valve preventing back pressure on the vaporizer which could result in erratic and inconsistent anesthetic agent concentrations.

o The patient air-outlet port on the ventilator also contains a nonreturn valve, preventing back flow into the ventilator from the patient side.

o Scavenging of waste gases can be accomplished by attaching corrugated anesthesia tubing to either the outlet port of the Ambu-E valve (induction circuit) or the exhalation port of the ventilator tubing (ventilator circuit) venting to the outside atmosphere.

o The following items are added to the circuit to improve this UPAC / Impact Uni-Vent Eagle 754 ventilator combination:

♦ Small and large circuit adapters to aid in attachment of various pieces.

♦ PALL Heat and Moisture Exchange Filter to conserve heat and limit patient contact with the circuit.

♦ Accordion circuit extender to move the weight of the circuit away from the patient connection.

♦ O_2 extension tubing to attach supplemental O_2.

o Two separate circuits should be constructed for use with the UPAC™/Uni-Vent Eagle 754 combination: one for induction and spontaneous ventilation and the second for controlled ventilation using the portable ventilator.

♦ This process can be complicated because switching circuit components requires several disconnections and reconnections, creating the potential for error. (Practice.)

• **Conventional plenum anesthesia machine.**

o Currently fielded models: Drager Narkomed and Magellan 2000.

o Compact version of standard OR machines, with comparable capabilities.

Chapter 10

Infections

Introduction

> **All wounds incurred on the battlefield are grossly contaminated with bacteria. Most will become infected unless appropriate treatment is initiated quickly.**

The battlefield environment is conducive to wound infection due to
- Absence of "sterile" wounding agents on the battlefield. All foreign bodies (wounding projectile fragments, clothing, dirt) are contaminated with bacteria.
- High-energy projectile wounding (devitalized tissue, hematoma, tissue ischemia).
- Delay in casualty evacuation.

Diagnosis of a Wound Infection
- The four "-ors:" dolor, rubor, calor, and tumor—**pain** and **tenderness**, **redness**, **warmth**, and **swelling**.
- Drainage or discharge, ranging from frank pus to the foul "dishwater" discharge of clostridial infection.
- Crepitus, radiographic evidence of soft-tissue gas, epidermal blistering, and/or epidermal necrosis are the hallmarks of necrotizing soft tissue infection, such as clostridial gas gangrene or necrotizing fasciitis.
- Systemic effects such as fever, leukocytosis, unexplained tachycardia, or hypotension.
- Confirm diagnosis by Gram stain and culture, if available, and/or tissue biopsy.

Common Microorganisms Causing Battlefield Infections

- Gram-positive cocci: staphylococci, streptococci, and enterococci.
- Gram-negative rods: *Escherichia Coli, Proteus*, and *Klebsiella*.
  - o *Pseudomonas, Enterobacter, Acinetobacter*, and *Serratia* are common nosocomial pathogens usually expected among casualties who have been hospitalized for an extended period, not those fresh off the battlefield.
- *Salmonella, Shigella*, and *Vibrio* should be suspected in cases of bacterial dysentery.
- Anaerobic Gram-positive and Gram-negative rods: *Clostridia, Bacteroides*, and *Prevotella* species.
- Fungal species: *Candida* species should be suspected in casualties hospitalized for prolonged periods, those malnourished or immunosuppressed, or those who have received broad spectrum antibiotics, adrenocortical steroids, or parenteral nutrition. Empiric therapy should be considered in appropriate patients with presumptive evidence of fungal infection.

The greatest threat of infection to the wounded battlefield casualty is the development of clostridial myonecrosis (gas gangrene), commonly due to *Clostridium perfringens*.

Common Patterns of Infection

- **Skin, soft tissue, muscle, and bone**: Primarily due to staphylococcal, streptococcal, and clostridial species. These infections include wound abscess, cellulitis, septic arthritis, osteomyelitis, necrotizing fasciitis, and gas gangrene.

Clostridium tetani **can enter through any wound—even minor burns and corneal abrasions. Prophylaxis is required to prevent tetanus toxemia.**

- **Intracranial**: Meningitis, encephalitis, and abscess, commonly due to staphylococci and Gram-negative rods, which are difficult to treat due to the impervious nature of the meninges to common antibiotics.

- **Orofacial and neck**: Gram-positive cocci and mouth anaerobes, generally responsive to surgery and clindamycin.
- **Thoracic cavity**: Empyema (usually staphylococcal) and pneumonia (*Staphylococcus*, *Streptococcus*, *Pseudomonas*), especially among those on prolonged mechanical ventilation or those casualties prone to aspiration (polymicrobial).
- **Intraabdominal**: Include posttraumatic or post-operative abscess, and peritonitis due to *Enterococcus*, Gram-negative rods, and anaerobic bacilli. *Clostridium difficile* is often responsible for a potentially severe diarrheal colitis that occurs following the administration of even one dose of antibiotic.
- **Systemic sepsis:** A syndrome caused by a bloodborne or severe regional infection resulting in a global inflammatory response (fever, leukocytosis, tachycardia, tachypnea, and possibly hypotension).
  - o A similar inflammatory response without infection can be caused by a focus of retained necrotic tissue, or the mere act of sustaining severe trauma.
  - o Culprit microorganisms will not be recovered in all cases of sepsis syndrome.
  - o Although typically associated with Gram-negative organisms, any bacterial or fungal agent can cause sepsis.

Prompt surgical debridement is the cornerstone of prophylaxis/treatment of war wound infections.

Treatment
General Principles
- Surgical and antibiotic treatment should begin early and be repeated in the prophylaxis of war wound infection.
- Optimally, surgical debridement should be achieved within 6 hours of injury.
- Following initial exploration and debridement, the wound should be sufficiently irrigated to ensure all dead material, bacterial contamination, and foreign material has been washed from the wound.

- Excessive irrigation, especially under pressure, should be avoided, because this can dilute the body's natural immune cellular defenses and contribute to bacteremia.
- The skin is left open, and a lightly moistened sterile gauze dressing is applied.
- Antibiotics should be started ASAP after wounding, then continued for 24 hours, depending on the size, extent of destruction, and degree of contamination of the wound.
  - o If time from wounding to initiation of antibiotics is > 6 hours, or time from wounding to surgery is > 12 hours, give antibiotics using regimen for established infection.
- The choice of empiric antibiotic is dependent on the part of the body injured (Table 10-1).
- Once a battlefield wound has become infected, treatment is two-fold—surgical and medical.
  - o Surgical strategy remains the same: Open the wound, remove infected and necrotic tissue, and inspect for foreign material.
  - o Drainage is generally employed in abscess cavities to prevent premature closure and reformation.
  - o Empiric broad-spectrum antibiotic therapy is initiated against likely pathogens and continued for 7 to 10 days.
  - o Ideally, obtain cultures and tailor therapy to cover the actual pathogens recovered on Gram stain and culture. Routine bacteriology is often not available in forward medical facilities.
  - o Because Bacteroides and Clostridia are difficult to culture, tailor antibiotic therapy to cover these organisms.
  - o If the debrided wound still has possibly ischemic tissue or retained foreign material, the patient is returned to the OR every 1 to 2 days for redebridement, until absolute assurance of healthy, clean tissue is achieved.

Specific Infections

- Tetanus.
  - o Battlefield wounds are "tetanus-prone" due to high levels of contamination with *Clostridium tetani*.
  - o Bacteria grow anaerobically and release a CNS toxin that results in muscle spasm, trismus, neck rigidity, and back arching.

Table 10-1. Empiric Antibiotic Coverage for War Injuries.

Site of Injury	Empiric Antibiotic	Covered Organisms
Cranium/penetrating injury	Ancef/Vanc + Flagyl brain injury	Gram positives + anaerobes
Maxillofacial	Ancef + clindamycin	Gram positives + anaerobes
Neck	Ancef	Skin flora
Chest	Ancef	Skin flora
Abdomen		
Liver	Fluoroquinolone/2nd generation cephalosporin	Gram negatives, gram positives, + anaerobes
Gastrointestinal tract	Carbapenam/penicillin (Zosyn) with gross contamination	"
Gastrointestinal tract	2nd generation cephalosporin without gross contamination	"
Genitourinary	Aminoglycoside + 2nd generation cephalosporin	"
Spleen	2nd generation cephalosporin + fluoroquinolone + immunize splenectomy patients later for encapsulated organisms	"
Pelvic		
With gastrointestinal injury	Carbepenam or combo penicillin	Gut flora + anaerobes
No gastrointestinal injury	2nd generation cephalosporin	Skin organisms
Extremity		
Soft tissue only	Ancef or 2nd generation cephalosporin + aminoglycoside	
Bone/vascular involvement	2nd generation cephalosporin + aminoglycoside and fluoroquinolone	

Treat gross contamination of any wound with debris from uniforms and the environment with broad spectrum Gram-negative and anaerobic coverage regardless of area of injury, eg, Ancef + penicillin + gentamicin; or Unasyn alone.

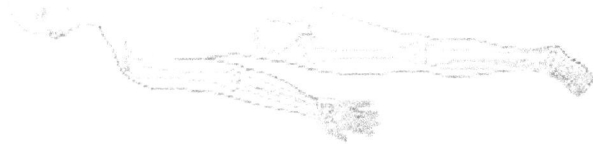

o **In addition to surgical debridement of war wounds, additional prophylactic measures for tetanus-prone wounds include**
  ◆ Administration of 0.5m L IM of **tetanus toxoid** if prior tetanus immunization is uncertain, less than three doses, or more than five years since last dose.
  ◆ Administration of 250–500 units IM of **tetanus immune globulin** in a separate syringe and at a separate site from the toxoid if prior tetanus immunization is uncertain or less than three doses.
o Treatment for <u>established</u> tetanus includes
  ◆ IV antibiotics (penicillin G, 24 million U/d; or doxycycline, 100 mg bid; or metronidazole, 500 mg q6h for 7 days).
  ◆ Tetanus immune globulin.
  ◆ Wound debridement as needed.
  ◆ IV diazepam to ameliorate the muscle spasm.
  ◆ Place patient in a dark, quiet room free of extraneous stimulation.
  ◆ May warrant endotracheal intubation, mechanical ventilation, and neuromuscular blockade.
- **Soft-tissue infections.**
  o **Cellulitis** is manifested by localized skin erythema, heat, tenderness, and swelling or induration.
    ◆ Treatment: IV antibiotics against streptococcal and staphylococcal species (IV nafcillin, cefazolin or, in the penicillin-allergic patient, clindamycin or vancomycin).
  o **Post-operative wound infections** become evident by wound pain, redness, swelling, warmth, and/or foul or purulent discharge, with fever and/or leukocytosis.
    ◆ Treatment: **Open the wound**, drain the infected fluid, and debride any necrotic tissue present.
    ◆ The wound is left open and allowed to close via secondary intention.
  o **Necrotizing soft tissue infections** are the most dreaded infections resulting from battlefield wounding. These include **clostridial myonecrosis (gas gangrene)** and **polymicrobial infections** caused by *Streptococcus, Staphylococcus, Enterococcus, Enterobacteriaceae, Bacteroides,* and *Clostridia.*

- The organisms create a rapidly advancing infection within the **subcutaneous tissues** and/or **muscle** by producing exotoxins that lead to bacteremia, toxemia, and septic shock.
- **All layers of soft tissue can be involved**, including skin (blistering and necrosis), subcutaneous tissue (panniculitis), fascia (fasciitis), and muscle.
- Clinical manifestations begin locally with severe pain, crepitus, and with clostridia, a thin, brown, foul-smelling discharge.
- The skin may be tense and shiny, showing pallor or a bronze color.
- Systemic signs include fever, leukocytosis, mental obtundation, hemolytic anemia, and hypotension, progressing rapidly to multiple organ failure and death in untreated or under-treated cases.
- The diagnosis is made by history of severe unexpected wound pain combined with palpable or radiographic soft tissue gas (air in subcutaneous tissue and/or muscle).
- Absence of soft-tissue gas does not exclude diagnosis of necrotizing infection.
- **Treatment is surgical**, including early, comprehensive, and repeated (every 24–48 hours) debridement of all dead and infected tissue, combined with **antibiotics**.
- **Excision** of affected tissue must be as radical as necessary (including amputation or disarticulation) to remove all muscle that is discolored, noncontractile, nonbleeding, or suspicious.
- Identification of causative organisms often problematic: Treatment must be aimed at all possible organisms.
- **IV antibiotic** therapy.
- **Clindamycin,** 900 mg q8h; **plus penicillin G**, 4 million U q4; **plus gentamicin,** 5–7 mg/kg qd.
  - ◊ As a **substitute for clindamycin**: metronidazole, 500 mg q6h.
  - ◊ As a **substitute for penicillin**: ceftriaxone, 2.0 g q12h, or erythromycin 1.0 g q6h.
  - ◊ As a **substitute for gentamicin**: ciprofloxacin, 400 mg q12h.

- ♦ Alternative regimen: penicillin G, 4 million U q4h **plus** imipenem, 500 mg q6h.
- ● **Intraabdominal infections.**
  - ♦ **Prevention**.
  - ♦ Regimens (start ASAP, continue x **24 hours** post-op).
    - ◊ Single agent: **cefotetan 1.0 g q12h**, or ampicillin/sulbactam, 3 g q6h, or cefoxitin, 1.0 g q8h.
    - ◊ Triple agent: ampicillin 2 g q6h; **plus** anaerobic coverage (metronidazole, 500 mg q6h; or clindamycin, 900 mg q8h); **plus** gentamicin 5–7 mg/kg qd.
  - ♦ **Established** intraabdominal infection (peritonitis or abscess).
  - ♦ Same regimen as above, except continue for 7 to 10 days.
  - ♦ Drain all abscesses.
- ● **Pulmonary infections.**
  - ♦ **Empyema** (generally Streptococcal) following penetrating thoracic trauma is typically due to contamination from the projectile, chest tubes, or thoracotomy.
  - ♦ Diagnosis: Loculations, air/fluid levels on radiograph, pleural aspirate.
  - ♦ Treatment.
    - ◊ Chest tube initially, and thoracotomy if unsuccessful.
    - ◊ Cefotaxime, or ceftriaxone, or cefoxitin, or imipenem.
  - ♦ **Pneumonia** is most frequently due to aspiration (eg, patients with head injury) and prolonged mechanical ventilation.
  - ♦ The diagnosis is made through radiograph finding of a new pulmonary infiltrate that does not clear with chest physiotherapy, combined with
    - ◊ Fever or leukocytosis.
    - ◊ Sputum analysis showing copious bacteria and leukocytes.
  - ♦ Empiric therapy is directed toward likely pathogens.
    - ◊ **Aspiration**: Streptococcal pneumonia, coliforms, and oral anaerobes are likely. IV antibiotics such as ampicillin/sulbactam, clindamycin, or cefoxitin have proven effective.
    - ◊ **Ventilator-associated pneumonia**: *staphylococcus*, *Pseudomonas*, and other nosocomial *Enterobacteriaceae*. Broad coverage is best with such agents as imipenem,

ciprofloxacin, vancomycin, and/or ceftazidime, plus an aminoglycoside.

Systemic Sepsis

Sepsis can be defined as infection combined with a prolonged systemic inflammatory response that includes two or more of the following conditions.

- Tachycardia.
- Fever or hypothermia.
- Tachypnea or hyperventilation.
- Leukocytosis or acute leukopenia.

Progression to septic shock is manifest by systemic hypoperfusion: profound hypotension, mental obtundation, or lactic acidosis. Treatment is a three-pronged approach:

- Identify and eradicate the source.
- Broad-spectrum intravenous antibiotics for the most likely pathogens.
- ICU support for failing organ systems, such as cardiovascular collapse, acute renal failure, and respiratory failure.

It is often difficult to identify the source of sepsis, but it is the **most important factor** in determining the outcome. Potential sources of occult infection include

- An undrained collection of pus such as a wound infection, intraabdominal abscess, sinusitis, or perianal abscess.
- Ventilator-associated pneumonia.
- Urinary tract infection.
- Disseminated fungal infection.
- Central intravenous catheter infection.
- Acalculous cholecystitis.

Intensive care support for sepsis involves vigorous resuscitation to restore perfusion to prevent multiple organ dysfunction. This requires optimization of hemodynamic parameters (pulmonary artery occlusion pressure, cardiac output, and oxygen delivery) to reverse anaerobic metabolism and lactic acidosis. Endpoints of resuscitation, such as urine output, base deficit, and blood lactate levels guide successful treatment. Until the source for sepsis is identified and actual pathogens isolated, empiric therapy with broad-spectrum intravenous antibiotics is warranted. Suitable regimens might include

- Imipenem, 500 mg q6h.
- Piperacillin and tazobactam (Zosyn), 3.375 g q6h; or ceftazidime, 2.0 g q8h; or cefepime, 2.0 g q12h; PLUS gentamicin, 5–7 mg/kg qd (based on once-daily dosing strategy and no renal impairment); or ciprofloxacin, 400 mg q12h.
- Addition of vancomycin, 1.0 g q12h if methicillin-resistant *Staphylococcus aureus* is a likely pathogen.
- Addition of linezolid, 600 mg q12h if vancomycin-resistant enterococcus (VRE) is a likely pathogen.

Conclusion

Battlefield casualties are at high risk for infection. In particular, war wounds are predisposed to infection due to environmental conditions on the battlefield, devitalized tissue, and foreign bodies in the wound. The key to avoiding wound infection is prompt and adequate wound exploration, removal of all foreign material, and excision of all dead tissue. All battlefield wounds and incisions should have the skin left open. Antibiotics play an adjunctive role in the prophylaxis of wound and other infections in the battlefield MTF. Knowledge of likely pathogens for particular infections and sites, as well as optimal antibiotics to eradicate those pathogens (Table 10-2), will aid the battlefield clinician in averting and treating infections.

Table 10-2. Spectrum and Dosage of Selected Antibiotic Agents.

Agent	Antibacterial Spectrum	Dosage
Penicillin G	*Streptococcus pyogenes*, penicillin-sensitive *Streptococcus pneumonia*, clostridial sp	4 mil U IV q4h
Ampicillin	Enterococcal sp, streptococcal sp, *Proteus*, some *E coli*, *Klebsiella*	2 g IV q6h
Ampicillin/ sulbactam	Enterococcal sp, streptococcal sp, *Staphylococcus*,* *E coli*, *Proteus*, *Klebsiella*, *Clostridial sp*, *Bacteroides*/*Prevotella* sp	3 g IV q6h
Nafcillin	Staphylococcal sp,* streptococcal sp	1 g IV q4h
Piperacillin/ tazobactam	Enterococcal sp, streptococcal sp, *Staphylococcus*,* *E coli*, *Pseudomonas* and other enterobacteriaceae, clostridial sp, *Bacteroides*/*Prevotella* sp	3.375 g IV q6h
Imipenem	Enterococcal sp, streptococcal sp, *Staphylococcus*,* *E coli*, *Pseudomonas* and other enterobacteriaceae, clostridial sp, *Bacteroides*/*Prevotella* sp	500 mg IV q6h
Cefazolin	Staphylococcal sp,* streptococcal sp, *E coli*, *Klebsiella*, *Proteus*	1.0 g IV q8h
Cefoxitin	Staphylococcal sp,* streptococcal sp, *E coli* and similar enterobacteriaceae, clostridial sp, *Bacteroides*/*Prevotella* sp	1.0 g IV q6h
Ceftazidime	Streptococcal sp, *E coli*, *Pseudomonas* and other enterobacteriaceae	2.0 g q8h
Ceftriaxone	Streptococcal sp, staphylococcal sp,* *Neisseria* sp, *E coli* and most enterobacteriaceae (NOT *Pseudomonas*), clostridial sp	2.0 g q12h
Ciprofloxacin	*E coli*, *Pseudomonas* and other enterobacteriaceae	400 mg q12h
Gentamycin	*E coli*, *Pseudomonas* and other enterobacteriaceae	5-7 mg/kg qd (based on once-daily dosing strategy and no renal impairment)
Vancomycin	Streptococcal, enterococcal, and staphylococcal species (including MRSA; not VRE)	1.0 g q12h
Erythromycin	Streptococcal sp, clostridial sp	0.5-1.0 g q6h
Clindamycin	*Streptococcus* sp, *Staphylococcus* sp,* clostridial sp, *Bacteroides*, and *Prevotella* sp	900 mg q8h
Metronidazole	Clostridial sp, *Bacteroides* and *Prevotella* sp	500 mg q6h

*Not methicillin resistant *Staphylococcus aureus* (MRSA)

Dosage and dosage intervals are average recommendations. Individual dosing may vary.

Chapter 11

Critical Care

Introduction
Each battlefield ICU should have a dedicated intensive care physician, due to the severity and lethality of blast and high-velocity wounds, and the need for ongoing resuscitation of casualties requiring damage control.

> **Damage control is the initial control of hemorrhage and contamination followed by intraperitoneal packing and rapid closure, then resuscitation to normal physiology in the intensive care unit and subsequent definitive re-exploration. This places large logistic requirements on the ICU. This may include rewarming, large-volume resuscitation, blood products, vasoactive drugs, and mechanical ventilation.**

The ICU physician should observe the following guidelines:
- **Reexamine** (possibly, retriage) the patient, using detailed primary and secondary surveys, with attention to the "ABCs," potential life-threatening injuries, and other injuries missed during the ER and OR phases of resuscitation (tertiary survey).

> **Trust no one's examination before your own because the patient's condition may have changed, or prior examinations may be inaccurate or incomplete.**

- Provide necessary available **monitoring** of physiology, with periodic assessment of pain control, level of consciousness, and intake and output.
- **Resuscitate** from shock, using appropriate endpoints.
- **Provide organ-specific support**, as is done for CNS injury, pulmonary failure, cardiovascular collapse, and renal dysfunction.

- Ensure adequate pain control.
  - o Use IV (not IM) narcotic agents in sufficient doses to alleviate pain.
  - o Patients on mechanical ventilation require **both** narcotics (morphine, fentanyl) and sedatives (propofol, lorazepam, midazolam).
- Prepare the patient for **transport** out of theater.
- Important caveats for the intensivist.
  - o **"Patients don't suddenly deteriorate; healthcare providers suddenly notice!"**
  - o The **organ system approach**, in which each organ system in turn is addressed in a mini-SOAP format, ensures that each of the body's physiologic systems is addressed in a complete, comprehensive, and integral fashion.
  - o The **systemic inflammatory response** (SIRS) is a common metabolic sequela of severe injury, not always associated with infection.

Fever or leukocytosis should prompt a thorough search for infection. Antibiotic discipline must be enforced, saving these medications for short-course prophylaxis, documented infection, or empiric treatment of rapid deterioration due to sepsis.

Resuscitation From Shock

Shock can be defined as an acute state of cardiovascular insufficiency resulting in life-threatening global hypoperfusion. Hemorrhagic shock is the most common form of shock following major trauma. Therefore, initial efforts should be directed toward correction of hypovolemia.

Hypoperfusion implies inadequate delivery of oxygen to the body's cells. Oxygen delivery is a function of cardiac performance, arterial hemoglobin content, and arterial oxygen saturation. All attempts to correct shock involve optimizing these three variables.

- Shock resuscitation is approached in two phases, based on endpoints of resuscitation:
  - o In the **first phase**, resuscitate to a mean arterial pressure of > 60 mm Hg, a urine output of 0.5 cc/kg/h (at least 30 ccs/h), and arterial oxygen saturation of > 92%.
  - o Pursue endpoints aggressively to eliminate hypoperfusion, ideally within 1 hour (see Chapter 7, Shock and Resuscitation).
  - o In the **second phase**, resuscitation is continued primarily with fluid, to eliminate metabolic acidosis (restore lactate to normal) within 24 hours.
  - o The resuscitative fluid of choice is a warmed, balanced crystalloid solution (normal saline or lactated Ringer's) and is preferable to colloid.
  - o Rate of infusion for resuscitation should be 500 mL to 1,000 mL bolus over 15–20 minutes and repeated as necessary.
  - o After 3 L of crystalloid, blood products should generally follow at similar rates.

> Vasopressor agents should **only** be considered for achieving minimal acceptable blood pressure **after** fluid boluses and confirmation of adequate intravascular volume.

  - o Dopamine, norepinephrine, and phenylephrine are the preferred vasoactive agents, starting in the lower dose range.
  - o Dobutamine should only be considered for demonstrated cardiac dysfunction, which may be seen in sepsis, the elderly, or myocardial infarction (MI).

Specific Organ Systems

Traumatic Brain Injury/CNS

> **Transient hypoxemia or hypotension in the patient with significant traumatic brain injury doubles the probability of death or poor neurologic outcome. The goal of treatment is to maintain cerebral perfusion pressure (CPP) and oxygenation.**

- Identify potential intracranial surgical lesions for possible emergent craniotomy.
- Prevent hypoxemia: Maintain O_2 sat > 92%, PaO_2 > 100, and intubate for GCS $\leq$ 8.
- Prevent hypotension.
  o Maintain SBP > 100 mm Hg, MAP > 80.
    ◆ MAP = DBP + $\frac{1}{3}$ (SBP - DBP).
- Prevent, monitor, and treat intracranial hypertension.
  o Maintain intracranial pressure (ICP) = 5–15 mm Hg.
  o Maintain CPP = 70–90 mm Hg.
    $$CPP = MAP - ICP$$
- **Measures to treat intracranial hypertension** include:
  o Elevation of head of bed 30° may be helpful.
  o Recognize that high levels of PEEP may raise ICP.
  o Control **serum osmolarity**.
    ◆ Normal saline is the preferred IV solution.
    ◆ Check serum sodium twice daily, and keep in the range of 145–150 mEq/dL.
    ◆ IV **mannitol** (not in anuric patients), 0.25–1.0 g/kg, every 6–8 hours to keep serum osmolarity optimal.
  o Control **$PaCO_2$**.

Hypercarbia should always be prevented. Modest therapeutic hyperventilation may be used ($PaCO_2$ 30–35 mm Hg) for brief periods in the deteriorating patient.

    ◆ Beneficial effects of hyperventilation/hypocarbia must be balanced: it reduces ICP through vasoconstriction, but also reduces cerebral blood flow.
    ◆ **Prophylactic hyperventilation should not be used.**
  o Removal of **cerebrospinal fluid** by placement of an intraventricular catheter.
  o Barbiturates have unproven benefit but may be considered in extreme cases.
  o **Craniotomy** with bone and brain removal is a drastic, lifesaving procedure of last resort in the moribund patient.

Steroids have <u>no role</u> in traumatic brain injury treatment.

---

o **Avoid hyperthermia,** because this raises ICP.
- General Considerations.
  o Appropriate precautions should be taken (H_2 blocker, heparin, and oral care) to prevent development of stress gastritis, deep venous thrombosis, and aspiration pneumonitis.
  o If **coagulopathy** develops, use blood products as necessary to correct an elevated prothrombin time.
  o Prevent and aggressively treat pain, agitation, shivering, and fever to avoid increased cerebral metabolism and oxygen consumption.
  o **Hyperglycemia** has an adverse effect on outcome and should be monitored and treated aggressively to keep glucose levels between 100–150 mg/dL.
  o Seizure prophylaxis. Phenytoin/phosphenytoin should be administered to therapeutic levels in the penetrating head-injured patient, and to blunt head-injury patients with seizure.

Pulmonary System and Ventilators

General Considerations
- **Supplemental oxygen** in the early phase of resuscitation is imperative. The maximum fraction of inspired oxygen (FIO_2) delivered by:
  o Nasal cannula approaches 0.35.
  o Venturi mask is 0.50.
  o Non-rebreathing reservoir mask approaches 0.90.
- **Monitoring**: May include portable chest radiographs, periodic ABGs, regular assessments of level of sedation, airway pressures, and functioning of ventilator alarms.

Airway Considerations
- **Indications for endotracheal intubation and mechanical ventilation include:**
  o Airway obstruction due to trauma, edema, excess secretions.
  o Apnea.

o Excessive work of breathing (eg, flail chest), as indicated by accessory muscle use, fatigue, diaphoresis, or tachypnea when respiratory failure is imminent.
o Decreased level of consciousness: GSC $\leq$ 8.
o Hypoxia: SaO_2 < 90%, PaO_2 < 60 mmHg on FIO_2 > 50%.
o Hypercarbia: $PaCO_2$ > 60 mm Hg acutely (lower threshold with tachypnea).
o Shock.
o **Caution**: Patients not meeting the above criteria may still require airway protection and mechanical ventilation preceding prolonged transport.
● **Field Ventilator.**
   o Impact Uni-Vent Eagle 754.
      ◆ Basic settings.
         ◊ Turn the ventilator on and set the mode using the **Mode Selector Switch** (lower right). Most patients can be well ventilated using SIMV (synchronized intermittent mandatory ventilation).
         ◊ Set FIO_2 using the **Air/Oxygen Mixer Control**, above the Mode Selector Switch. Generally, ICU patients should be started at an FIO_2 of 1.0, and weaned as appropriate to a level of 0.40.
         ◊ Set minute ventilation using **Tidal Volume** and **Ventilation Rate** controls. The tidal volume is set at 6–10 mL/kg. Initial rate is set at 10–14 breaths/minute and titrated to normalize $PaCO_2$.
         ◊ Set positive end-expiratory pressure (PEEP) using the **PEEP Control** located on the upper left of the control panel. Initial PEEP is usually set at 5 cm H_2O. Higher values can be set in severe respiratory failure such as adult respiratory distress syndrome (ARDS), although generally not higher than 15 cm H_2O.

Summary of typical initial settings for mechanical ventilator: FIO_2 1.0, SIMV mode, rate 12, tidal volume 800 mL, PEEP 5 cm H_2O.

ARDS
- ARDS can start within days of injury, and should be suspected in any casualty with:
  - o Acute hypoxemia (PaO_2/FIO_2 ratio < 200).
  - o Progressive fall in pulmonary compliance (stiff lungs, increasing airway pressures).
  - o Bilateral alveolar infiltrates on chest radiograph, with no clinical evidence of volume overload.

Mechanical Ventilation Priorities in ARDS
- Maintain patient analgesia and sedation to prevent agitation and ventilator/patient asynchrony.
- Keep SaO_2 > 90% by increasing FIO_2 and/or PEEP (maximum 15–18 cm H_2O).
- Avoid prolonged FIO_2 > 0.60 due to O_2 toxicity.
- Avoid respiratory acidosis. Keep $PaCO_2$ 35–45 mm Hg, and arterial blood pH > 7.25.
- Keep peak inspiratory pressure (PIP) < 40 cm H_2O to prevent iatrogenic pneumothorax and destruction of normal lung tissue.
  - o Decrease tidal volume to 5–7 mL/kg.
  - o Increase ventilator rate.
  - o If other measures are unsuccessful, allow **permissive hypercapnia** by accepting a respiratory acidosis ($PaCO_2$ 55–70 mm Hg). Use bicarb to maintain pH > 7.2.

Respiratory acidosis is less dangerous than ventilator-induced lung injury caused by high PIP and high tidal volumes.

Cardiovascular System
- The patient who exhibits **cardiovascular deterioration** after a period of apparent stability should be evaluated to rule out the following:
  - o Hypoxia or loss of airway.
  - o Tension pneumothorax.
  - o Recurrent bleeding from sites of injury or surgery.
  - o Cardiac tamponade or direct myocardial injury.

o Tachyarrhythmia.
o Fluid loss due to "third-spacing," burns, fever, diarrhea, or vomiting.
o Undiagnosed injury: intestinal injury, pancreatitis, or infection.
o Vasodilatation due to spinal shock, epidural anesthesia/analgesia, and sepsis.
o Side effect from medication.
o GI bleeding.
o Pulmonary embolus.
o Abdominal compartment syndrome.
o Excessive airway pressures from mechanical ventilation can directly decrease cardiac ventricular function and decrease venous preload.

- Management.
  o Support cardiovascular system by monitoring end-organ perfusion (urine output, capillary refill) and using four parameters of hemodynamic performance:
    ◆ **Preload** (Best index: pulmonary capillary wedge pressure – PCWP).
    ◆ **Afterload** (systemic vascular resistance [SVR] = [MAP – CVP]/ CO • 80).
    ◆ **Heart rate**.
    ◆ **Cardiac contractility** (best index: stroke volume; SV = CO/h).
    ◆ "Make do" with the best information available—use CVP when PA catheter unavailable.
    ◆ For hypovolemia and cardiovascular instability due to sepsis:
      ◊ Assure adequate preload by volume repletion before adjusting other variables (eg, adding inotropes for low cardiac output).
      ◊ In other states of cardiovascular instability, the variable manipulated is the one indicative of the major problem.

Sinus tachycardia may be a sign of an underlying problem (eg, hypoxia, hypovolemia, infection, or pain). Seek and treat the primary problem, not the tachycardia.

- **Myocardial ischemia/infarction (MI)** is an uncommon battlefield problem.
  - o Suspicion is aroused when the patient exhibits angina-like chest pain or unexplained cardiac instability (arrhythmias or hypotension).
  - o The diagnosis of an acute myocardial event is made by the presence of ST segment elevation or depression on 12-leak ECG and/or an abnormal elevation of serum markers of myocardial injury (myoglobin [MB] fraction of creatine phosphokinase, Troponin I).
- **Emergency treatment for MI.**
  - o Supplemental O_2.
  - o Morphine for pain, rest.
  - o Aspirin 325 mg tablet chewed and swallowed (then one tablet PO qd).
  - o NTG SL (0.4 mg tablet every 5 minutes until pain relieved, maximum 3 doses) or IV infusion depending on severity of condition.
  - o Beta-blocker such as metoprolol (5–15 mg IV slowly q6h or 50–100 mg PO q12h) or atenolol (50–100 mg PO) on diagnosis and daily.
  - o As resources and patient condition permit for MI with diagnostic ECG: Optimal therapy would also include, within 6 hours of symptoms, IV heparin and a thrombolytic such as tissue plasminogen activator.

Renal System and Electrolytes

- Monitor urine output, blood urea nitrogen (BUN), serum creatinine, and serum electrolytes.
- Acute renal failure (ARF) is manifested by oliguria (< 0.5 cc/kg/h) and a rise in BUN and creatinine. The most frequent causes for ARF are:
  - o Hypovolemia.
  - o Acute tubular necrosis (ATN) due to:
    - ◆ Hypovolemia.
    - ◆ Sepsis, IV contrast agents, aminoglycoside antibiotics, or NSAIDs.
  - o Crush, massive, soft-tissue injury or compartment syndrome, with resultant rhabdomyolysis and myoglobinuria.

♦ In ARF due to rhabdomyolysis, consider administering large volumes of IV fluid (300–800 mL/h), combined with 50 mEq $NaHCO_3$/L, to alkalinize the urine with the goal of achieving a urine output of 2.0 cc/kg/h.
♦ Bilateral renal or ureteral trauma.

> **Two hours of oliguria (< 20cc/h) in an ICU patient (almost always due to inadequate resuscitation) warrants aggressive, immediate action.**

● Algorithm for hemodynamically stable ICU patient with profound **oliguria** or **anuria**:
  o **Irrigate or replace Foley** catheter to ensure function.
  o After ensuring no signs of intravascular volume overload (diffuse pulmonary crackles, S3 heart sound), administer **bolus** of 1–2 L IV saline over 30 minutes.
  o Review medication list and medical history to elicit potential factors causing ARF; **stop any agents** that could contribute.
  o Send any urine to lab with serum sample to calculate fractional excretion of sodium $(\textbf{FENA}) = (U_{NA} \bullet P_{CR})/(P_{NA} \bullet U_{CR})$; FENA < 1.0 indicates prerenal cause (eg, hypovolemia); FENA > 2.0 points to renal insult (ATN; myoglobinuria) or postrenal cause (obstruction).
  o Consider **sonogram** of kidneys to rule out bilateral renal obstruction.
  o Consider **pulmonary artery catheter** to optimize preload (PCWP).
  o Once PCWP > 16–18 mm Hg, and urine output minimal/nonexistent, administer **furosemide** in escalating doses IV bolus: 40, 80, 160, 240 mg max (> 100mg = ototoxic). Combine last dose with single dose 1.0 g chlorothiazide IV, or administer 10 mg metolazone PO given 30 minutes before last dose. Also consider furosemide drip or metolazone drip.
● If ineffective or if other complications of ARF occur, arrange for **dialysis** as a temporizing renal support until spontaneous renal recovery occurs. This means the physician must optimize the casualty for transport out of theater, with special attention to volume status, potassium, and acid base status.

- o **Indications for dialysis in the casualty with ARF:**
    - ♦ Anuria beyond 8–12 hours.
    - ♦ Hypervolemia.
    - ♦ Hyperkalemia.
    - ♦ Acidosis.
    - ♦ Complications of uremia: mental status changes, pericardial rub.
    - ♦ Toxic levels of drugs/medications (eg, digoxin).
- **Hyperkalemia.**
    - o Verify again **hyperkalemia (serum K > 6 mEq/L) and serum pH.**
    - o Give IV calcium chloride, 10 mL of 10% solution over 5 minutes.
    - o Give IV $NaHCO_3$, 50 mEq over 5 minutes.
    - o Give IV Dextrose (50g D50) 50 grams + 10 units regular insulin IV over 10 minutes.
    - o Recheck K^+.
    - o Give beta-agonist albuterol 10–20 mg over 15 minutes by inhalation.
    - o Consider enteral K-binding with enema of sodium polystyrene sulfonate, 25–50 g, in sorbitol.
- **Hypokalemia**: Treatment: 10–20 mEq KCL IV/hour in monitored setting; difficult to treat hypokalemia unless concomitant hypomagnesemia is first corrected.
- **Hypernatremia**: Usually indicative of free water deficit. Water deficit (L) = 0.6 • weight (kg) • [(measured serum Na)/(normal serum Na of 140) – 1]. Half of this deficit should be replaced over first 12–24 hours, and the remainder over the next 1–2 days.
- **Hyponatremia**: Indicative of excess of free water or vasopressin (SIADH). Levels of serum sodium < 125 mEq/L are associated with mental status changes or seizures. Treatment should involve **free water restriction** or use of IV normal saline, with goal of correction of sodium level no more than 15 mEq/L over 24 hours, to prevent complication of central pontine myelinolysis.
- **Hypophosphatemia**: Phosphate is important as an energy source, and should be repleted to level of 2.5 mg/dL with IV KPO_4 or $NaPO_4$, 30 mMol over 1 hour.

- **Hyperphosphatemia** (usually associated with ARF): Phosphate levels over 6.0 mg/dL should be treated by enteral binding agents, such as calcium acetate or sucralfate.
- **Hypomagnesemia**: Administer 2 g magnesium sulfate IV in solution over 60 minutes to goal of serum level of 2.0 mEq/dL.
- **Metabolic acidosis**: Primarily lactic (**most commonly due to hypovolemia**) and ketoacidosis. Neither should be treated with sodium bicarbonate (it is contraindicated in lactic acidosis). **Sodium bicarbonate has very limited role** in ICU disorders: hyperkalemia, alkalinization of urine in myoglobinuria, bicarbonate-responsive renal tubular acidosis (RTA), and for massive gastrointestinal losses of bicarbonate (profound diarrhea, enterocutaneous fistula).
- **Metabolic alkalosis**: NG **suction of stomach acid** causes a hypochloremic alkalosis, responsive to replacement of NG losses with crystalloid. **Excessive loop diuretic use** can also cause metabolic (contraction) alkalosis. If further diuresis is needed, use a carbonic anhydrase inhibitor (acetazolamide 250 mg IV every 6 h) for 1–2 days.

Hematologic System
- Most common coagulation disorder: **dilutional coagulopathy**.
  - o Others include heparin-induced thrombocytopenia, disseminated intravascular coagulation, coagulopathy due to hypothermia or diffuse hepatic damage, and thrombocytopenia.
  - o Most require replacement transfusion of appropriate blood products.
- To prevent trauma-related deep venous thrombosis (DVT) and pulmonary embolism, prophylactic measures (subcutaneous heparin or sequential compression devices) are required.

Gastrointestinal System and Nutrition
- Prolonged shock can lead to GI dysfunction.
  - o **Stress gastritis**: Increased risk of severe head injuries or burns, mechanical ventilation, systemic anticoagulation therapy, or sepsis. Prevention: sucralfate, histamine-2 receptor antagonist (eg, ranitidine) or a proton pump inhibitor (eg, omeprazole).

o **Acalculous cholecystitis**: Suspect with right upper quadrant abdominal pain, abnormalities in liver function tests, or fever/leukocytosis of unclear cause. Ultrasound shows gallbladder inflammation with wall thickening or pericholecystic fluid. Treatment: broad-spectrum antibiotics and ultrasound-guided percutaneous drainage or operation.

o **Hepatic failure** portends a dire prognosis. Initial signs include hyperbilirubinemia, elevation of the prothrombin time, hypoalbuminemia, profound hypoglycemia, obtundation. Massive amounts of fresh frozen plasma are required to prevent exsanguination from coagulopathy.

- **Nutrition** can prove problematic in the battlefield ICU patient.
  o Systemic inflammation induced by severe injury often results in catabolism and protein wasting, making early nutritional support imperative.
  o Nutrition should commence within 24–48 hours of injury.
  o Enteral feedings are superior to parenteral nutrition (TPN), offering a lower infection rate and shorter ICU stays.
  o The following goals serve to guide nutritional management:
    ♦ Caloric requirement: 25–30 kcal/kg/d.
    ♦ Protein requirement: 1.0–1.5 g/kg/d.
    ♦ 30%–40% of total caloric intake per day should be as fat.
  o Nutrition should include a balanced electrolyte solution containing supplemental potassium, calcium, magnesium, phosphate, multivitamins and trace elements (zinc, copper, manganese, and chromium).
  o The two most common problems associated with enteral nutrition are diarrhea and aspiration.
    ♦ Aspiration can be associated with severe pneumonitis, but can be prevented by:
      ◊ Keeping the head of the bed up.
      ◊ Feeding into the jejunum or duodenum rather than the stomach.
      ◊ Checking gastric residuals every 4 hours (feedings should be stopped if residual greater than 200 mL).
    ♦ Diarrhea can be alleviated by:
      ◊ Decreasing the osmolarity of the enteral solution.
      ◊ Adding fiber.
      ◊ Agents such as loperamide in small doses.

Immune System and Infections
- Differential diagnosis of ICU infections.
  - Pneumonia (nosocomial or aspiration).
  - Central venous catheter infection – if considered, remove catheter.
  - UTI.
  - Wound or soft-tissue infection.
  - Intra-abdominal abscess (especially following laparotomy).
  - Systemic fungal infection.
  - Sinusitis.
  - Acalculous cholecystitis.
  - Pancreatitis.
- Prophylactic antibiotics.
  - A short course of prophylactic antibiotics (24–48 h) is warranted after penetrating injury on the battlefield.
  - After this, antibiotics should be withheld unless a documented infection is confirmed, or a severe deterioration in clinical status suggestive of sepsis is encountered.
  - Sepsis warrants a short course of broad spectrum IV antibiotics, but they must be stopped in 72 hours if no microbiologic pathogens are confirmed by culture.
  - **Fever and leukocytosis, by themselves, are not sufficient justification for antibiotics.**

Endocrine System
- Hyperglycemia.
  - Control, to prevent ketoacidosis, hyperosmolar coma, and intravascular volume loss due to osmotic diuresis.
  - The two most common causes are uncontrolled or unrecognized infections and the use of TPN.
  - The best technique for control of hyperglycemia is a constant IV infusion of insulin, usually 1.0–10 units per hour.
    - Due to frequent problems with patient perfusion, subcutaneous injections are less reliable in the ICU patient.
    - Patients with profound hyperglycemia (serum glucose > 800 mg/dL) and volume depletion, due to osmotic diuresis, should receive fluid resuscitation with crystalloid

before receiving insulin, to prevent further shifts in intravascular volume as the glucose shifts intracellularly.
- ◆ Limit correction rate to 100 mg/dL per hour (700 mg/dL takes 7 h to correct) and assess for resultant hypokalemia.
- Corticosteroids are rarely indicated after major trauma.
  - o There is no proven benefit to steroid treatment for closed head injury or sepsis.
  - o Steroids are indicated for proven adrenocortical deficiency (a rare occurrence among battlefield casualties) and spinal cord injury with neurologic deficit.

Musculoskeletal System
- Monitor for the development of compartment syndrome, vascular ischemia, and rhabdomyolysis.
- Distal extremities should be assessed regularly for neurovascular status: **presence of pulses**, sensation, motor function, warmth, and skin color.

Preparation for Evacuation
- Optimally, the combat casualty will be medically stabilized before transport out of theater.
  - o Native or mechanical airway is maintained.
  - o Sufficient blood pressure, to allow organ perfusion, that has been stable for at least 8 hours.
  - o Both primary and secondary phases of shock resuscitation have been completed.
  - o All sources of bleeding have been identified and controlled.
  - o Life-saving or definitive surgery not required for the next 24 hours.
- Transfer out of a battlefield ICU requires a USAF Critical Care Air Transport Team (CCATT) with physician-to-physician and nurse-to-nurse communication to summarize condition of the patient, operations performed, treatment being given, and support required during flight (in particular, need for oxygen, mechanical ventilation, suction, blood products, and monitoring).
- Copies of medical records, radiographs, 3 days of IV fluid, and all medications should accompany the patient.

Chapter 12

Damage Control Surgery

Introduction

The traditional approach to combat injury care is surgical exploration with definitive repair of all injuries. This approach is successful when there are a limited number of injuries. Prolonged operative times and persistent bleeding lead to the lethal triad of coagulopathy, acidosis, and hypothermia, resulting in a mortality of 90%.

> **Damage control is defined as the rapid initial control of hemorrhage and contamination, temporary closure, resuscitation to normal physiology in the ICU, and subsequent re-exploration and definitive repair. This approach reduces mortality to 50% in some civilian settings.**

- What might increase the life and limb salvage rate in troops in the field setting is the application of the damage control concepts described above in patients with favorable physiology.
- Tactical Abbreviated Surgical Control (TASC).
  - o Damage control techniques in a tactical environment.
  - o Abbreviated, focused operative interventions for peripheral vascular injuries, extensive bone and soft tissue injuries, and thoracoabdominal penetrations in patients expected to survive, instead of definitive surgery for every casualty.
  - o This may conserve precious resources, such as time, operating table space, and blood.
- This TASC philosophy relies on further definitive surgical care at the next echelon of care.

Damage control techniques should be considered in all multi-system casualties at the onset of surgical therapy. When initially rejected, reconsideration should occur when unexpected findings are discovered or natural breaks in the surgical therapy occur, following an initial decision to perform a definitive repair.

The goal of damage control is to restore normal physiology rather than normal anatomy. It is used for the multiple injured casualty with combinations of abdominal, vascular, genitourinary, neurologic, orthopedic, and/or thoracic injury in **three separate and distinct phases**:

1. **Primary Operation and Hemorrhage Control** – surgical control of hemorrhage and removal of contamination; laparotomy terminated, abdomen packed and temporary closure; definitive repair is deferred.
2. **Critical Care Considerations** – normal physiology restored in ICU by core rewarming, correction of coagulopathy, and hemodynamic normalization.
3. **Planned Reoperation** – re-exploration to complete the definitive surgical management or evacuation.

General Considerations

- Philosophy of damage control is "a live patient above all else."
  - o Avoid hypothermia.
  - o Rapidly achieve hemostasis.
  - o Perform only essential bowel resections.
  - o Close or divert all hollow viscus injuries, only performing reconstruction at the second operation after the patient has stabilized and can tolerate a prolonged operation.
- **When to employ damage control.**
  - o Use damage control in patients who are present with or at risk for developing:
    - ◆ Multiple life-threatening injuries.
    - ◆ Acidosis (pH < 7.2).
    - ◆ Hypothermia (temp < 34°C).
    - ◆ Hypotension and shock on presentation.
    - ◆ Combined hollow viscus and vascular or vascularized organ injury.
    - ◆ Coagulopathy (PT > 19 sec and/or PTT > 60 sec).

♦ Mass casualty situation.
o Take into account ability to control hemorrhage, severity of liver injury, and associated injuries.
o Pack **before** massive blood loss (10–15 units of pRBCs) has occurred.
o Injuries that typically require damage control techniques.
   ♦ Upper abdominal injuries that are not isolated spleen injuries (duodenal, large liver injuries, pancreas, and so forth).
   ♦ Major penetrating pelvic trauma of more than one system.
   ♦ Any retroperitoneal vascular injury.

To reiterate, damage control is practiced in three phases:
1. Primary operation and hemorrhage control.
2. Critical care resuscitation.
3. Planned reoperation.

Phase 1: Primary Operation and Hemorrhage Control
Phase 1 of damage control includes 5 distinct steps:
1. Control of hemorrhage.
2. Exploration to determine extent of injury.
3. Control of contamination.
4. Therapeutic packing.
5. Abdominal closure.

● Control of hemorrhage/Vascular injury repair.
   o Control of hemorrhage is best done with ligation, shunting, or repair of injured vessels as they are encountered.
   o The primary goal is hemorrhage control, not maintenance of blood flow.
   o For the patient in extremis, clamping or shunting of major vessels is recommended over repair.
      ♦ THINK: ligate/shunt ⇒ fasciotomy.
   o Additional methods of hemorrhage control include balloon catheter tamponade of vascular or solid viscus injuries.
● Exploration to determine extent of injury.
   o Damage control laparotomy.
      ♦ Rapidly achieve hemostasis.

- ♦ Perform only essential resections or pack solid organs to diminish blood loss.
- ♦ Close or divert all hollow viscus injuries.
- ♦ Rapidly terminate the procedure to correct hypovolemia, hypothermia, and acidosis to prevent coagulopathy.
- ♦ Perform definitive reconstruction only after the patient has stabilized and can tolerate a prolonged operation.
- Control of Contamination.
  - o Contamination control also proceeds as injuries are encountered, utilizing clamps, primary repair or resection without reanastomosis.
  - o With multiple enterotomies, if the area of injury represents less than 50% of the length of the small bowel, a single resection can be undertaken.
  - o At this stage of the operation, the surgeon must decide whether or not to proceed with definitive repair of the identified and controlled injuries. Careful communication with the anesthesiologist is critical to this decision.
    - ♦ If aggressive resuscitation has been successful in maintaining normal temperature, coagulation, and acid base status, then definitive repair may proceed.
    - ♦ If any of these interrelated factors are abnormal, the procedure should be terminated (contamination controlled without reanastomosis) and the patient taken to the ICU for further resuscitation.
    - ♦ The presence and status of extra-abdominal injuries needs to be taken into consideration when deciding how much physiologic reserve the patient has left.
- Therapeutic Packing.
  - o Resuscitative vs Therapeutic Packing.
    - ♦ Resuscitative packing is manual compression of the bleeding site as an initial measure in controlling or minimizing blood loss.
    - ♦ Therapeutic packing provides long-term tamponade of liver, pelvic, and retroperitoneal bleeding.
  - o Do not use the "pack and peek" technique wherein the liver is packed and the patient resuscitated; the packs are removed to identify the source of bleeding, but rebleeding

occurs before the site can be identified; the liver is packed again; the patient is resuscitated again; and the entire cycle is repeated.

o Definitive therapeutic packing is based on three basic principles.

♦ Pressure stops bleeding.

♦ Pressure vectors should recreate tissue planes (attempt to recreate the pressure vectors created by the capsule of a solid organ or fill the space of that organ, not random pack placement).

♦ Tissue viability must be preserved.

o 6–12 laparotomy pads are the best commonly available packing material.

o An intervening layer, such as a bowel bag, sterile drape, absorbable mesh, or omentum, can be placed between packs and the tissue to aid in easy pack removal at relaparotomy.

- Abdominal Closure.

o Leave the fascia open.

o Vacuum pack (preferred technique — easy, keeps patient dry, allows for expansion).

♦ With fascia open, place fully plastic-covered (bowel bag, X-ray cassette bag, Ioban drape) sterile operating room (OR) towel circumferentially under the fascia to cover the viscera. Place a small number of central perforations to allow fluid to egress to the drains.

♦ Place closed-suction drains (Jackson-Pratt, modified Foley, small chest tube) above the plastic at the level of the subcutaneous tissue brought out through separate stab wounds or the inferior portion of the wound.

♦ Place lap sponges to fill in the wound.

♦ Cover the entire wound with a large Ioban drape.

♦ Place drains on low suction and secure to the skin.

o A silastic sheet or 3-liter IV bag, sewn to the skin or fascia, can accomplish abdominal closure in virtually every instance.

o Skin closure is not recommended, but may be quickly accomplished with skin staples, towel clips (reliably stronger), or running monofilament suture.

> Skin closure may lead to abdominal compartment syndrome.

Thoracic injuries
- **The goal of abbreviated thoracotomy is to stop the bleeding and restore a survivable physiology; contamination is usually not a problem.**
- In the exsanguinating patient, formal lung resection gives way to using large staplers in a nonanatomic wedge resection to rapidly achieve hemostasis and control of air leaks.
- In pulmonary tractotomy, the lung bridging the wound tract is opened between long clamps or with a linear stapler. The tract can thus be directly inspected, bleeding points selectively ligated, and air leaks controlled.
- Vascular injuries can be treated with intraluminal shunts or Fogarty balloons to achieve distal control in inaccessible areas.
- Tracheal injury can be treated with airway control placed through the site of injury.
- Extensive bronchial repairs are not feasible in the patient in extremis; therefore, rapid resection of the affected lobe or lung would be best.
- When dealing with esophageal injury, diversion, and wide drainage, not definitive repair, is the best course of action.
- A single en masse suture closure of the chest wall is best because wound closure of skin with towel clips may result in significant blood loss from the musculature.

Phase 2: Critical Care Considerations
- Physiologic support in the post-op TASC patient is paramount to survival.
  - **Core rewarming**: warmed resuscitative fluids, blankets, ventilator air, and environment, or commercially available products such as Bair Hugger, Chill Buster.
  - **Reversal of acidosis**: appropriate/aggressive resuscitation with crystalloid, colloid, and blood products.
  - **Reversal of coagulopathy**: at many locations, only ultra-fresh whole blood is available to correct coagulopathy.
- Abdominal compartment syndrome.

o Abdominal compartment syndrome is a condition in which **increased intra-abdominal pressure adversely affects the circulation and threatens the function and viability of the viscera**.
o Measurement is performed using urinary bladder pressure (normal = zero).
  ♦ Several methods are available for performing bladder pressure.
    ◊ Place 100–150 cc of sterile saline in the bladder and clamp the foley.
    ◊ Access the needle port on the catheter and attach to a pressure monitor (central venous pressure transducer).
    ◊ Access the needle port and create a column of water via plain IV tubing held vertically or use of the pressure gauge from a lumbar puncture kit.
    ◊ If there is no needle port, clamp the foley proximal and the distal end of regular IV tubing in the usual drainage end of the catheter until firmly in place.
  ♦ Measurement of bladder pressure is a good variable to test and follow; however, intervention for abdominal compartment syndrome (ACS) should occur when suspected or clinically indicated.
o Occurs in abdominal trauma accompanied by visceral swelling, hematoma, or abdominal pack use.
o Physiology of abdominal compartment syndrome.
  ♦ Cardiac output and venous return are decreased.
  ♦ Reduction in blood flow to liver, intestines, and kidneys can result in anuria.
  ♦ The two hemidiaphragms push upward, decreasing thoracic volume, and compliance leading to elevated peak airway pressures.
  ♦ Central venous, pulmonary capillary wedge, and right atrial pressures increase with intra-abdominal pressure (can lead to false PA catheter pressures).
  ♦ PO_2 is decreased due to increases in airway pressures and ventilation/perfusion abnormalities that worsen with positive end-expiratory pressure (PEEP).

Abdominal Pressure	Degree of Elevation	Clinical Effect
10–20 mm Hg	Mild	Insignificant
20–40 mm Hg	Moderate	Oliguria and organ dysfunction
>40 mm Hg	Severe	Requires immediate attention

Phase 3: Planned Reoperation

- Packs should be left in place until the patient's hemodynamics are stable and all major sites of hemorrhage have had time to clot.
- Reoperation should be scheduled when the probability of achieving definitive organ repair and complete fascial closure are highest.
- Timing must coincide with reversal of hypotension, acidosis, hypothermia, and coagulopathy. Typically occurs 24–48 hours following the primary insult when brisk diuresis, negative fluid balance, diminishing abdominal girth, and decreasing peripheral edema indicate reduction in visceral and parietal edema.
- **This surgery may occur at the next echelon of care.**
  - o Stratovac should be weighed carefully because transit operative care is minimal. Surgical expertise is generally not available and transit times are often greater than 24 hours.
- Timing can, however, be dictated by other pressing clinical concerns such as abdominal compartment syndrome, limb ischemia, and suboptimal control of spillage at primary operation.
- In cases of a packed and drained duodenum, pancreas, kidney or bladder, or liver injuries with gross bowel contamination, packs should be retrieved within 36–48 hours.
- It is sometimes necessary to perform this type of operation at the bedside, as the patient's cardiopulmonary status does not allow a trip to the OR.

Conduct of Relaparotomy

- It is to be presumed that injuries were missed.
- **A complete laparotomy must be performed in search of missed injury.**

- The surgeon must exercise caution and sound judgment before performing full reconstruction of the GI tract because the patient is typically still critically ill and catabolic, making the patient less likely to heal anastomoses and even less likely to tolerate a leak or uncontrolled fistula.
- Feeding tube placement, either transabdominal or naso-enteric, should be placed at this time.
- Repacking may be re-employed if other measures fail to control hemorrhage.
- An abdominal film should be obtained to insure all packs have been removed from the abdomen. Sponge counts should be considered unreliable in this situation.

- **Unplanned Reexploration.**
  - o Emergent, unplanned reexploration should be performed in any:
    - ♦ Normothermic patient with unabated bleeding (> 2 units of PRBCs/h).
    - ♦ Patient who develops severe intra-abdominal compartment syndrome.
    - ♦ Patient requiring postoperative transfusion of > 10 units of PRBCs.
    - ♦ Patient with persistent lactic acidosis.

Austere Field and Military Surgical Considerations
- Due to severe physiological insult, the typical civilian damage control patient requires 2 surgeons and 1 nurse, at a minimum, at the bedside for the first 6 hours. An example of the magnitude of the ICU problem that may be encountered is a casualty who requires a pulmonary artery catheter, 3 operations, 33 units of PRBCs, and an ICU stay of 23 days. In mass casualty scenarios, this patient would likely be triaged as expectant.

> Tactical Abbreviated Surgical Control philosophy allows the surgeon to apply damage control techniques when the limitations of reserve exist outside the patient, in the tactical environment, not just to patients about to exhaust their physiological reserve (classic damage control scenario).

Summary Points

- Damage control is not a procedure of last resort. The consideration of damage control techniques should be made at the initiation of operative intervention in any multitrauma casualty and reconsidered during any case where extensive injuries are involved.
- Consider damage control in patients with severe liver injury, combined vascular and hollow viscus injuries, multiple sites of hemorrhage, diminished physiological reserve, and combinations of severe injury involving multiple organ systems (eg, CNS, orthopedic, vascular, or thoracoabdominal).
- Consider damage control early, ISS > 35, pH < 7.2, temperature < 34°C, shock, or coagulopathy.
- Avoid: hypothermia, 'pack and peek', tight abdominal closure, abdominal compartment syndrome, delayed relaparotomy for surgical bleeding, and getting stuck in a conventional thinking mode.
- Think: vascular shunts/fasciotomy, abdominal packing, external fixators, angiographic embolization (when available), temporary closure, nonanatomic resections, and missed injury.
- Plan sequence of operation in stable patients to allow for use of damage control if instability develops.

Chapter 13

Face and Neck Injuries

Introduction

> **Immediate recognition and appropriate management of airway compromise is critical to survival.**

- Face and neck injuries can be the most difficult-to-manage wounds encountered by health care providers in the combat zone. **Focusing on ABC priorities is vital.**
- During **airway** control, maintain cervical spine immobilization in bluntly injured patients. (Unstable C-spine injury is very rare in neurologically intact penetrating face and neck wounds.)
- **Bleeding** should be initially controlled with direct pressure. If bleeding cannot be controlled, immediate operative intervention is necessary.
- **Complete assessment** of remaining injuries (fractures, lacerations, esophageal injury, ocular injuries).

Immediate Management of Facial Injuries
- Airway.
  - o Airway distress due to upper airway obstruction above the vocal cords is generally marked by inspiratory stridor:
    - ◆ Blood or edema resulting from the injury.
    - ◆ Tongue may obstruct the airway in a patient with a mandible fracture.
    - ◆ A fractured, free-floating maxilla can fall back, obstructing the airway.
    - ◆ Displaced tooth fragments may also become foreign bodies.
  - o Maneuvers to relieve upper airway obstruction:

- ◆ Remove foreign bodies (strong suction, Magill forceps, among others).
- ◆ Anterior jaw-thrust maneuver.
- ◆ Place adjunctive airway device (nasal trumpet or oropharyngeal airway).
- ◆ Endotracheal intubation and assisted ventilation.
- ◆ Cricothyroidotomy or emergent tracheotomy may become necessary.
- ● Cervical spine.
  - o Up to 10% of patients with significant blunt facial injuries will also have a C-spine injury.
    - ◆ In awake patients, the C-spine can be cleared clinically by palpating for point tenderness.
    - ◆ Obtunded patients with blunt facial trauma should be treated with C-spine immobilization.
- ● **Vascular Injury.**
  - o Injuries to the face are often accompanied by **significant bleeding**.
  - o Control of facial vascular injuries should progress from simple wound compression for mild bleeding to vessel ligation for significant bleeding.

Vessel ligation should only be performed under direct visualization after careful identification of the bleeding vessel. Blind clamping of bleeding areas should be avoided, because critical structures such as the facial nerve and parotid duct are susceptible to injury.

- ◆ Foley catheter inserted blindly into a wound may rapidly staunch bleeding.
- o Intraoral bleeding must be controlled to ensure a patent and safe airway.
  - ◆ Do not pack the oropharynx in an awake patient due to risk of airway compromise: first secure the airway with an endotracheal tube.
  - ◆ Copious irrigation and antibiotics with gram-positive coverage should be used liberally for penetrating injuries of the face.

- Evaluation.
  - o Once the casualty is stabilized, cleanse dried blood and foreign bodies gently from wound sites in order to evaluate the depth and extent of injury.
  - o The bony orbits, maxilla, forehead, and mandible should be palpated for stepoffs or mobile segments suggestive of a fracture.
  - o A complete intraoral examination includes inspection and palpation of all mucosal surfaces for lacerations, ecchymosis, stepoffs, and malocclusion as well as dental integrity.
  - o **In the awake patient, abnormal dental occlusion indicates probable fracture.**
  - o Perform a cranial nerve examination to assess vision, gross hearing, facial sensation, facial muscle movement, tongue mobility, extraocular movements, and to rule out entrapment of the globe.
  - o Consult an ophthalmologist for decreased vision on gross visual field testing, diplopia, or decreased ocular mobility.
  - o If the intercanthal distance measures > 40 mm (approximately the width of the patient's eye), the patient should be evaluated and treated for a possible naso-orbito-ethmoid (NOE) fracture.
- If a NOE fracture is present, do not instrument the nose if possible. There may be a tear in the dura, and instrumentation may contaminate the CSF via the cribiform.

Facial Bone Fracture Management

The goals of fracture repair are realignment and fixation of fragments in correct anatomic position with dental wire (inferior, but easier) or plates and screws.

With the exception of fractures that significantly alter normal dental occlusion or compromise the airway (eg, mandible fractures), repair of facial fractures may be delayed for two weeks.

- Fractures of the mandible.
  - o Second most commonly fractured bone of the face.
  - o Most often fractured in the subcondylar region.

o Multiple mandible fracture sites present in 50% of cases.
o Patients present with limited jaw mobility or malocclusion.
o Dental Panorex is the single best plain film (but is unavailable in the field environment); mandible serves as a less reliable but satisfactory study (might overlook subcondylar fractures).
o Fine cut (1–3 mm) (CT scan will delineate mandibular fractures).
o Treatment is determined by the location and severity of the fracture and condition of existing dentition.
  ♦ Remove only teeth that are severely loose or fractured with exposed pulp.
  ♦ Even teeth in the line of a fracture, if stable, and not impeding the occlusion, should be maintained.
o Nondisplaced subcondylar fractures in patients with normal occlusion may be treated simply with a soft diet and limited wear of Kevlar helmet and protective mask.
o Immediate reduction of the mandibular fracture and improvement of occlusion can be accomplished with a bridle wire (24 or 25 gauge) placed around at least 2 teeth on either side of the fracture.
o More severe fractures with malocclusion will require immobilization with maxillary-mandibular fixation (MMF) for 6–7 weeks.
o Place commercially made arch bars onto the facial aspect of the maxillary and mandibular teeth.
  ♦ The arch-bars are then fixed to the teeth with simple circumdental (24 or 25 gauge) wires (Fig. 13-1).
  ♦ After proper occlusion is established, the maxillary arch bar is fixed to the mandibular arch bar with either wire or elastics.
  ♦ If the patient's jaws are wired together, it is imperative that **wire cutters be with the patient at all times.**
  ♦ If portions of the mandible have been avulsed or the mandibular fragments are extremely contaminated, an external biphase splint should be placed to maintain alignment.

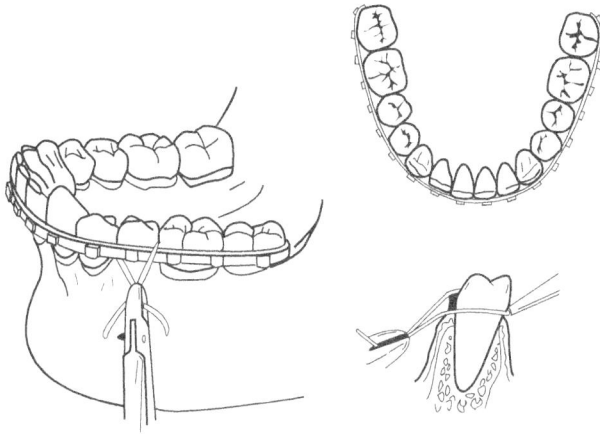

Fig. 13-1. Arch bar applications.

    o Open reduction and internal fixation with a mandibular plate across fracture sites may obviate the need for MMF.

• **Nasal fractures.**
    o Most common fracture.
        ♦ Control of epistaxis: anterior pack-gauze/balloon/tamponade.
    o Diagnosed clinically by the appearance and mobility of the nasal bones.

> The patient's septum should be evaluated for the presence of a septal hematoma, which if present, must be immediately drained by incision, followed by packing.

    o Treat by closed reduction of the fractured bones and/or septum into their correct anatomic positions up to 7 days after fracture.

   ◆ Place a blunt elevator (Sayer) into the nasal cavity in
     order to elevate the depressed bony segment while
     simultaneously repositioning the bone with the
     surgeon's thumb placed externally.
   o The nose may then be fixed with tape or a splint in order
     to maintain the reduction (Fig. 13-2).

a   b

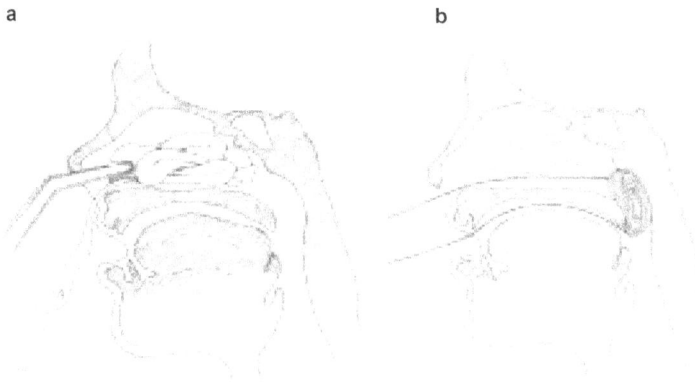

Fig. 13-2. (a) Anterior and (b) posterior packing of the nose.

- **Maxillofacial Trauma.**
  o Life-threatening due to loss of airway, hemorrhage, or
    spinal injury.
  o Fragment wound of maxillary sinus is commonly seen and
    requires surgical removal of retained fragments (can delay
    until specialist is available).
- Bleeding.
  o Common from epistaxis, oral hemorrhage or combination
    bleeding.
  o Nasal fracture—most common fracture.
    ◆ Control Epistaxis with Anterior Pack (gauze/balloon/
      tampon).
  o Mandibular fracture fixation (wires/archbars, **with wire
    cutters at bedside**).
  o Facial and scalp lacerations.
  o Mid-face fracture (Le Fort)—The most difficult bleeding
    to control.

- ♦ Requires "significant" trauma.
- ♦ Be aware of associated CNS and orbital injury.
- ♦ Significant hemorrhage due to laceration of IMA and branches.
  - ◊ Is difficult to control.
  - ◊ May be life-threatening.
  - ◊ Treat by controlling airway, reducing fracture, and placing a pressure dressing such as packing or balloon.
- ♦ Edema may cause loss of airway, which may be immediate or delayed.
- ♦ Can be difficult to diagnose. Criteria:
  - ◊ Mobile hard palate and mid-face while stabilizing the skull.
  - ◊ Penetrating injury may not follow classic Le Fort patterns but may have a significant soft tissue injury component (base of tongue, soft palate).
- Treatment.
  - o ABCs.
  - o Check CNS and vision.
  - o Can immobilize maxilla by using the mandible as a splint (wires/archbars, **with wire cutters at bedside**).
  - o Control hemorrhage by tamponade.
    - ♦ Nasopharynx, nasal cavity.
    - ♦ Oropharynx.
- Surgical Repair.
  - o **Not** an **emergency** once hemorrhage is controlled.
  - o Requires ENT, oral, plastic, and ophthalmology surgical expertise.
  - o Time consuming.
  - o Open and closed reductions with hardware that is usually unavailable in the field.
- Fractures of Facial Bones.
  - o Potentially life-threatening due to loss of airway, hemorrhage, or spinal injury.
  - o Fragment wound of maxillary sinus is commonly seen, and requires surgical removal of retained fragments (can delay until specialist available).
  - o Mid-face fracture (Le Fort)—**The** most difficult bleeding to control.
    - ♦ Requires "significant" trauma.

- ◆ Be aware of associated CNS and orbital injury.
- ◆ Significant hemorrhage due to laceration of IMA and branches.
  - ◊ Is difficult to control.
  - ◊ May be life threatening.
  - ◊ Treat by controlling the airway, reducing fractures, and placing pressure dressings such as packing or balloon tamponade.
- ◆ Edema may cause loss of airway, which may be immediate or delayed.
- ◆ Can be difficult to diagnose.
  - ◊ Mobilize the hard palate and mid-face while stabilizing the skull. Place thumb and forefinger of one hand on nasal bridge to stabilize, then with the other hand, determine mobility of maxilla by placing the thumb on alveolus and forefinger on the palate and attempting gentle distraction in an anterior-posterior direction.
  - ◊ Penetrating injury may not follow classic Le Fort patterns but may have a significant soft tissue injury component (base of tongue, soft palate).
  - ◊ Apply principles of systemic palpation and inspection, looking for crepitus, tenderness, internal and external ecchymosis, and subconjunctival hemorrhage that might suggest fractures.
- o Classification by Le Fort (Fig. 13-3).

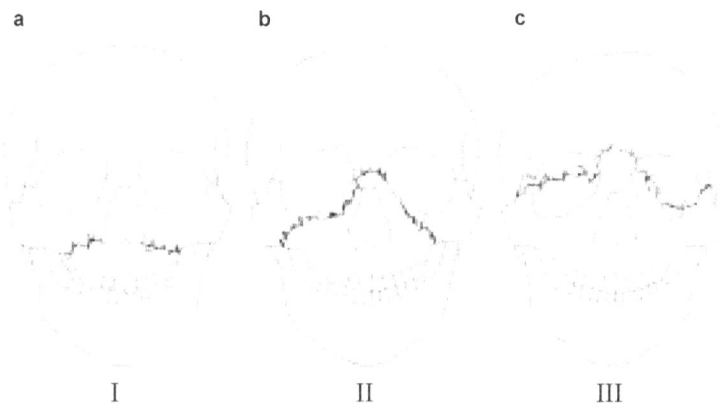

Fig. 13-3. Le Fort facial fracture classifications.

- ◆ I–Fracture separates the entire alveolar process from maxilla.
- ◆ II–Separation of mid-face, including the nasal bone, from the orbit (pyramidal).
- ◆ III–Detachment of the face from the skull (craniofacial disarticulation).
  - o Treatment.
    - ◆ ABCs.
    - ◆ If nasal intubation is used, **extremely careful placement** is mandatory to avoid cribriform plate or anterior cranial fossa penetration.
    - ◆ Classification by Le Fort.
    - ◆ Check CNS and vision.
    - ◆ Can immobilize maxilla by using the mandible as a splint (wires/arch bars, **with wire cutters at bedside**). It is much easier to place patient into micromodilator or fixation if either a nasal airway or tracheostomy is employed.
    - ◆ Control hemorrhage by tamponade as previously described.
      - ◊ Nasopharynx, nasal cavity.
      - ◊ Oropharynx.
  - o Definitive Surgical Repair.
    - ◆ **Not** an **emergency** once hemorrhage is controlled.
    - ◆ Requires expertise in ENT, oral and maxillofacial, plastic, and ophthalmology surgery.
    - ◆ Time consuming.
    - ◆ Open and closed reductions require hardware usually unavailable in the field.

Soft Tissue Injuries
- ● **General principles.**
  - o Avoid injury to surrounding structures such as the facial nerve or parotid duct.
  - o Wounds should be gently cleansed with saline and light scrub solutions; foreign bodies should be meticulously cleaned from wounds prior to closure.
  - o Sharply debride devascularized wound edges **minimally.**
  - o **Facial lacerations should be closed in layers within 24 hours.**
    - ◆ Use 4-0 or 5-0 absorbable suture for subcutaneous/ dermal layers.

        ◆ Use 5-0 or 6-0 nonabsorbable sutures on the skin of the face.

        ◆ Remove sutures in 5–7 days.

● **Facial nerve injuries.**

    o Carefully examine for facial nerve function in all **five** branches (Fig. 13-4).

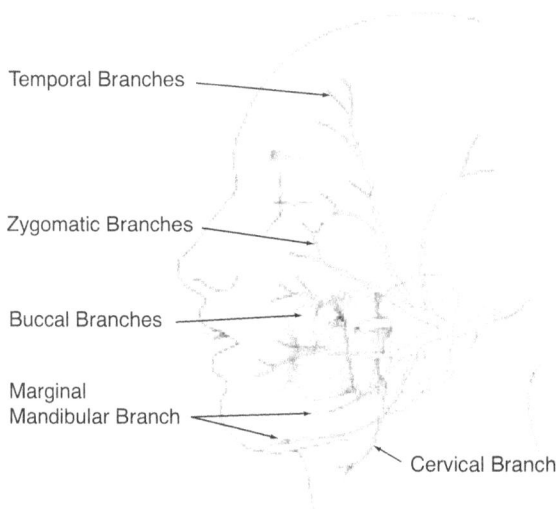

Temporal Branches

Zygomatic Branches

Buccal Branches

Marginal Mandibular Branch

Cervical Branch

Fig. 13-4. Branches of the facial nerve parotid duct injury.

Facial nerve branches that are lacerated at a site anterior to a vertical line drawn down from the lateral canthus of the eye do not need to be surgically reapproximated because these branches are very small and will spontaneously regenerate with good return of facial function.

---

    o The severed ends of the nerve may be located in the wound with a nerve stimulator, for up to 3 days.

    o Cut nerve ends should be reapproximated primarily with three or four fine (9-0) nylon sutures placed through the epineurium.

    o If a gap exists between severed ends of the facial nerve due to tissue loss, an interposition graft may be placed using a section of the great auricular nerve to bridge the gap.

o If the wound is heavily contaminated and cannot be closed primarily, the severed ends of the nerve should be located and tagged for identification and repair at the time of wound closure.

● Parotid duct injuries.

  o Evaluate penetrating wounds of the parotid/buccal regions of the face for salivary leakage due to a lacerated parotid duct (see Fig 13-5).

    ♦ The wound may be manually compressed and inspected for salivary leakage.

    ♦ If the parotid duct is injured by a facial laceration, the distal end of the duct may be identified by placing a lacrimal probe through the intraoral opening of the duct located near the maxillary second molar (see Fig. 13-4).

    ♦ The proximal end may be identified by compressing the wound and identifying any areas of salivary leakage.

  o Repair with absorbable (6-0) sutures (Fig. 13-5).

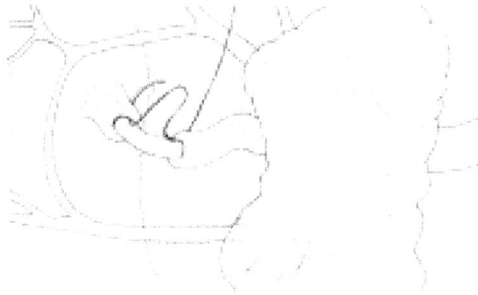

Fig. 13-5. Repair of parotid duct.

o A stent may be placed into the duct to facilitate the closure and prevent stenosis.

    ♦ Possible stents include lacrimal stents, large (size 0) polypropylene sutures, or long angiocaths.

    ♦ Stents may be sutured to the buccal mucosa and removed after seven days.

Penetrating Neck Trauma
- Introduction.
  - o Vascular injuries occur in 20% and aerodigestive tract in 10% of cases.
  - o Mortality is primarily due to exsanguinating hemorrhage.
  - o Esophageal injury, which results in mediastinitis and intractable sepsis, may also be fatal.
- **Anatomy.**

The neck is divided into three zones to aid decision making for diagnostic tests and surgical strategy. In each zone, the primary structures at risk of injury are different (Fig. 13-6).

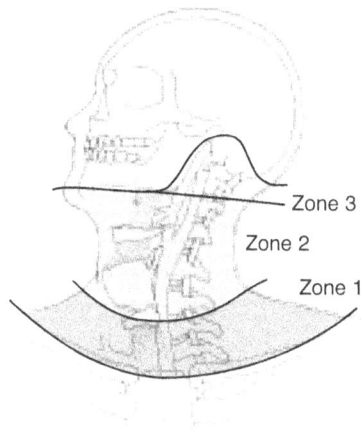

Fig. 13-6. Zones of the neck.

- o Zone 1 (clavicle to cricoid membrane): The structures of concern include large vessels of the thoracic outlet (subclavian artery and vein, common carotid artery), the lung, and the brachial plexus.
- o Zone 2 (cricoid membrane to angle of mandible): Structures of concern include the common carotid artery, internal jugular vein, esophagus, and trachea.
- o Zone 3 (angle of mandible to base of skull): The structure of concern is primarily the internal carotid artery.

- Immediate management.
  - o Initially, same as above.
  - o Obtain chest and soft tissue neck radiographs.
  - o Address tetanus and antibiotic prophylaxis.
- Operative strategy.
  - o If no platysma violation, surgical intervention is not indicated.
  - o Zone 2 injuries that penetrate the platysma should undergo routine exploration to rule out life threatening vascular, esophageal or tracheal injuries via an incision along the anterior border of the sternocleidomastoid muscle (Fig. 13-7).

Fig. 13-7. Neck exposure of zone 2.

  - o Zone 1 and 3 injuries require selective management, based on clinical signs and chest radiograph findings, making an incision dependent on the vascular structure most probably injured.
    - ◆ Zone 1 and 3 penetrations without clinical signs of injury (see below) may be evacuated without operative intervention.
  - o The most important clinical signs pointing to probable injuries (pertinent to all 3 zones):

♦ Signs of vascular injury.
  ◊ Current or history of significant bleeding.
  ◊ Expanding hematoma.
  ◊ Bruit or thrill in the neck.
  ◊ Hypotension.
  ◊ Dyspnea, hoarseness, or stridor.
  ◊ Absent or decreased pulses in neck or arm.
  ◊ Focal neurologic deficit or mental status change.
  ◊ Chest radiograph findings of hemothorax or mediastinal widening.
♦ Signs of aerodigestive injury (esophagus, trachea, larynx).
  ◊ Crepitus or subcutaneous emphysema.
  ◊ Dyspnea or stridor.
  ◊ Air bubbling from wound.
  ◊ Tenderness or pain over trachea; odynophagia.
  ◊ Hoarse or abnormal voice.
  ◊ Hematemesis or hemoptysis.

Surgical Principles
- The groin and upper thigh should be surgically prepped for greater saphenous vein interposition graft or patch angioplasty.
- Exsanguinating hemorrhage from injured vessels at the base of the skull (Zone 3) can often be controlled with inflation of a directed catheter (Fogarty, Foley), left in place and inflated for 48–72 hours, then deflated in the OR under controlled visualization for rebleeding.
- Repair esophageal injuries in a single-layer and place closed suction drains. The drain tip should not be placed near a concomitantly repaired carotid artery. A muscle flap should be interposed between repaired esophageal and tracheal injuries to prevent fistula. Obtain an oral contrast swallow radiograph seven days after repair before feeding.
- Repair laryngotracheal injuries with single-layer monofilament absorbable suture. Must search for concomitant esophageal injuries.
- Unreconstructable (significant segmental loss, or > 50% diameter loss) tracheal injuries should be managed with an endotracheal tube placed through the defect.

- **Vertebral artery injury.**
  - o Suspect if bleeding continues from a posterolateral neck wound despite pressure on the carotid artery.
  - o Preoperative angiography localizes site of injury and establishes the existence of a patent contralateral vertebral artery, aplasia of which is most commonly located on the left side.
  - o Exposure of vertebral artery may be difficult. When contralateral vertebral artery is intact, ligation proximal and distal to the injury will likely be necessary.
  - o Bone wax or a Foley catheter may be useful for control of bleeding.
- **Intraoral injuries**
  - o Penetrating injuries to the oral cavity LATERAL to the tonsillar fossa are at a significant risk of causing occult internal carotid injury. Neurologic testing/monitoring is critical and CT scanning and/or angiography should be considered. If after a penetrating lateral oral injury the patient bleeds a small amount only to stop, this may signify a "sentinel" bleed. A carotid blowout may follow.
- **Internal carotid artery injury.**
  - o Should be repaired primarily unless there is profound hemiplegia with deep coma Glasgow Coma Scale (GCS < 8). All other carotid branches can be ligated.
  - o The use of carotid shunts during repair has no proven benefit.
  - o In small perforations, debride minimally, and close with 6-0 polypropylene.
  - o With loss of vascular tissue, vein angioplasty is required.
  - o If there is extensive destruction, segmental resection and restitution of flow is established by:
    - ♦ End-to-end anastomosis (if the vessel is sufficiently elastic to permit).
    - ♦ Interposition vein graft.
    - ♦ External carotid swing-over and interposition.
    - ♦ Temporary (24–48 h) shunt as part of damage control maneuver.
  - o The mortality is high in patients with severe neurologic deficit; carotid ligation is justifiable in complete occlusion of the entire carotid system and depending on the triage situation.
  - o Distal clot may be removed by extremely gentle use of a balloon catheter prior to shunt insertion or repair.

- **Internal jugular vein injury.**
  - o Preferably repaired by lateral suture.
  - o Ligation OK, if the contralateral internal jugular is patent.
  - o Larynx.
  - o After immediate control of the airway has been achieved by intubation or tracheotomy (not through the wound in the larynx!), a complete airway evaluation by direct laryngoscopy and bronchoscopy must be performed.
  - o Debridement of laryngotracheal injuries must be careful and conservative. A fragmented larynx or trachea should be reapproximated and sutured with extraluminal, absorbable sutures for tracheal injuries and nonabsorbable sutures or micro-plates used for laryngeal fractures.
  - o The management of laryngeal trauma includes accurate reduction and stabilization of fractures, mucosa-to-mucosa closure of lacerations, and use of a soft stent if there is extensive cartilaginous damage and structural support is decreased or the anterior commissure is involved. The stent may need to be temporarily placed for 4–6 weeks to maintain correct anatomic architecture and requires a complementary tracheotomy.
  - o The excessive removal of cartilage and mucosa must be avoided to prevent tracheal or laryngeal stenosis.
- **Laryngotracheal injuries.**
  - o If laryngotracheal separation is suspected (massive crepitis over the larynx/trachea) in an otherwise "stable" airway, endotracheal intubation should not be undertaken as this may cause a partial separation to become a complete separation and/or blind passage of the endotracheal tube may occur with resulting impending airway emergency.
  - o It is best to perform an awake tracheotomy/cricothyroidotomy under local anesthesia without paralysis. Good anesthesia can be achieved with a 4% (40mg/cc) lidocaine nebulizer, 2cc in 3cc of saline, and direct administration of 4% lidocaine into the trachea for an awake tracheotomy (in addition to local anesthetic infiltration into the skin and subcutaneous tissues). When instilling anesthesia into the airway, aspirate and ensure air enters the syringe before injecting.

- **Tracheal injury and reconstruction.**
  - o Small anterior wounds can have tracheostomy tube placed through them after debridement.
  - o Repair simple lacerations with absorbable monofilament suture.
  - o Up to 5 cm can be resected with proximal and distal mobilization.
  - o Mobilize anteriorly and posteriorly to preserve lateral blood supply.
  - o Remove endotracheal tube as soon as possible post-op.
  - o May need to suture chin to chest for 10 days to avoid extension injury.
- **Esophageal injury and repair.**
  - o Difficult to diagnose.
  - o 25% may be asymptomatic.
  - o Missed injury is a major source of late morbidity/mortality.
  - o Insufflation with air may aid in identification during exploration.
  - o Debride devitalized tissue.
  - o Wound closure in two layers with absorbable sutures.
  - o Viable muscle flap to protect repairs from leak.
  - o Drainage with closed suction drain.
  - o Barium swallow 7 days post-op, prior to oral intake.
  - o Oral intake prior to drain removal.
  - o Extensive injuries may require lateral cervical esophagostomy.
  - o Cervical esophagostomy is preferred to closure under tension.
- **Combined injuries.**
  - o All esophageal injuries combined with airway or vascular injury require separation with healthy tissue. Strap muscles are ideal, but can use pedicle of sternocleidomastoid if straps are devitalized.
- **Esophageal fistula.**
  - o 10%–30% incidence.
  - o Due to inadequate debridement, devascularization of remaining esophageal wall, closure under tension, or infection.
  - o Treatment.

◆ Maintain nutrition.
◆ Assure control with drains.
◆ Weekly barium swallow to assess closure.
◆ Oral intake prior to removing drain.

Skull Base, Temporal Bone and Otologic Injury

● Ensure that the facial nerve is assessed and documented on an awake patient and at the earliest convenience in a patient who has regained consciousness. Delineation between delayed onset and acute facial paralysis is critical for management and outcome of facial nerve injuries. Also critical is delineation between a distal and proximal nerve injury. If a distal injury is present, one or more branches may be affected.

o Be as concise as possible in describing facial motion even if not technically accurate; be complete in the description. A more proximal injury (proximal to the *Pes Anserinus*) will most likely result in all branches being equally affected. Accurate documentation may spare the patient from unwarranted surgical intervention to explore the entire length of the facial nerve. It is desirable to accurately describe the motion of EACH branch of the facial nerve. Eyelid movement does not ensure that the facial nerve is intact since the levator palpebrae is innervated by the occulomotor nerve and will remain intact despite facial nerve injury.

o If there is no contraindication for systemic steroids, they should be administered for suspected facial nerve paralysis. Crush injuries to the facial nerve may present with delayed onset paralysis and the severity and course of the paresis may be improved with systemic administration of steroids.

● Skull base fractures are often occult. Assess the patient for evidence of basilar skull fractures (Battle's sign, raccoon eyes).

● Ensure that the external auditory canal is examined. Do not instrument the external auditory canal, however. If a temporal bone fracture is present and the dura is not intact, instrumentation may introduce bacteria and/or a foreign body into the CSF.

- The external auditory canal should be inspected for a tear of the lining of the canal. A tear of the lining of the canal suggests a temporal bone fracture.
  - o If a temporal bone fracture is suspected, it is critical that the facial nerve be assessed.
- Tympanic membrane perforations can be managed expectantly. The vast majority of them will heal spontaneously, but the patient should be followed for evidence of cholesteatoma formation from traumatic implantation of the squamous epithelium. This may occur months to years after the injury. Acutely, application of otic antibiotic drops will prevent the perforation from desiccating, but this is not required. The patient should be instructed to keep the ears dry (avoid water contamination).
- Hemotympanum may be seen with acoustic & temporal bone trauma. These patients will have hearing loss. If available, perform a gross audiological evaluation with tuning forks. Hemotympanum with hearing loss (conductive) should resolve in about 6 weeks.
  - o Examination for hearing in the field can be accomplished with a single 512 tuning fork.
    - ◆ With the tuning fork placed on the mastoid tip and then alternately in front of the external canal (Rinne). Documentation as A>B (air > bone) or B>A is sufficient – do not report as "positive" or "negative":
      - ◊ Air conduction greater than bone conduction with a 512 tuning fork is normal.
      - ◊ Bone conduction greater than air is suggestive of a conductive hearing loss.
    - ◆ With the 512 tuning fork on the frontal bone/ nasal dorsum/ or central incisors (best) (Weber):
      - ◊ If the Rinne test suggests a conductive hearing loss – the 512 should lateralize to the side with the conductive loss.
      - ◊ If the Rinne is NORMAL (A>B) – the 512 should lateralize to the ear with a sensorineural loss
- Any otologic blast injury or injury to the temporal bone may result in tinnitus. Management is expectant and it may resolve

spontaneously. Accurate documentation is critical for future management of these patients, however.

- If sensorineural hearing loss is suspected and documented after a blast injury or noise trauma, steroids are indicated. 1mg/kg of prednisone is appropriate. If after five days there is no improvement, the patient can be taken off of the steroids. If improvement is noted, a taper over 3–4 weeks is indicated. Be mindful that steroids may affect a patient's affect and impair judgment.

- Dizziness and vertigo may result from acoustic trauma. If true vertigo exists after an otologic injury (observed nystagmus), the patient may have a perilymphatic fistula from depression of the stapes into the oval window or rupture of the round window. These patients may have tinnitus and hearing loss with vertigo. If a perilymphatic fistula is suspected, this patient should be seen by an Otolaryngologist as soon as possible to prevent further damage to the inner ear.

Chapter 14

Ocular Injuries

Introduction
The preservation of the eyes and eyesight of service personnel is an extremely important goal. Despite comprising as little as 0.1% of the total body surface area, injuries to the eye are found in 5–10% of all combat casualties. In the Vietnam War almost 50% of casualties with penetrating eye wounds eventually lost vision in the injured eye. Improvements in ophthalmic care in the last 30 years offer hope that blindness in combat casualties will be less common in future wars.

Triage of Patients With Eye Injuries
- ABCs (airway, breathing, and circulation) and life-threatening injuries have priority, then treat eyesight and limbs.
- Soldiers with mild eye injuries may be treated and returned to duty by nonspecialized personnel.
- Soldiers with more severe injuries should be evacuated to save vision.
- Distinguishing major ocular injuries from minor ones may be difficult.
- At the FST level, due to time and equipment restraints, surgeons will likely 'patch and evacuate'.

Identifying Severe Eye Injuries
- Associated injuries.
  - o Shrapnel wounds of the face — think intraocular foreign body (IOFB).
  - o Lid laceration — check for underlying globe laceration.
- Vision.

o Use book print, medication labels, finger counting, and the like, to evaluate vision.
o Compare sight in the injured eye to the uninjured eye.
o Severe vision loss is a strong indicator of serious injury.
- Eyeball structure.
  o Obvious corneal or scleral lacerations.
  o Subconjunctival hemorrhage — may overlay an open globe.
  o Dark uveal tissue presenting on the surface of the eye indicates an open globe.
  o Foreign body — did it penetrate the eye?
  o Blood in the anterior chamber (hyphema) indicates severe blunt trauma or penetrating trauma.
- Proptosis — may indicate a retrobulbar hemorrhage.
- Pupils.
  o Pupillary distortion — may be associated with an open globe.
- Motility.
  o Decreased motility on one side may be caused by an open globe.
  o Other causes include muscle injury, orbital fracture, and orbital hemorrhage.

Open Globe
- May result from penetrating or blunt eye trauma.
- May cause loss of vision from either disruption of ocular structures or secondary infection (endophthalmitis).
- Biplanar radiographs or a CT (computed tomagraphy) scan of the head may help to identify a metallic intraocular fragment in a casualty with severe vision loss, a traumatic hyphema, a large subconjunctival hemorrhage, or other signs suspicious for an open globe with an IOFB.

Immediate Treatment of an Open Globe
- Tape a rigid eye shield (NOT a pressure patch) over the eye.
- Do not apply pressure on or manipulate the eye.
- Do not apply any topical medications.
- Start quinolone antibiotic PO or IV (eg, ciprofloxacin 500 mg bid).

- Schedule an urgent (within 24–48 h) referral to an ophthalmologist.
- Administer tetanus toxoid if indicated.
- Prevent emesis (Phenergan 50 mg or Compazine 10 mg IM/IV).

Treatment of Other Anterior Segment Injuries
Subconjunctival Hemorrhage
- Small subconjunctival hemorrhages (SCH) may occur spontaneously or in association with blunt trauma. These lesions require no treatment.
- SCH may also occur in association with a rupture of the underlying sclera.
- Warning signs for an open globe include a large SCH with chemosis (conjunctiva bulging away from globe) in the setting of blunt trauma, or **any** SCH in the setting of penetrating injury. Casualties with blast injury and normal vision do not require special care.
- Suspected open globe patients should be treated as described above.

Treatment of Chemical Injuries of the Cornea
- Immediate copious irrigation (for 30 minutes) with normal saline (NS), lactated Ringer's (LR), or balanced salt solution.
- Nonsterile water may be used if it is the only liquid available.
- Use topical anesthesia before irrigating, if available.
- Measure the pH of tears to ensure that if there is either acid or alkali in the eye, the irrigation continues until the pH returns to normal. Do not use alkaline solutions to neutralize acidity or vice versa.
- Remove any retained particles.
- Using fluorescein test, look for epithelial defect.
    - o If none, then mild chemical injuries or foreign bodies may be treated with artificial tears.
    - o If an epithelial defect is present, use a broad-spectrum antibiotic ophthalmic ointment (Polysporin, erythromycin, or bacitracin) 4 times per day.
- Noncaustic chemical injuries usually resolve without sequelae.

- More severe chemical injuries may also require treatment with prednisolone 1% drops 4–9 times per day and scopolamine 0.25% drops 2–4 times per day.
- Pressure patch between drops or ointment if a large epithelial defect is present.
- Monitor (daily topical fluorescein evaluation) for a corneal ulcer until epithelial healing is complete.
- Severe acid or alkali injuries of the eye (recognized by pronounced chemosis, limbal blanching, and/or corneal opacification) can lead to infection of the cornea, glaucoma, and possible loss of the eye. Refer to an ophthalmologist within 24–48 hours.
- Treat mustard eye injuries with ophthalmic ointments, such as 5% boric acid ointment, to provide lubrication and minimal antibacterial effects. Apply sterile petrolatum jelly between the eyelids to provide additional lubrication and prevent sealing of the eyelids.
- Treat nerve agent ocular symptoms with 1% atropine sulfate ophthalmic ointment, repeat as needed at intervals of several hours for 1–3 days.

Corneal Abrasions
- Diagnosis.
  - o Be alert for the possibility of an associated open globe.
  - o The eye is usually very symptomatic with pain, tearing, and photophobia.
  - o Vision may be diminished from the abrasion itself or from the profuse tearing.
  - o Diagnose with topical fluorescein and cobalt blue light (Wood's lamp).
  - o A topical anesthetic may be used for diagnosis, but should NOT be used as an ongoing analgesic agent — this delays healing and may cause other complications.
- Treatment.
  - o Apply broad spectrum antibiotic ointment (Polysporin, erythromycin, or bacitracin) qid.
  - o Options for pain relief.
    - ◆ Pressure patch (usually sufficient for most abrasions).
    - ◆ Diclofenac 0.1% drops qid.

- ◆ Larger abrasions may require a mild cycloplegic agent (1% Mydriacyl or Cyclogyl) and a pressure patch.
- ◆ More severe discomfort can be treated with 0.25% scopolamine one drop bid, but this will result in pupil dilation and blurred vision for 5–6 days.
- o Small abrasions usually heal well without patching.
- o If the eye is not patched
  - ◆ Antibiotic drops (fluoroquinolone or aminoglycoside) may be used qid in lieu of ointment.
  - ◆ Sunglasses are helpful in reducing photophobia.
- o Casualties who wear contact lenses should have the lens removed and should not be treated with a patch because of the higher risk of developing a bacterial corneal ulcer.
- o Abrasions will normally heal in 1–4 days.
- o Initial treatment of thermal burns of the cornea is similar to that for corneal abrasions.

All corneal abrasions need to be checked once a day until healing is complete to ensure that the abrasion has not been complicated by secondary infection (corneal ulcer, bacterial keratitis).

Corneal Ulcer and Bacterial Keratitis
- Diagnosis.
  - o **Corneal ulcer and bacteria keratitis are serious conditions that may cause loss of vision or even loss of the eye!**
  - o A history of corneal abrasion or contact lens wear.
  - o Increasing pain and redness.
  - o Decreasing vision.
  - o Persistent or increasing epithelial defect (positive fluorescein test).
  - o White or gray spot on the cornea seen on examination with penlight or direct ophthalmoscope.
- Treatment.
  - o Quinolone drops (eg, Ocuflox), 1 drop every 5 minutes for 5 doses initially, then 1 drop every 30 minutes for 6 hours, then 1 drop hourly around the clock thereafter.
  - o Scopolamine 0.25%, one drop bid may help relieve discomfort caused by ciliary spasm.

o Patching and use of topical anesthetics for pain control are contraindicated (see pain control measures above).
o Expedited referral to an ophthalmologist within 3–5 days unless patient is not improving within 48 hours. Infection may worsen, leading to permanent injury.

Conjunctival and Corneal Foreign Bodies
- Diagnosis.
  o Abrupt onset of discomfort and/or history of suspected foreign body.
  o If an open globe is suspect, treat as discussed above.
  o Definitive diagnosis requires visualization of the offending object, which may sometimes be quite difficult.
    ♦ A hand-held magnifying lens or pair of reading glasses will provide magnification to aid in the visualization of the foreign body.
    ♦ Stain the eye with fluorescein to check for a corneal abrasion.
  o The casualty may be able to help with localization if asked to indicate the perceived location of the foreign body prior to instillation of topical anesthesia.
  o Eyelid eversion with a cotton-tipped applicator helps the examiner identify foreign bodies located on the upper tarsal plate.
- Treatment.
  o Superficial conjunctival or corneal foreign bodies may be irrigated away or removed with a moistened sterile swab under topical anesthesia.
  o Objects adherent to the cornea may be removed with a spud or a sterile 22-gauge hypodermic needle mounted on a tuberculin syringe (hold the needle **tangential** to the eye).
  o If no foreign body is visualized, but the index of suspicion is high, vigorous irrigation with artificial tears or sweeps of the conjunctival fornices with a moistened cotton-tipped applicator after topical anesthesia may be successful in removing the foreign body.
  o If an epithelial defect is present after removal of the foreign body, treat as discussed above for a corneal abrasion.

Hyphema: Blood in the Anterior Chamber
- Treatment (to prevent vision loss from increased intraocular pressure).
  - o Be alert for a possible open globe and treat for that condition if suspected.
  - o Avoidance of rebleeds is a major goal of management.
    - ◆ **Avoid** aspirin or nonsteriodal antiinflammatory drugs (NSAID).
    - ◆ No strenuous activity (bedrest) for 14 days.
    - ◆ No reading for 7 days.
  - o Prednisolone 1% drops 4 times a day.
  - o Scopolamine 0.25% drops twice a day.
  - o Cover eye with protective shield.
  - o Elevate head of bed to promote settling of red blood cells (RBC) in anterior chamber.
  - o Provide a 24–48 hour referral to an ophthalmologist to monitor for increased intraocular pressure (which may cause permanent injury to the optic nerve) and to evaluate for an associated open globe.
  - o If evaluation by an ophthalmologist is delayed (> 24 hrs), treat with a topical B-blocker (timolol or levobunolol) bid to help prevent intraocular pressure elevation.
  - o If intraocular pressure is found to be markedly elevated (above 30 mm Hg) with a tonopen or other portable tonometry device, other options for lowering intraocular pressure include acetazolamide 500 mg PO or IV and mannitol 1–2 g/kg IV over 45 minutes.

Retrobulbar (Orbital) Hemorrhage
- Keys to recognition: Severe eye pain, proptosis, vision loss, decreased eye movement.
  - o Marked lid edema may make the proptosis difficult to appreciate.
  - o Failure to recognize may result in blindness from increased ocular pressure.
- Perform an immediate lateral canthotomy.
- Provide an urgent referral to an ophthalmologist, within 24–48 hours.

- If evaluation by an ophthalmologist is delayed (>24 hrs), treat with a topical B-blocker (timolol) bid to help lower intraocular pressure elevation.
- If intraocular pressure is found to be elevated (>30 mm Hg), treat as discussed above.

Lateral Canthotomy/Cantholysis

Do not perform such procedures if the eyeball structure has been violated. If the eye is sliced open, apply a Fox shield for protection and seek immediate ophthalmic surgical support.

- Inject 2% lidocaine with 1:100,000 epinephrine into the lateral canthus (Fig. 14-1a).
- Crush the lateral canthus with a straight hemostat, advancing the jaws to the lateral fornix (Fig. 14-1b).
- Using straight scissors make a 1-cm long horizontal incision of the later canthal tendon, in the middle of the crush mark (Fig. 14-1c).
- Grasp the lower eyelid with large toothed forceps pulling the eyelid away from the face. This pulls the inferior crus (band of the lateral canthal tendon) tight so it can be easily cut loose from the orbital rim (Fig.14-1d).
  - o Use blunt tipped scissors to cut the inferior crus.
  - o Keep the scissors parallel (flat) to the face with the tips pointing toward the chin.
  - o Place the inner blade just anterior to the conjunctiva and the outer blade just deep to the skin.
  - o The eyelid should pull freely away from the face, releasing pressure on the globe.
  - o Cut residual lateral attachments of the lower eyelid if it does not move freely.
  - o Do not worry about cutting $1/2$ cm of conjunctiva or skin.
  - o The lower eyelid is cut, relieving orbital pressure. If the intact cornea is exposed, apply, hourly, copious erythromycin ophthalmic ointment or ophthalmic lubricant ointment to prevent devastating corneal dessication and infection. Relief of orbital pressure must be followed by lubricating protection of the cornea and urgent ophthalmic surgical support. Do NOT apply absorbent gauze dressings to the exposed cornea.

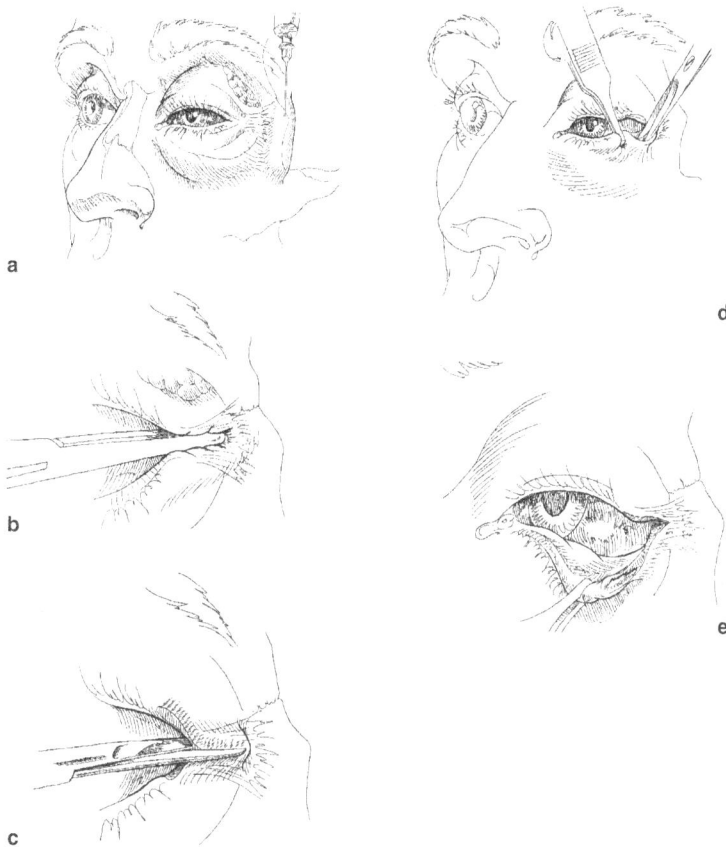

Fig. 14-1. Lateral canthotomy and inferior catholysis are indicated for casualties presenting with serious orbital hemorrhage.

Orbital Floor (Blowout) Fractures

These fractures are usually the result of a blunt injury to the globe or orbital rim, often associated with head and spine injuries. Blowout fractures may be suspected on the basis of enophthalmos, diplopia, decreased ocular motility, hypoesthesia of the V2 branch of the trigeminal nerve, associated subconjunctival hemorrhage, or hyphema. Immediate treatment includes pseudoephedrine 60 mg q 6 hours and a broad-spectrum antibiotic for 7 days, ice packs, and instructing the casualty not to blow his nose. Definitive diagnosis requires CT scan of orbits with axial and coronal views. Indications for repair include severe enophthalmos and diplopia in the primary or reading gaze positions. The surgery may be performed 1–2 weeks after the injury.

Lid Lacerations
Treatment guidelines for lid lacerations not involving the lid margin
- Excellent blood supply — delayed primary closure is not necessary.
- Eyelid function (protecting the globe) is the primary consideration.
- Begin with irrigation, antisepsis (any topical solution), and a check for retained foreign bodies.
- Superficial lacerations of the eyelid, not involving the eyelid margin, may be closed with running or interrupted 6-0 silk (preferred) or nylon sutures.
- Horizontal lacerations should include the orbicular muscle and skin in the repair.
- If skin is missing, an advancement flap may be created to fill in the defect. For vertical or stellate lacerations, use traction sutures in the eyelid margin for 7–10 days.
- Antibiotic ointments qid.
- Skin sutures may be removed in 5 days.

Treatment guidelines for lid lacerations involving the lid margin
- Repair of a marginal lower-eyelid laceration with less than 25% tissue loss (Fig. 14-2).
  - o The irregular laceration edges may be freshened by creating a pentagonal wedge — remove as little tissue as possible (Fig. 14-2b).
  - o A 4-0 silk or nylon suture is placed in the eyelid margin (through the meibomian gland orifices 2 mm from the wound edges and 2 mm deep) and is tied in a slipknot. Symmetric suture placement is critical to obtain post-op eyelid margin alignment (Fig. 14-2c).

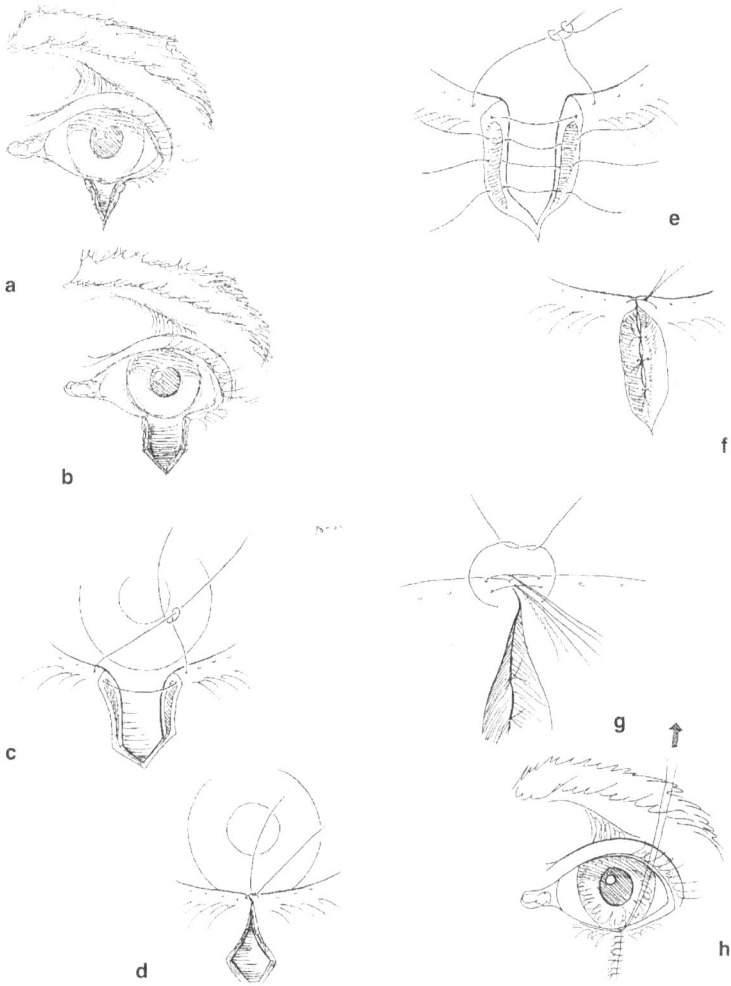

Fig. 14-2. Lid margin repair.

o The slipknot is loosened and approximately two or three absorbable (Vicryl or gut) 5-0 or 6-0 sutures are placed internally to approximate the tarsal plate. The skin and conjunctiva should not be included in this internal closure (Fig. 14-2d).

o Anterior and posterior marginal sutures (6-0 silk or nylon) are placed in the eyelid margin just in front and behind the previously placed 4-0 suture (Fig. 14-2e).

o The middle and posterior sutures are left long and tied under the anterior suture. Ensure that the wound edges are everted (Fig. 14-2f).

o The skin is closed with 6-0 silk or nylon sutures. The lid is placed on traction for at least 5 days. The skin sutures are removed at 3–5 days and the marginal sutures are removed at 10–14 days (Fig. 14-2g).

Additional Points in Lid Laceration Repair

- Tissue loss greater than 25% will require a flap or graft.
- If there is orbital fat in the wound or if ptosis is noted in an upper lid laceration, damage to the orbital septum and the levator aponeurosis should be suspected.
- If the eyelid is avulsed, the missing tissue should be retrieved, wrapped in moistened Telfa, and preserved on ice. The tissue should be soaked in a dilute antibiotic solution prior to reattachment. If necrosis is present, minimal debridement should occur in order to prevent further tissue loss. The avulsed tissue should be secured in the anatomically correct position in the manner described for lid margin repair above.
  o Damage to the canilicular system can occur as a result of injuries to the medial aspect of the lid margins. Suspected canalicular injuries should be repaired by an ophthalmologist to prevent subsequent problems with tear drainage. This repair can be delayed for up to 24 hours.

Laser Eye Injuries

- Battlefield lasers may be designed to cause eye injuries or may be part of other weapons or sensor systems.
- **Prevention is the best option!** Wear eye protection designed for the appropriate light wavelengths if there is a known laser threat.
- The type of ocular damage depends on the wavelength of the laser — retinal injuries are most common.

- The primary symptom of laser injury is loss of vision, which may be preceded by seeing a flash of light. Pain may not be present.
- Immediate treatment of corneal laser burns is similar to that for corneal abrasions.
- Laser retinal burns have no proven immediate treatment, although improvement with corticosteroids has been reported.
- Routine evacuation for evaluation by an ophthalmologist is required.

Enucleation

A general surgeon in a forward unit should not remove a traumatized eye unless the globe is completely disorganized. Enucleation should only be considered if the patient has a very severe injury, no light perception using the brightest light source available, and is not able to be evacuated to a facility with an ophthalmologist. Sympathetic ophthalmia is a condition that may result in loss of vision in the fellow eye if a severely traumatized, nonseeing eye is not removed, but it rarely develops prior to 21 days after an injury. **Delaying the enucleation until the patient can see an ophthalmologist is thus relatively safe.**

Chapter 15

Head Injuries

Introduction
The prognosis of brain injuries is good in patients who respond
to simple commands, are not deeply unconscious, and do not
deteriorate. The prognosis is grave in patients who are rendered
immediately comatose (particularly those sustaining penetrating
injury) and remain unconscious for a long period of time. Any
subsequent neurologic improvement may indicate
salvageability and should prompt reevaluation.

**Neurosurgical damage control includes early intracranial
pressure (ICP) control; cerebral blood flow (CBF) preservation;
and prevention of secondary cerebral injury from hypoxia,
hypotension, and hyperthemia.**

A motor examination of the most salvageable severely brain-
injured patients will demonstrate localization to central
stimulation and these patients will require expedited treatment.
Immediate intubation with adequate ventilation is the most
critical first line of treatment for a severely head-injured patient.
Evacuation to the nearest neurosurgeon, avoiding diagnostic
delays, and initiating cerebral resuscitation allow for the best
chance for ultimate functional recovery.

Combat Head Injury Types
- Blunt (closed head injury).
- Penetrating.
  o Penetrating with retained fragments.
  o Perforating.
  o Guttering (grooving the skull).
  o Tangential.
  o Cranial facial degloving (lateral temple, bifrontal).

- Blast over-pressure CNS injuries.
  - o A force transmitted by the great vessels of the chest to the brain; associated with unconsciousness, confusion, headache, tinnitus, dizziness, tremors, increased startle response, and occasionally (in the most severe forms) increased ICP. Bleeding may occur from multiple orifices including ears, nose, and mouth.

A combination of multiple injury types are typically involved in combat-related brain injuries. Those injuries generally involve the face, neck, and orbit; entry wounds may be through the upper neck, face, orbit, or temple (Fig. 15-1).

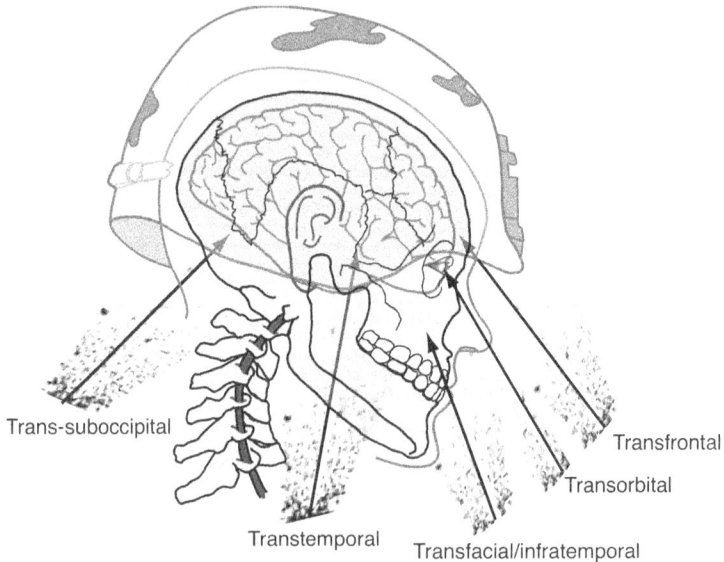

Fig. 15-1. Common vectors of penetrating injury.

The subocciput, occiput, and retroauricular regions are overlooked most. Injuries to these areas can indicate underlying injury to the posterior fossa, major venous sinus, or carotid artery, as fragments pass through the skull base. Reconstructing the fragment path based on combination of plain films and computed tomography (CT) can be challenging. In transorbital, transtemple, or penetrating injuries that cross the midline, an underlying injury to intracranial vessels should be suspected with associated psuedoaneurysms, dissections, or venous sinus injury.

Explosion results in flying fragments, with possible vehicular-collision–associated blunt injuries. Depending on the proximity to the explosion, a blast over-pressure phenomenon may also result. In a severely brain-injured patient, more deficits than indicated by the CT scan may be due to possible underlying injury to brachiocephalic vessels, shear injury, or the effects of blast over-pressure with resulting cerebral vasospasm. Plain films, more useful in penetrating than blunt trauma, may reveal a burst fracture of the skull indicating the tremendous perforating force of a penetrating missile. Transventricular bihemispheric fragment tracts portend a poor prognosis.

Severe head injuries are often seen in combination with significant chest, abdomen, and extremity injuries. Very rapid hemorrhage control is the priority in the noncranial injuries; utilizing damage control concepts and focusing attention on the head injury. All efforts should be directed toward early diagnosis and intervention of the head injury.

Traditional Classification of Head Injuries
- **Open** injuries are the most commonly encountered brain injuries in combat.
- **Closed** injuries, seen more often in civilian settings, may have a higher frequency in military operations other than war.
- **Scalp** injuries may be closed (eg, contusion) or open (eg, puncture, laceration, or avulsion).
  - o Any scalp injury may be associated with a skull fracture and/or underlying brain injury.
  - o Open scalp injuries bleed profusely, even to the point of lethal blood loss, but usually heal well when properly repaired.
- **Skull fractures** may be open or closed, and are described as linear, comminuted, or depressed.
  - o Skull fractures are usually associated with some degree of brain injury, varying from mild concussion, to devastating diffuse brain injury, to intracranial hematomas.

o Open skull fractures are prone to infection if not properly treated.

Mechanisms of Injury
- **Primary injury** is a function of the energy transmitted to the brain by the offending agent.
  - o Very little can be done by healthcare providers to influence the primary injury.
  - o Enforcement of personal protective measures (eg, helmet, seatbelts) by the command is essential prevention.
- **Secondary injury** results from disturbance of brain and systemic physiology by the traumatic event.

Hypotension and hypoxia are the two most acute and easily treatable mechanisms of secondary injury.

---

o Other etiologies include seizures (seen in 30%–40% of patients with penetrating brain injuries), fever, electrolyte disturbances (specifically, hyponatremia or hyperglycemia), and infection.

o **All of the above conditions can be treated.**

o Elevations of ICP may occur early as a result of a space-occupying hematoma, or develop gradually as a result of brain edema or hydrocephalus.

o Normal ICP is 5–15 mm Hg, with normal cerebral perfusion pressure (CPP = MAP-ICP) usually around 70–80 mm Hg.

o Decreases in perfusion pressure as a result of systemic hypotension or elevated ICP gradually result in alteration of brain function (manifested by impairment of consciousness), and may progress to global brain ischemia and death if not treated.

Patient Assessment and Triage
During the primary and secondary assessment, attention should be placed on a complete examination of the scalp and neck. Fragments that enter the cranial vault with a transtemple, transorbital, or cross midline trajectory should be suspected as having associated neurovascular injuries. Wounds are typically contaminated by hair, dirt, and debris

and should be copiously irrigated clean with control of scalp hemorrhage **but not at the expense of delaying definitive neurosurgical treatment**! Scalp hemorrhage can be controlled with a head wrap, scalp clips, or surgical staples; a meticulous plastic surgical closure is only appropriate after intracranial injuries have been ruled out.

- The most important assessment is the **vital signs.**
- Next is the **level of consciousness**, best measured and recorded by the Glasgow Coma Scale (GCS) (see below).

GLASGOW COMA SCALE

Component	Response	Score
Motor Response (best extremity)	Obeys verbal command	6
	Localizes pain	5
	Flexion-withdrawal	4
	Flexion (decortication)	3
	Extension (decerebration)	2
	No response (flaccid)	1
	Subtotal	**(1–6)**
Eye Opening	Spontaneously	4
	To verbal command	3
	To pain	2
	None	1
	Subtotal	**(1–4)**
Best Verbal Response	Oriented and converses	5
	Disoriented and converses	4
	Inappropriate words	3
	Incomprehensible sounds	2
	No verbal response	1
	Subtotal	**(1–5)**
	Total	**(3–15)**

- Triage decisions in the patient with craniocerebral trauma should be made based on **admission GCS** score.
  - o A GCS ≤ 5 indicates a dismal prognosis despite aggressive comprehensive treatment and the casualty should be considered expectant.

o A GCS $\geq$ 8 indicates that a casualty may do well if managed appropriately.
  ♦ In general, neurologically stable patients with penetrating head injury can be managed effectively in the ICU with airway and ventilatory support, antibiotics, and anticonvulsants while awaiting surgery.
  ♦ An exception to this would be a deteriorating patient with a large hematoma seen on CT—this should be considered a surgical emergency.
o **Casualties with GCS 6–8 can be the most reversible, with forward neurosurgical management involving control of ICP and preservation of CBF.**
● Another important assessment is **pupillary reactivity**.

> **A single dilated or nonreactive pupil adds urgency and implies the presence of a unilateral space-occupying lesion with secondary brain shift. Immediate surgery is indicated.**

o The presence of bilateral dilated or nonreactive pupils is a dismal prognostic sign in the setting of profound alteration of consciousness.
● **Radiographic evaluation.**
o Deployable CT scanners in standard ISO shelters are increasingly available in the field environment. **To keep the scanner operational, a qualified maintenance chief should be married to the scanner ("crew-chief" concept).**
  ♦ CT is the definitive radiographic study in the evaluation of head injury, and should be employed liberally as it greatly improves diagnostic accuracy and facilitates management.
o Skull radiographs still have a place in the evaluation of head injury (**especially penetrating trauma**).
  ♦ In the absence of CT capability, AP and lateral skull radiographs help to localize foreign bodies in cases of penetrating injuries and can also demonstrate skull fractures.
  ♦ This can help direct otherwise "blind" surgical intervention initially to the side of the head where the fracture is identified.

o Cervical spine injury is uncommon in the setting of penetrating head injury.
   ♦ Closed head injury is commonly associated with injury of the cervical spine.
   ♦ Assume the presence of cervical spine injury and keep the cervical spine immobilized with a rigid collar until standard AP, lateral, and open-mouth radiographs can be obtained to exclude injury.
   ♦ CT once again is useful in evaluating casualties with a high suspicion for spinal injury.

Management
● **Medical.**
   o Primary tenets are basic but vital; clear the airway, ensure adequate ventilation, and assess and treat for shock (excessive fluid administration should be avoided).
   o In general, patients with a GCS ≤ 12 should be managed in the ICU.
   o **ICU management should be directed at the avoidance and treatment of secondary brain injury.**
      ♦ Pa_{O_2} should be kept at a minimum of 100 mm Hg.
      ♦ P_{CO_2} maintained between 35 and 40 mm Hg.
      ♦ The head should be elevated approximately 30°.
      ♦ Sedate patient and/or pharmacologically paralyze to avoid "bucking" the ventilator and causing ICP spikes.
      ♦ Broad-spectrum antibiotics should be administered to patients with penetrating injuries (a third-generation cephalosporin, vancomycin or Ancef, Unasyn or meropenen if acinetobacter suspected).
      ♦ Anaerobic coverage with metronidazole should be considered for grossly contaminated wounds or those whose treatment has been delayed more than 18 hours.
      ♦ Phenytoin should be administered in a 17-mg/kg load, which may be placed in a normal saline piggyback and given over 20–30 minutes (no more than 50 mg/min, because rapid infusion may cause cardiac conduction disturbances).

◊ A maintenance dose of 300–400 mg/d, either in divided doses or once before bedtime, should be adequate to maintain a serum level of 10–20 µg/L.

♦ Measure serum chemistries daily to monitor for hyponatremia.

♦ Monitor and treat coagulopathy aggressively.

♦ Monitoring of ICP is recommended for patients with GCS≤ 8 (in essence, it is a substitute for a neurologic examination).

◊ A simple fluid-path monitor usually works well and allows CSF drainage. It may then be coupled to a manometer or to a multifunction cardiac monitor similar to a central venous catheter or arterial line.

▪ Administer prophylactic antibiotic.

▪ Make an incision just at or anterior to the coronal suture, approximately **2.5–3 cm** lateral to the midline (Fig. 15-2a,b).

▪ A twist drill craniostomy is performed, the underlying dura is nicked, and a ventricular catheter placed into the frontal horn of the lateral ventricle (encountered at a depth of 5 to 6 cm) (see Fig. 15-2b,c). Catheter should be directed toward the medial epicanthis on the coronal plane, and the tragus in the sagittal plane.

▪ Even small ventricles can be easily cannulated by aiming the tip of the catheter toward the nasion in the coronal plane.

▪ Ventricular catheters are highly preferable; acceptable substitutes are an 8 F Robinson catheter or pediatric feeding tube.

▪ A key feature of this technique is to tunnel the drain out through a separate incision 2–3 cm from the primary one, thus reducing the risk of infection.

◊ The goal of management is to maintain a CPP of 60–90 mm Hg.

◊ A sustained ICP > 20 mm Hg should be treated (Fig. 15-3).

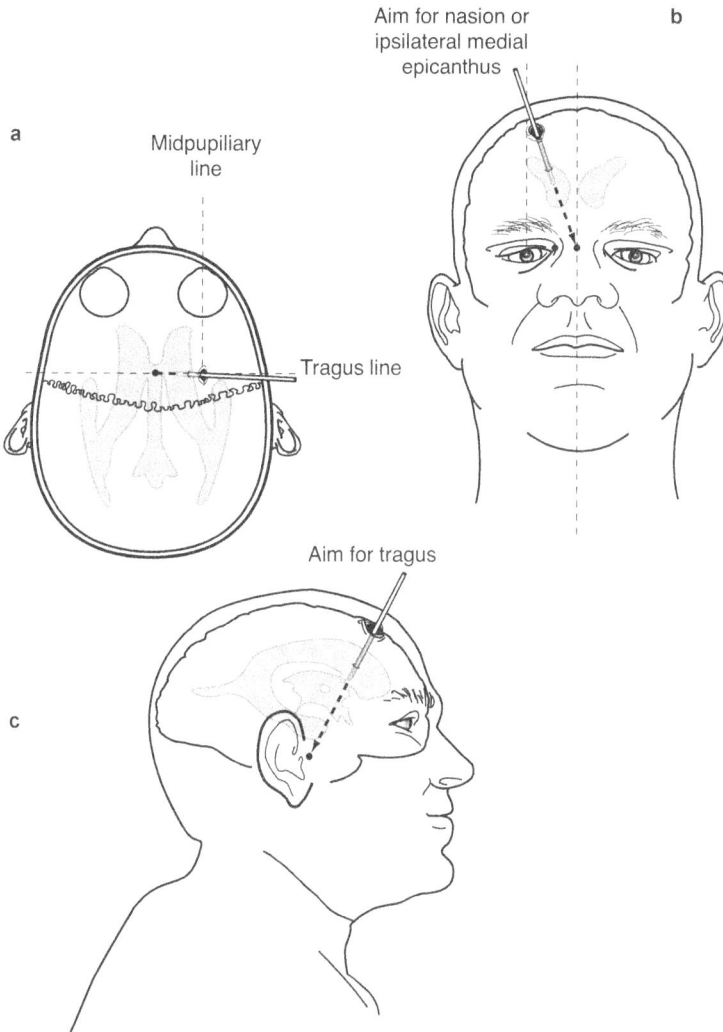

Fig. 15-2. Placement of intracranial ventricular catheter.

```
┌─────────────────────────────────────┐
│        Levels of Intervention        │
└─────────────────────────────────────┘

             Pentobarbital
            or Thiopental Load

          Hemicraniectomy/Duraplasty

      Mild Hypothermia (34°–36°C) should be
             considered in isolated head
      injury but should be avoided in multi-trauma

     Mannitol/Lasix (possible 3.0% Hypertonic Saline)

          CSF Drainage via Ventricutostomy

          Moderate Head-Up Posture (30°)

  Adequate Sedation/Analgesia (Versed, Fentanyl, Morphine, Propofol)
```

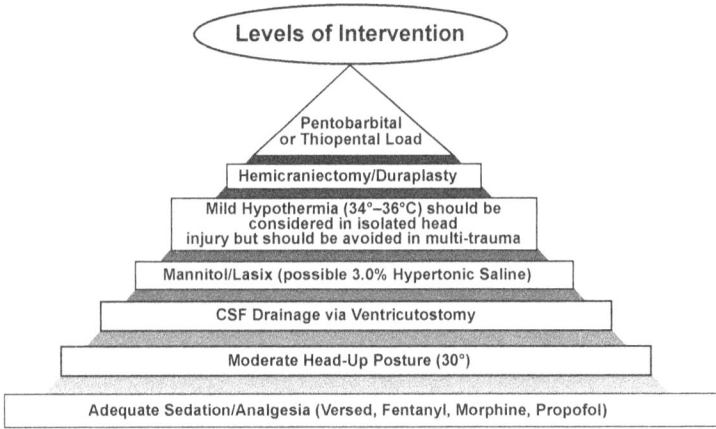

Fig. 15-3. Levels of intervention to reduce ICP.

- Sedation, head elevation, and paralysis.
- CSF drainage if a ventricular catheter is in place.
- **Hyperventilation to a P_{CO_2} of 30 to 35 mm Hg only until other measures take effect.** (Prolonged levels below this are deleterious as a result of small vessel constriction and ischemia.)
- Refractory intracranial hypertension should be managed with an initial bolus of 1g/kg of **mannitol** and intermittent dosing of 0.25–0.5 g/kg q4h as needed.
  - Aggressive treatment with mannitol should be accompanied by placement of a CVP line or even a PA catheter because hypovolemia may ensue.
- Any patient who develops intracranial hypertension or deteriorates clinically should undergo prompt repeat CT.
- ◊ Mild hypothermia may be considered in isolated head injury, but avoid in the multitrauma patient.
- ♦ Treat hypovolemia with albumin, normal saline, hypertonic saline, or other volume expanders to create a euvolemic, hyperosmolar patient (290–315 mOsm/L).
- ♦ Blast over-pressure CNS injuries.

◊ Supportive medical therapy is usually sufficient. Only in rare cases is an ICP monitor, ventriculostomy, or cranial decompression necessary. In the absence of hematomas the use of magnesium has been beneficial. Structures particularly sensitive include optic apparatus, hippocampus, and basal ganglia. Delayed intracranial hemorrhages have been reported. Additionally, these patients have a higher susceptibility to subsequent injury and should be evaluated at a level 4/5 facility. Repetitive injury and exposure to blast over-pressure may result in irreversible cognitive deficits.

- **Surgical**
  o Goals: prevent infection and relieve/prevent intracranial hypertension.
  o Indications for emergent exploration.
    ♦ Space-occupying lesions with neurological changes (eg, acute subdural/epidural hematoma, abscess).
    ♦ Intracranial hematoma producing a > 5 mm midline shift or similar depression of cortex.
    ♦ Compound depressed fracture with neurological changes.
    ♦ Penetrating injuries with neurological deterioration.
  o Relief of ICP with hemicraniectomy/duraplasty/ventriculostomy.
    ♦ A large trauma flap should be planned for the evacuation of a mass lesion with significant underlying edema in the supratentorial space.
    ♦ The flap should extend a minimum of 4 cm posterior to the external auditory canal and 3–4 cm off midline. Exposing the frontal, temporal, and parietal lobes allows for adequate cerebral swelling and avoids brain herniation at the craniotomy edge.
    ♦ A capacious duraplasty should be constructed with a subdural ICP/ventricular catheter in place, allowing monitoring and drainage from the injured hemisphere.
  o Shave hair widely and scrub and paint the scalp with betadine.
  o General anesthesia for major cases.

o Administer empiric antibiotics (third-generation cephalosporin).
o Positioning can be adequately managed with the head in a doughnut or horseshoe-type head holder. For unusual positioning of the head, such as to gain access to the subocciput, use a standard three-point Mayfield fixation device.
o Make a generous scalp incision to create an adequate flap.
   ◆ The flap should have an adequate pedicle to avoid ischemia.
   ◆ Retraction of the scalp flap over a rolled laparotomy sponge will avoid kinking the flap, which also may lead to ischemia.
o The skull should be entered through a series of burr holes (Fig. 15-4) that are then joined to create a craniotomy flap (Fig. 15-5a).

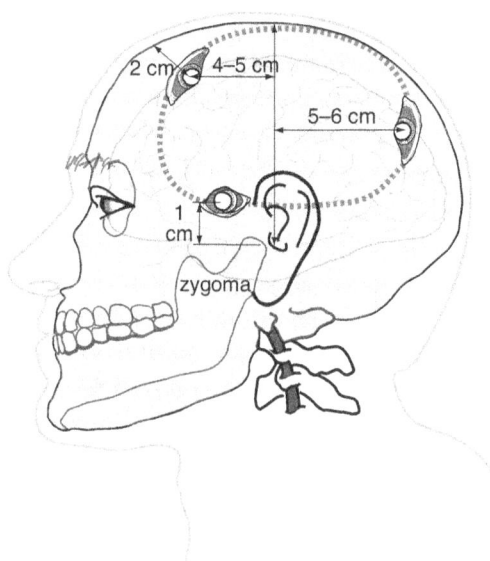

Fig. 15-4. Cranial landmarks and location of standard burr holes.

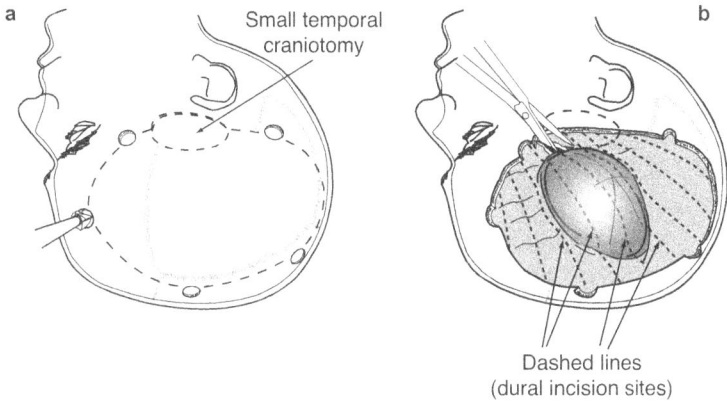

Fig. 15-5. Craniotomy flap and exposed hematoma.

◆ **Burr holes alone are inadequate to treat acute hematomas**, but are of diagnostic utility in the absence of CT scanner. Exploratory burr holes may miss subfrontal or interhemispheric hematomas (Fig. 15-6).

Fig. 15-6. Hematomas missed with routine exploratory burr holes.

15.13

- ♦ The bone work may be done with a Hudson brace and Gigli's saw, though a power craniotome is certainly preferable if available (see Fig. 15-5a).
- o A dural opening, using the entire expanse of the cranial opening (with enough edge left to close the dura at the end of the case), should be created.
  - ♦ The base of the dural opening should be on the side near any neighboring major venous sinus to avoid injury to large draining veins and aggravation of cerebral edema.
- o The hematoma should then be gently evacuated with a combination of suction, irrigation, and mechanical removal (see Fig. 15-5b).
- o Meticulous hemostasis should be achieved and the dura closed.
- o Approach to **penetrating injury with neurologic changes** is aimed at removal of devitalized brain and easily accessible foreign bodies.
  - ♦ Perform copious irrigation with an antibiotic solution (such as bacitracin) and a concerted attempt made to achieve watertight dural closure (again, using pericranium, among others, as needed).
  - ♦ Tension-free scalp closure is also essential, but replacement of multiple skull fragments in an attempt to reconstruct the skull defect is not appropriate in the battlefield setting.
    - ◊ Excellent results can be achieved with cranioplasty after evacuation out of the theater and a sufficient delay to minimize risk of infection.
- o If a duraplasty is required, pericranium, temporalis fascia, or tensor fascia lata may be used.
- o Tack-up sutures should be placed around the periphery and in the center of the dural exposure to close the dead space and discourage post-operative epidural hematoma formation.
- o Replace bone flap and secure with wire or heavy suture.
  - ♦ If severe brain swelling precludes replacement of the bone flap it can be discarded or preserved in an abdominal-wall pocket.

o The galea of the scalp should generally be closed separately with an absorbable suture, and with staples used to close the skin.

 ♦ A single layer closure with heavy monofilament nylon is acceptable but should definitely include the galea, with the sutures remaining in place at least 10 days.

 ♦ A subgaleal or epidural drain may be used at the discretion of the surgeon.

o Apply a snug dressing using roller bandages around the entire head.

Evacuation of the Severely Head-Injured Patient

The trip is always longer than advertised. Transport only patients who can be expected to survive 12–24 hour movements, due to unexpected delays, route changes, or diversion in the tactical situation. A post-operative, craniotomy patient should first be observed for 12–24 hours prior to transport. Evacuating immediately may lead to the inability to treat delayed post-operative hematomas that may occur.

o All patients with GCS < 12 are ventilated.

o Patients with GCS < 8T require ICP monitoring.

o Ventriculostomies should be placed, position confirmed, secured, and working prior to departure.

o The critical care evacuation team must be confident in the ability to medically treat increased ICP and troubleshoot the ventriculostomy.

o Medical management of ICP in flight is limited to the use of head-of-bed elevation (30°–60°), increased sedation, thiopental, ventricular drainage, and mild hyperventilation. Loading a patient head-of-bed first limits the effect of takeoff on ICP.

o The escort of a severely head-injured patient must be able to manage the airway, ventilator, IV pumps, IV medicines, suction, in addition to ICP and CBF.

o Patients with possible intracranial pathology who may deteriorate inflight should be neurosurgically maximized on the ground prior to departure (eg, placement of a ventriculostomy or evacuation of a hematoma).

o If a head-injured patient (GCS > 12) deteriorates in flight and is not already intubated, intubation should be performed and planned. Ensure rapid sequence intubation medicines, IV access, and airway equipment (especially Ambu bag, ventilator) are working and available.

o The most difficult part of an evacuation is from the CSH to the CASF/MASF. Typically, battery life of the ventilator and monitors, and supplies of oxygen can be depleted before the exchange of the patient to the CASF/MASF. Although electric power is available on Black Hawks and FLA (ground ambulance), it is rarely used.

o Prior to departure from the CSH the following precautions must be taken by the escort:

♦ Ensure knowledge of patient injuries and clinical course. (Have narrative summary and pertinent radiographs in hand.)

♦ Ensure adequate medicines for minimum of 3 days.

♦ Ensure monitors, ventilators, and suction and IV pumps all have adequate battery life.

♦ Ensure adequate oxygen supplies, and that the escort has the familiarity with and the ability to switch oxygen tanks.

♦ Have an alternate battery-operated, tactical light source to read monitors during transport.

♦ Assemble patients on the stretcher to avoid iatrogenic injuries to limbs, organizing tubes, lines, electrical leads, and wires so as not to become snared during movements. (When available, a SMEED shelf attached to the stretcher allows monitors to be secured and elevated off the patient's body.)

♦ Ensure that limbs (toes and fingers) and torso are covered and insulated during the trip to prevent hypothermia.

♦ During movements ensure central lines, a-lines, and ventricular catheters do not become dislodged. Ensure lines and tubes are sutured or otherwise secured.

♦ Ensure the ventriculostomy does not develop an air-lock. Venting the tublet can be performed with a 21-gauge needle.

Chapter 16

Thoracic Injuries

Introduction

About 15% of war injuries involve the chest. Of those, 10% are superficial (soft tissue only) requiring only basic wound treatment. The remaining 90% of chest injuries are almost all penetrating.

Those injuries involving the central column of the chest (heart, great vessels, pulmonary hilum) are generally fatal on the battlefield. Injuries of the lung parenchyma (the vast majority) can be managed by the insertion of a chest tube and basic wound treatment. Although penetrating injuries are most common, blunt chest trauma may occur and can result in disruption of the contents of the thorax as well as injury to the chest wall itself. Blast injuries can result in the rupture of air-filled structures (the lung) as well as penetrating injuries from fragments.

> **The immediate recognition and treatment of tension pneumothorax is the single most important and life-saving intervention in the treatment of chest injuries in combat. Distended neck veins, tracheal shift, decreased breath sounds, and hyperresonance in the affected hemithorax, and hypotension are the cardinal signs. None or all may be present. Immediate decompression is lifesaving.**

With the advent of body armor, it is hoped that the majority of thoracic injuries seen in past conflicts will be avoided. Unfortunately, there will be individuals who will not have such protection, as well as others who will sustain chest injuries despite protection.

Anatomic Considerations

- Superior border is at the level of the clavicles anteriorly and the junction of the C7-T1 vertebral bodies posteriorly. The thoracic inlet at that level contains major arteries (common carotids, vertebrals), veins (anterior and internal jugulars), trachea, esophagus, and spinal cord.
- Within or traversing the container of the chest itself are found the heart and coronary vessels, great vessels including arteries (aorta, arch, inominate, right subclavian, common carotid, left subclavian, and descending aorta), veins (superior and inferior vena cava, azygous vein, brachiocephalic vein), pulmonary arteries and veins, distal trachea and main stem bronchi, lungs, and esophagus.
- The inferior border is described by the diaphragm, attached anteriorly at the T6 level and gradually sloping posteriorly to the T12 level.

> **Penetrating thoracic injuries below the T4 level (nipple line) have a high probability of involving abdominal structures (Fig. 16-1).**

Evaluation and Diagnosis

Knowledge of the mechanism of injury (eg, blast, fragment, among others) may increase the index of suspicion for a particular injury. A complete and accurate diagnosis is usually not possible because of the limited diagnostic tools available in the setting of combat trauma. Nonetheless, because injuries to the chest can profoundly affect breathing and circulation (and on rare occasion, the airway), a complete and rapid assessment of each injury is mandatory.

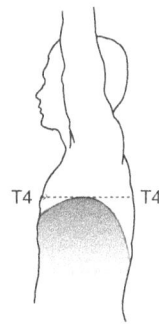

Fig. 16-1. Thoracic incision of abdominal contents.

- If the casualty is able to talk, there is reasonable assurance that the airway is intact.

Life-Threatening Injuries

> **Injuries not immediately obvious, yet requiring urgent attention, include tension pneumothorax, massive hemothorax, and cardiac tamponade.**

- **Tension Pneumothorax.**
  - A patient with a known chest injury presenting with an open airway and difficulty breathing has a tension pneumothorax until proven otherwise and requires rapid decompression and the insertion of a chest tube.
- **Massive Hemothorax.**
  - The return of blood may indicate a significant intrathoracic injury. Generally, the **immediate return of 1,500 cc of blood mandates thoracotomy** (especially if the wound was sustained within the past hour). With less blood initially, but a continued loss of **200 cc/hour for over 4 hours**, thoracotomy is indicated.
  - Casualties with massive thoracic hemorrhage require damage control techniques (see Chapter 12, Damage Control Surgery).
- **Cardiac Tamponade.**
  - Distended neck veins (may be absent with significant blood loss) in the presence of clear breath sounds and hypotension indicate the possibility of life-threatening cardiac tamponade.
  - Fluid resuscitation may temporarily stabilize a patient in tamponade.
  - Perform an ultrasound (US) with a **stable** patient.
    - ♦ If **positive,** proceed to the OR (pericardial window, sternotomy, thoracotomy). Any pericardial blood mandates median sternotomy/thoracotomy.
    - ♦ A **negative** US requires either repeat US or pericardial window, depending on level of clinical suspicion.
  - Pericardiocentesis is only a stopgap measure on the way to definitive surgical repair.

- **Open pneumothorax** (hole in chest wall) is treated by placing a chest tube and sealing the hole. Alternatives include one-way valve chest dressings or a square piece of plastic dressing taped to the chest on three sides.
- **Flail chest** (entire segment of the chest wall floating due to fractures of a block of ribs, with two fractures on each rib) will require treatment (either airway intubation or observation) based on the severity of the underlying lung injury. In cases where intubation is not required, repeated intercostal nerve blocks with a long-acting local anesthetic such as Marcaine may be very helpful in relieving pain and limiting atelectasis and other pulmonary complications.

Surgical Management

> **Most penetrating chest injuries reaching medical attention are adequately treated with tube thoracostomy (chest tube) alone.**

Tube thoracostomy (chest tube).
- Indications.
  - o Known or suspected tension pneumothorax.
  - o Pneumothorax (including open).
  - o Hemothorax.
  - o Any penetrating chest injury requiring transport (mandatory in case of aeromedical evacuation).
- Procedure (Fig. 16-2).
  - o In cases of tension pneumothorax, **immediate decompression with a large bore needle is lifesaving**. An IV catheter (14/16/18 gauge at least 2–3 inches in length) is inserted in the midclavicular line in the second interspace (approximately 2 fingerbreadths below the clavicle on the adult male). Entry is confirmed by the sound of air passing through the catheter. **This must be rapidly followed by the insertion of a chest tube.**
  - o In a contaminated environment, a single gram of IV cefazolin (Ancef) is recommended.
  - o If time allows, prep the anterior and lateral chest on the affected side with povidone-iodine.

o Identify the incision site along the anterior axillary line, intersecting the 5th or 6th rib.
o Inject a local anesthetic in the awake patient, if conditions allow.
o Make a transverse incision, 3–4 cm in length, along and centered over the rib, carrying it down to the bone.

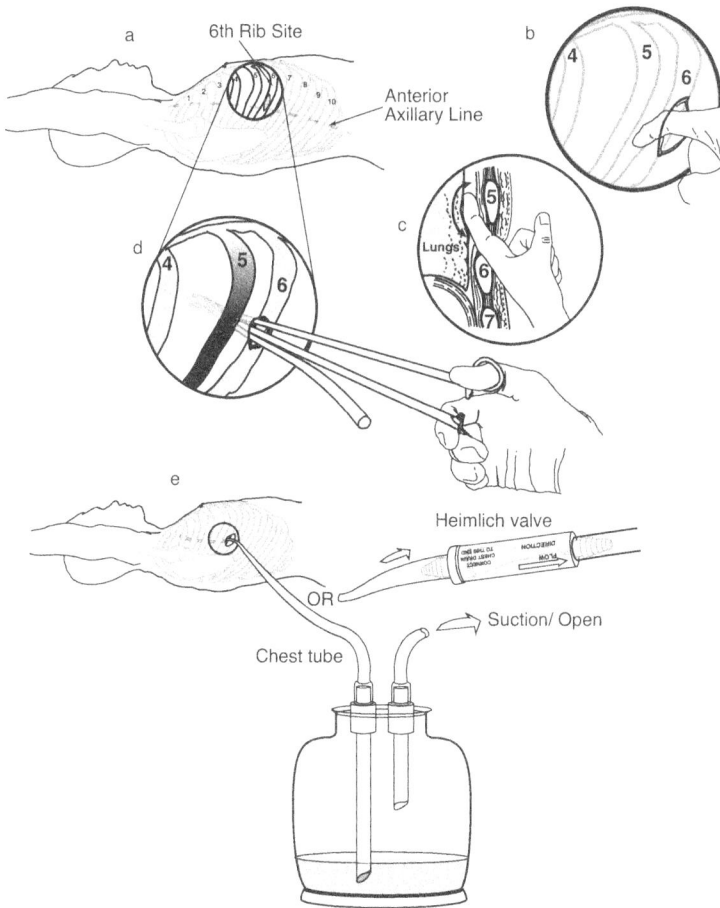

Fig. 16-2. Procedure for tube thoracostomy.

o Insert a curved clamp in the incision, directed over the top of the rib, and push into the chest through the pleura. A distinct pop is encountered when entering the chest and a moderate amount of force is necessary to achieve this entry. A rush of air out of the chest will confirm a tension pneumothorax. Insertion depth of the tip of the clamp should be limited by the surgeon's hand to only 3 or 4 cm to make sure that the clamp does not travel deeper into the chest, resulting in damage to underlying structures.

o Spread the clamp gently and remove. The operator's finger is then inserted to confirm entry.

o Insert a chest tube (24 to 36 French) into the hole. All chest tube side-holes must be in the chest. If no chest tubes are available, an adult endotracheal tube may be used.

o Attach a chest tube to a Heimlich valve, sealed pleurovac, or bottles. In a resource constrained environment, a cut-off glove or Penrose drain may be attached to the end of the chest tube.

o Secure the tube with suture, if possible, and dress to prevent contamination.

Resuscitative Thoracotomy

- **Only indicated in penetrating chest injury in extremis or with recent loss of vital signs.**
- **These patients are generally unsalvageable, even with unlimited resources and no other significant casualties.**
- **If performed, a rapid assessment of injuries should be made, and in the case of unsalvageable injuries, the procedure should be immediately terminated.**

Procedure

- With the patient supine, make an incision in the left inframammary fold starting at the lateral border of the sternum extending to the midaxillary line (Fig. 16-3).
- The procedure should be abandoned upon the discovery of devastating injuries to the heart and great vessels.

- If no injury is found in left chest, rapidly extend the incision across the midline, crossing through the sternum with a Lebsche sternum knife, performing a mirror-image thoracotomy (clamshell, Fig. 16-4). When doing this procedure you will cut across both internal mammary arteries, which will be a significant source of bleeding.

Fig. 16-3. Incision for resuscitative thoracotomy.

- Elevating the anterior chest wall will expose virtually all mediastinal structures.
- Open the pericardium and assess the heart.
- **Priorities are to stop bleeding and restore central perfusion.**
  - o Holes in the heart and/or great vessels should be temporarily occluded.
    - ◆ Temporary occlusion can be achieved with fingers, side-biting clamps or Foley catheters with 30 cc balloons. Any other sterile device of opportunity is acceptable.
  - o Major pulmonary hilar injuries should be cross-clamped en masse.
  - o Descending aorta located, cross-clamped, and cardiac function restored via defibrillation or massage. (Make sure to open the mediastinal pleura over the aorta to securely apply the vascular clamp.)
  - o If unable to restore cardiac function rapidly, abandon the operation.
- With successful restoration of cardiac function, injuries should be more definitively repaired.

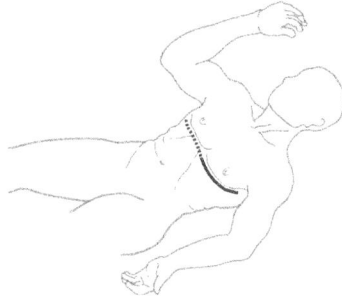

Subxiphoid Pericardial Window

> **Subxiphoid pericardial window should not be attempted in an unstable patient. Unstable patients with penetrating injuries suspicious for cardiac injury should undergo immediate median sternotomy/thoracotomy.**

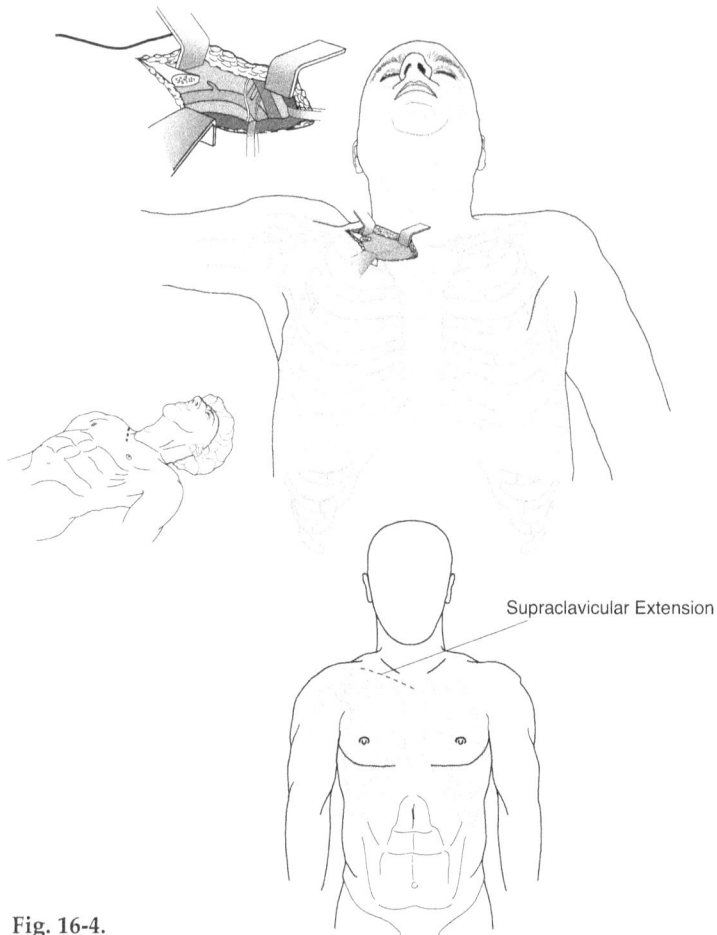

Fig. 16-4.
Supraclavicular approach.

Procedure
- With the patient supine, make a 4–5 cm longitudinal incision just on and below the xiphoid process through the skin and fascia.
- Bluntly dissect superiorly toward the heart exposing the phrenopericardial membrane below the heart.

- Place two stay sutures into the membrane and sharply incise between them, with care to avoid the heart, opening the pericardial sac and exposing the underlying beating heart.

Median Sternotomy
- Indications.
  - o Suspected cardiac injury in an unstable patient.
  - o Positive pericardiocentesis/subxiphoid pericardial window.
  - o Suspected injury to the great vessels in the chest.
  - o Suspected distal tracheal injury.
- Procedure.
  - o In the supine position, make a midline skin incision from the sternal notch to just below the xiphoid.
  - o Through blunt/sharp dissection, develop a plane for several centimeters both superiorly and inferiorly beneath the sternum.
  - o Divide the sternum with a sternal saw or Lebsche knife. Keep the foot of the knife/saw tilted up toward the undersurface of the sternum to avoid cardiac injury. Bone wax can be used to decrease bleeding on the cut edges of the sternum.
  - o Separate the halves of the sternum using a chest retractor.
  - o Carefully divide the pericardium superiorly, avoiding the innominate vein, exposing the heart and base of the great vessels.

In general, exposure to the heart and great vessels is best achieved through a median sternotomy. For proximal left subclavian artery injuries, additional exposure (trap door) may be necessary.

  - o Close with wire suture directly through the halves of the sternum, approximately 2 cm from the edge, or around the sternum through the costal interspaces using wire sutures.
  - o Place one or two mediastinal tubes for drainage, exiting through a midline stab wound inferior to the mediastinal skin incision.

Other Approaches
- **Supraclavicular.**
    - o Indication.
        - ♦ Mid to distal subclavian artery injury.
    - o Procedure.
        - ♦ Make an incision 2 cm above and parallel to the clavicle, beginning at the sternal notch and extending laterally 8 cm.
- **Trap door** (Fig. 16-5).
    - o Indication.
        - ♦ Proximal left subclavian artery injury.
    - o Procedure.

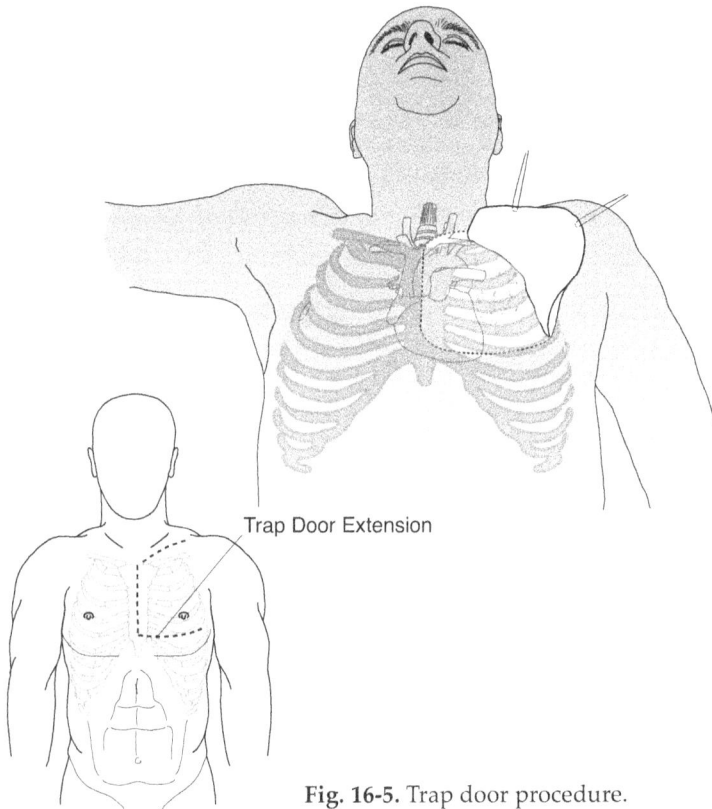

Trap Door Extension

Fig. 16-5. Trap door procedure.

- ◆ Perform supraclavicular approach as above.
- ◆ Perform a partial median sternotomy to the fourth intercostal space.
- ◆ At the fourth intercostal interspace, incise the skin laterally in the submammary fold to the anterior axillary line.
- ◆ Divide the sternum laterally and continue in the 4th intercostal space (ICS) to the anterior axillary line. The internal mammary artery will be divided and must be controlled.
- ◆ It may be necessary to either fracture or remove a section of clavicle to gain adequate exposure of the proximal left subclavian artery.
- ◆ Approach distal left subclavian artery injuries through a supraclavicular incision.
- ● **Thoracoabdominal.**
  - o Indication.
    - ◆ Combined thoracic and abdominal injuries.
  - o Procedure.
    - ◆ The resuscitative thoracotomy can be continued medially and inferiorly across the costal margin into the abdominal midline to complete a thoracoabdominal incision.
    - ◆ Alternatively, a separate abdominal incision can be made.
    - ◆ With right-sided lower chest injuries, the liver and retrohepatic vena cava can be exposed well using a right thoracoabdominal approach.

Specific Injuries
- ● **Vascular.**
  - o Initially, holes in vessels should be digitally occluded. Stopgap measures include placing Fogarty or Foley catheters, side-biting clamps, or in the case of venous injuries, sponge sticks.
  - o Total occlusion or clamping may temporarily be necessary to allow resuscitation to continue and restore cardiac function.

o If cardiac function cannot be restored within 5 to 10 minutes, the procedure should be abandoned (on-the-table triage).

o Repair of vessels should follow the principles detailed in vascular repair: attempting primary repair if possible, with the use of prosthetics if primary repair is not feasible. Consider shunting as an alternative.

● **Heart.**

> **The usual result of high-velocity injuries to the heart is irreparable destruction of the muscle.**

o Isolated punctures of the heart should be exposed (opening the pericardium) and occluded by finger pressure. Other methods include the use of a Foley catheter or skin staples.

o Use pledgeted horizontal mattress sutures (2-0 prolene) on a tapered needle for definitive repair. **Care must be taken to avoid additional injury to coronary vessels.** Extreme care must be taken to avoid tearing the cardiac muscle.

o Atrial repairs may include simple ligature, stapled repair, or running closures (Fig. 16-6).

o Temporary inflow occlusion may prove helpful in repair.

o More complex repairs are impractical without cardiac bypass.

● **Lung.**

o **Tube thoracostomy alone is adequate treatment for most simple lung parenchymal injuries.**

o **Large air leaks not responding to chest tubes** or that do not allow adequate ventilation will require open repair (see tracheobronchial tree below).

o **Posterolateral thoracotomy is preferred for isolated lung injuries.** Anterior thoracotomy may also be used.

o Control simple bleeding with absorbable suture on a tapered needle. Alternatively, staples (TA-90) may be used for bleeding lung tears.

o **Tractotomy**: Open any bleeding tracts (through and through lung penetrations) with a GIA stapler and ligate bleeding points.

Do not simply close the entrance and exit points of penetrating tracts in the lung. With positive pressure ventilation, the risk is air embolism. The more central the injury, the higher the risk.

---

o Resection for bleeding may be indicated with severe parenchymal injury. Anatomic resections are **not** indicated and simple stapled wedge excisions recommended.
o Uncontrolled parenchymal/hilar bleeding, or complex hilar injuries with massive air leak should be controlled with hilar clamping and repair attempted. Pneumonectomy is performed as a last resort (90% mortality).

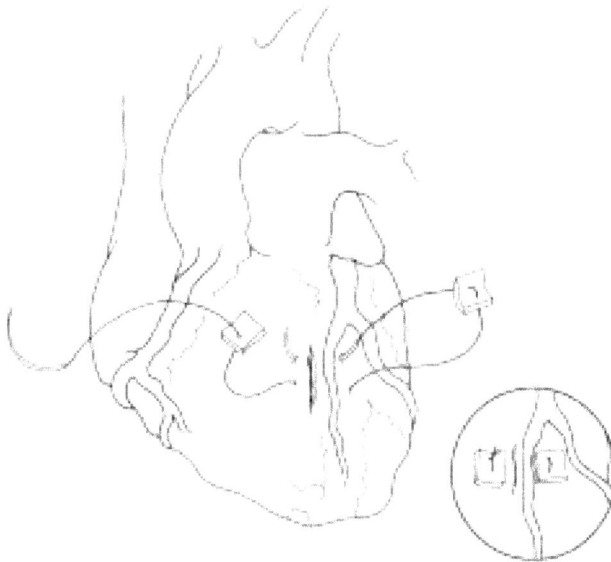

Fig. 16-6. Repair of penetrating cardiac injury.

- **Tracheobronchial tree.**
  - o Suspect the diagnosis with massive air leak, frothy hemoptysis, and pneumomediastinum.
  - o Confirm by bronchoscopy.
  - o Airway control is paramount.
  - o Median sternotomy is best approach.
  - o Repair over endotracheal tube with absorbable suture — may require segmental resection. Bolster with pleural or intercostal muscle flap.
  - o Temporizing measures include:
    - ♦ Single lung ventilation.
    - ♦ Control the airway through the defect.

- **Esophagus.**
  - o Isolated thoracic esophageal injuries are exceedingly rare. They will usually be diagnosed incidentally associated with other intrathoracic injuries.
  - o Diagnostic clues include pain, fever, leucocytosis, cervical emphysema, Hamman's sign, chest X-ray (CXR) evidence of pneumothorax, mediastinal air, and pleural effusion. Contrast swallow may confirm the diagnosis.
  - o Start IV antibiotics as soon as the diagnosis is suspected, and continue post-op until fever and leucocytosis resolve. This is an adjunctive measure only. **Surgery is the definitive treatment.**
  - o For stable patients in a forward location, chest tube drainage and a nasogastric tube placed above the level of injury is a temporizing measure. Ideally, primary repair is performed within 6–12 hours of injury. Beyond 12 hours, isolation of the injured segment may be necessary.

> **The preferred approach for intrathoracic esophageal injuries is posterolateral thoracotomy; right for upper esophagus and left for lower esophagus.**

  - o Locate the injury by mobilizing the esophagus. Primarily repair with a single layer of 3-0 absorbable suture and cover with pleural or intercostal muscle flap.

o Drainage with chest tubes (one apical, one posterior) is recommended.
o If unable to primarily repair (as with a large segmental loss or severely contaminated/old injury), staple above and below the injury, place a nasogastric (NG) tube into the upper pouch and place a gastrostomy tube into the stomach. Drain the chest as indicated above. Complex exclusion procedures are not indicated in a forward operative setting.
o An alternative when the esophageal injury is too old for primary repair is to close the injury over a large T-tube, which converts the injury to a controlled fistula. The mediastinum is then widely drained using chest tubes or closed suction catheters placed nearby. After a mature fistula tract is established, slowly advance the T-tube and later the mediastinal drains can be slowly advanced.

- **Diaphragm.**
  o All injuries of the diaphragm should be closed.
    ◆ Simple small lacerations (< 2 cm) should be reapproximated with interrupted nonabsorbable 0 or 1-0 horizontal mattress sutures.
    ◆ Lacerations larger than 2 cm should be approximated as above, then reinforced with a running suture to assure an airtight closure.
    ◆ Care should be exercised in the central tendon area to avoid inadvertent cardiac injury during the repair.
  o If there is significant contamination of the pleural space by associated enteral injuries, anterior thoracotomy and plueral irrigation and drainage with two well-placed chest tubes should strongly be considered.
    ◆ Inadequate irrigation and drainage leads to a high incidence of empyema, especially of the fungal variety.

Chapter 17

Abdominal Injuries

Introduction
Changing patterns of warfare together with improvements in protective body armor combine synergistically to minimize truncal trauma incidence, severity, and mortality, despite increasingly lethal weapons systems. Despite these advances, penetrating abdominal trauma still occurs and treatment of these injuries will always be an important component of war surgery.

Trauma to the abdomen, both blunt and penetrating, can lead to occult injury that can be devastating or fatal if not treated. In the unstable patient with abdominal injury, the decision to operate is usually straight forward and should be acted on as soon as it is made. In a few rapidly hemorrhaging patients with thoracoabdominal injuries, a rapid decision must be made as to which cavity to enter first. This chapter addresses some of these issues.

> **Penetrating injuries below the nipples, above the symphysis pubis, and between the posterior axillary lines must be treated as injuries to the abdomen and mandate exploratory laparotomy.**

- Posterior truncal penetrating injuries from the tip of the scapula to the sacrum may also have caused retroperitoneal and intra-abdominal injuries. A low threshold for exploratory lapartotomy in these patients is warranted when there are not other diagnostic modalities available.

Diagnosis of Abdominal Injury
- Document a focused history to include time of injury, mechanism of injury, previous treatments employed, and any drugs administered.

17.1

- Inspection of the chest and abdomen will be the most reliable part of the physical examination, especially regarding penetrating injuries.
- Determine if the patient requires laparotomy, not the specific diagnosis.

Indications for Laparotomy – Who, When, and Where
First imperative is to determine **who** needs surgery.
- Patients **who** have
  o Penetrating abdominal wounds as described in box above.
  o Other penetrating truncal injuries with potential for peritoneal penetration and clinical signs/symptoms of intraperitoneal injury.
  o Blunt abdominal injuries presenting in shock.
- **When** and **Where.**
  o When aeromedical evacuation is uncertain and will involve substantial distance, unstable patients with life or limb threatening circumstances should undergo laparotomy at the nearest forward surgical team (FST).
  o Stable patients who can tolerate transport and delay of 6 hours or so, should undergo initial controlled resuscitation, presurgical care (including antibiotics), and be transported to the next level of care for surgery.

> When the tactical situation is static, aeromedical evacuation effective, and the distance between FST and combat support hospital (CSH) or higher level hospitals is short, all casualties, including those who are unstable, should bypass the FST and be taken directly to a higher level hospital.

Diagnostic Adjuncts
Minimally invasive adjuncts to diagnosis—computed tomography (CT) scan, diagnostic peritoneal lavage (DPL), and ultrasound (US)—have been used to decrease the number of negative laparotomies in stable, blunt abdominal trauma patients in peace-time settings with good follow-up of patients. Some have been used in lieu of laparotemy to evaluate those with penetrating injuries, when the suspicion is high that no intra-abdominal injury has occurred. This practice has the

potential of missing injuries. These diagnostic screening procedures are primarily used in stable patients with a mechanism of injury suggesting abdominal injury, but without an obvious operative indication. They should be relied on only when good follow up is possible. US and, to a limited extent, DPL have some use in the unstable patient to indicate which cavity should be entered first. US and DPL may also serve as triage tools in the mass casualty situation.

Abdominal Ultrasound
- Advantages: Noninvasive, may repeat frequently, quick, easy, identifies fluid in the abdomen reliably.
- Disadvantages: Operator dependant, may miss small amounts of fluid associated with hollow-viscus injuries.
- Sonography (focused abdominal sonography for trauma [FAST]) has become an extension of the physical examination of the abdomen and should be performed whenever available and when abdominal injury is suspected.
  o 3.5 to 5 MHz curved probe is optimal.
  o The abdomen is examined through four standard sonographic windows.
- A FAST examination assists the surgeon to determine the need for laparotomy in blunt-injured patients but does NOT identify specific injuries.
  o A FAST examination does not identify or stage solid organ or hollow-viscous injury, but reliably identifies free intraperitoneal fluid.
- FAST aids in prioritization of penetrating injury patients for the OR.
- FAST aids in identifying which cavity to open first in patients with thoracoabdominal injuries.
- A FAST examination identifies pericardial fluid, and may assist in the diagnosis of hemopneumothorax.

Ultrasound Views
A typical portable sonography device is shown in Fig. 17-1. The standard locations for "sonographic windows" are shown in Fig. 17-2. Examples of positive and negative sonographic examinations are shown in Figs. 17-3 through 17-6.

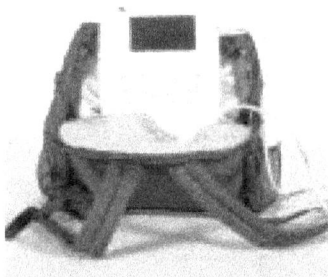

Fig. 17-1. Typical sonography device.

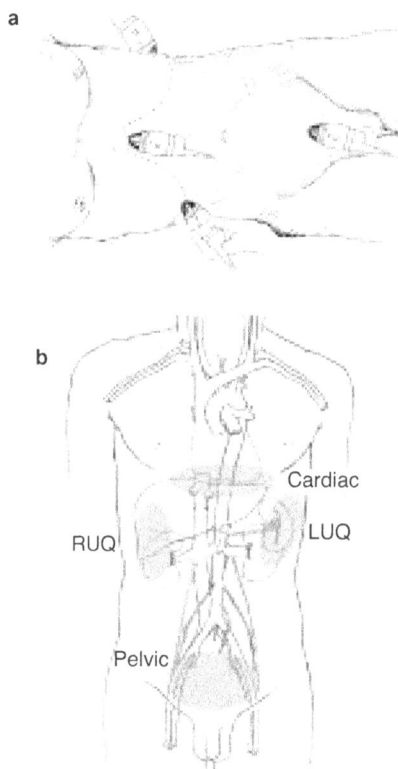

Fig. 17-2 a,b. The standard four locations for sonographic windows.

a

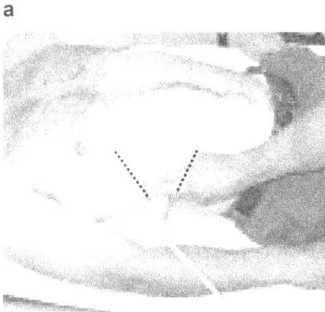

a

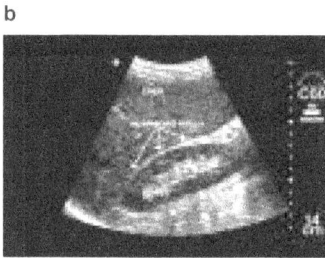

b

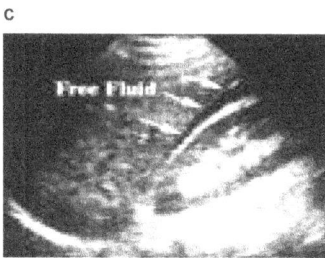

normal

b

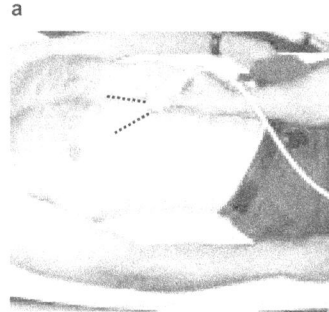

normal

c

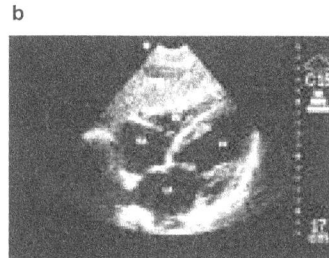

abnormal

c

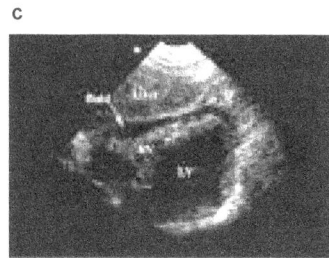

abnormal

Fig. 17-3 a,b,c. Normal and abnormal negative sonographic examinations for the right upper quadrant.

Fig. 17-4 a,b,c. Normal and abnormal negative sonographic examinations for the cardiac window.

17.5

a

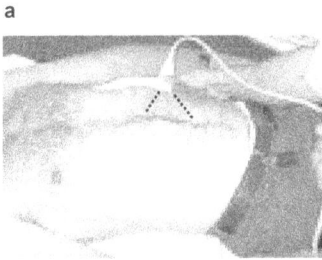

b

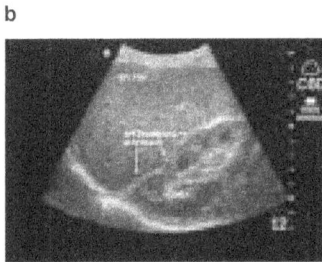

normal

c

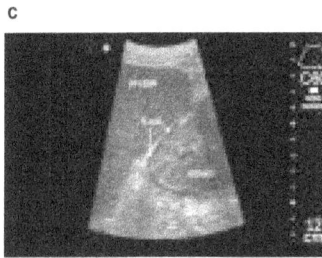

abnormal

Fig. 17-5 a,b,c. Normal and abnormal negative sonographic examinations for the left upper quadrant.

⟶

Fig. 17-6 a,b,c,d. Normal and abnormal negative sonographic examinations for the pelvic window.

a

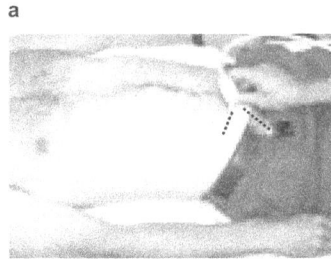

b

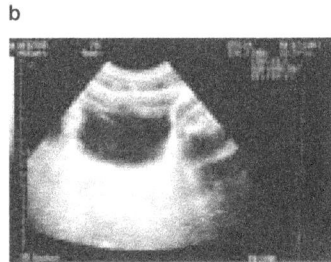

normal

c

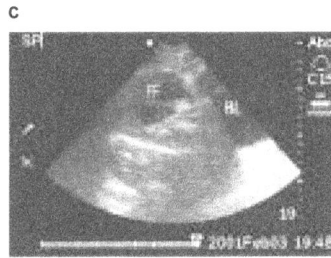

abnormal, male

d

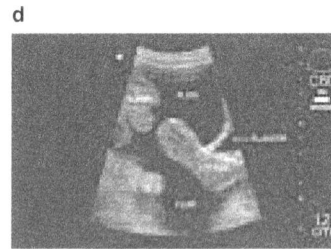

abnormal, female

Diagnostic Peritoneal Lavage

DPL has been a mainstay of blunt abdominal trauma diagnosis for many years. Unfortunately, in-theatre combat medical units from Level 1 to Level 3 are not routinely outfitted with microscopic laboratory functions to provide cell counts or fluid enzyme determinations. Thus, the only reliable information obtained from DPL is the aspiraton of 10 cc of gross blood. Gross blood aspiration is the most infrequently positive criterion of DPL, and its value is probably supplanted by FAST.

- May be useful when US or CT are not available, or as triage tool.
- Requires laboratory for most sensitivity.
  - o Blunt: Aspiration of 10 cc of gross blood, RBCs > 1,000,000/mL, WBCs > 500/mL, fecal material.
  - o Penetrating: not recommended to ruling out (R/O) injury in penetrating combat wound.
- May help determine which body cavity to enter first in an unstable patient with truncal injury.
- Advantages: Sensitive to small amounts of fluid, including hollow-visceral leaks; fairly quick.
- Disadvantages: Invasive, not repeatable, slower than US.
- Kits allow Seldinger technique.
  - o Arrow (AK-09000).
  - o Baxter Lazarus-Nelson (MLNK9001).
- Field Expedient substitution: Open technique with small, vertical infraumbilical incision and any tubing (IV, straight or balloon catheter). Cut at least a dozen extra side holes.

CT Scan
- Advantages: Defines injured anatomy in **stable** patients.
- Disadvantages: Slow; requires contrast use and equipment availability; may miss small hollow organ leaks; requires transport away from emergency care area; operator/interpreter dependant; difficult to repeat.

Wound Exploration

- Blast injuries and improvised explosive devices (IEDs) create many low-velocity fragments that may penetrate the skin but not the abdominal cavity. Operative wound exploration in the stable patient with a normal or equivocal examination can help determine the need for formal exploratory laparotomy.
    - o When possible wound exploration should be performed in the operating room with adequate instruments and lighting.
    - o Finding the fragment in the abdominal wall precludes laparotomy.
    - o If the tract is not adequately identified or the fragment seen on plain film cannot be identified, formal laparotomy should be performed.

Operative Planning and Exposure Techniques

- Give broad spectrum antibiotic pre-op, continue for 24 hours.
    - o Redose short half-life antibiotics intraoperatively and consider redosing antibiotics with large amounts of blood loss.
- Perform laparotomy through a midline incision.
    - o When wide exposure is needed, extend the incision superiorly just lateral to the xiphoid process and inferior to the symphysis pubis.
- Quickly pack all 4 quadrants while looking for obvious injuries.
- Control hemorrhage.
- **Assess physiologic status.**
    - o Considering casualty physiology, create operative plan to control contamination and complete operation.
        - ◆ Consider damage control (see Chapter 12, Damage Control Surgery) early and often.
        - ◆ If stabilized/improving, proceed with definitive surgery.
- Identify all organ and hollow-viscus injuries.

- Eviscerate the small bowel to increase workspace.
- Divide the ligamentous attachments of the liver to improve exposure in the right upper quadrant or upper midline.
- Fold the left lateral segment of the liver down and to the right to improve exposure at the gastroesophageal junction.
- Improve exposure to the liver by extending the incision into the inferior sternum and across into the lower right chest (thoracoabdominal).

Stomach Injuries
- The stomach is a vascular organ and will do well after almost any repair.
  o Always enter the lesser sac to determine posterior wall injuries.
- Encircle the distal esophagus with a Penrose drain to provide traction and improve visibility in high midline injuries.
- Minimally debride and primarily close stomach defects.

Duodenum Injuries
Injuries to the Duodenum are associated with massive upper abdominal trauma. Early consideration for damage control surgery should be considered (see Chapter 12, Damage Control Surgery).
- Missed injuries of the duodenum have devastating morbidity.
- Bile staining or hematoma in the periduodenal tissues mandates full exploration of the duodenum (Kocher maneuver).
- Minor injuries can be repaired primarily.
- Major injuries should be repaired if the lumen will not be narrowed by more than 50%. Options for closing injuries of greater than 50%:
  o Close duodenal wall around a tube duodenostomy.
    ♦ Use a No. 2-0 absorbable suture (Vicryl).
    ♦ Use the largest malecot catheter available.
  o Bring up a Roux-en-Y jejunal limb and create an anastamosis between the limb and the injury (Fig. 17-7).
  o The procedure of last resort is pancreaticoduodenectomy.

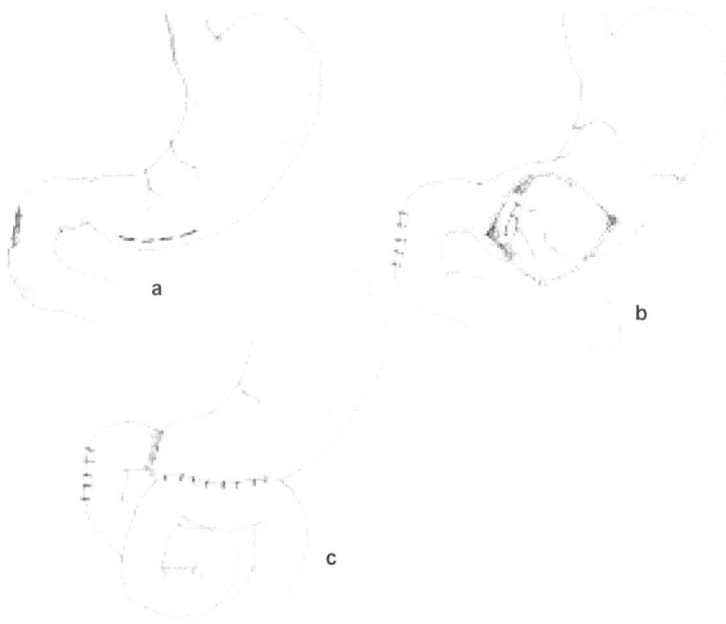

Fig. 17-7. (a) Ligation of pylorius, (b) Duodenal injury, (c) Roux-en-Y anastomosis.

- For major injuries, divert the gastric stream with a gastrostomy and close the pylorus—two options:
  - o Through a gastrotomy, ligate the pylorus with No. 0 absorbable suture.
  - o Using a noncutting stapling device, staple but **do not divide** the pylorus. Place a feeding jejunostomy for nutrition at this controlled reconstruction.
- Widely drain all injuries with closed-suction drains.
- Any method used to close the pylorus will last only 14–21 days. The possibility of injury to the biliary and pancreatic ducts should be considered when injuries involve the 2nd portion of the duodenum or the pancreatic head.

Pancreas Injuries
- Any injury to the pancreas/duct requires drainage.

17.10

o Even if ductal injury is not identified, it should be presumed and drained.
o Resect clearly nonviable pancreatic body/tail tissue.
- Transection or near-transection of the pancreatic duct can be treated by
  o Distal end of proximal pancreas segment oversewn/stapled.
  o Proximal end of distal segment oversewn/stapled and entire distal segment left in-situ.
  o Distal segment resection (typically requires splenectomy).
  o Distal segment drainage by Roux-en-Y anastomosis to small bowel.

> Major injuries to the head of the pancreas may require pancreaticoduodenectomy, which SHOULD NEVER BE ATTEMPTED in an austere environment but instead treated by the principles of damage control surgery—DRAIN, DRAIN, DRAIN.

Liver Injuries
- Most liver injuries can be successfully treated with direct pressure and packing followed by aggressive resuscitation and correction of coagulopathy.
- Generous exposure is required and should be gained early and aggressively.
  o Mobilize triangular and coronary ligaments for full exposure
  o Use extension into right chest if needed.
  o Place several laparotomy pads above the dome of the liver to displace it down into the field of view.
- Short duration clamping of hepatic artery and portal vein (Pringle maneuver) may be required to slow bleeding while gaining other control. If bleeding continues despite Pringle maneuver, especially from behind the liver, this indicates a retrohepatic venous injury or retrohepatic vena caval injury. The injuries should be approached in only the most advanced settings with extraordinary amounts of resources. On table retriage or aggressive packing and intensive care unit (ICU) resuscitation should be employed.
- Use finger fracture of liver parenchyma to expose deep bleeding vessels.

- Large exposed injuries of the liver parenchyma can be controlled in a number of ways:
  - o Exposed large vessels and ducts should be suture-ligated.
  - o Overlapping mattress sutures of No. 0-Chromic on a blunt liver needle is fast and effective for controlling raw surface bleeding.
  - o Placement of Surgicel on the raw surface and high-power electrocautery to "weld" it in place is also effective.
- Bleeding tracts through the liver can be controlled by tying off the end of a Penrose drain, placing it through the tract, and "inflating" it with saline to tamponade the tract.
- Urgent surgical resection is **strongly discouraged**:
  - o Indicated only when packing/pressure fails.
  - o Follows functional or injury pattern, not anatomic lines.
- Use a pedicle of omentum in a large defect to reduce dead space.

Avoidance of coagulopathy, hypothermia and acidosis is essential in successful management of major liver injuries. APPLY DAMAGE CONTROL TECHNIQUES EARLY.

- Retrohepatic vena cava and hepatic vein injuries require a tremendous amount of resources (blood products, OR time, equipment) typically unavailable in a forward surgery setting (on-table triage in mass casualty).
  - o Packing is most successful option.
  - o If packing fails, consider an atrio-caval shunt. (see Figure 17-8).
- Provide generous closed suction drainage around major liver injuries.

Biliary Tract Injuries
- Injuries to the gall bladder are treated by cholecystectomy.
- Repair common bile duct injuries over a T-tube.

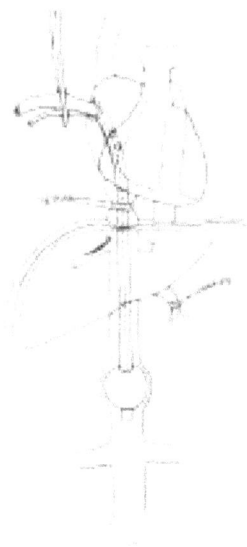

Fig. 17-8. Atrio-caval shunt.

o A No. 4-0 or smaller absorbable suture is used on the biliary tree.
- Extensive segmental loss requires choledochoenterostomy or tube choledochostomy (depending on time and patient physiology).
- Drain widely.

Splenic Injuries
- Splenic salvage has no place in combat surgery.
- Drains should not be routinely placed postsplenectomy if the pancreas is uninvolved.
- Splenic injury should prompt exploration for associated diaphragm, stomach, pancreatic, and renal injuries.
- Immunize post-op with pneumococcal, haemophilus, and meningococcal vaccines (may defer until Level 3/CONUS MTF, **but must not be forgotten**).

Small-Bowel Injuries
- Debride wound edges to freshly bleeding tissue.
- Close enterotomies in one or two layers (skin stapler is a rapid alternative).
- With multiple enterotomies to one segment of less than 50% of small-bowel length, perform single resection with primary anastomosis. Avoid multiple resections.

Colon Injury
Simple, isolated colon injuries are uncommon. In indigenous populations and enemy combatants (eg, patients who cannot be readily evacuated), diversion with colostomy should be the procedure of choice, especially at Level 2. The often poor nutritional status of these populations does not support primary repair. The presence of any of the complicating factors listed below mandates colostomy.
- Simple, isolated colon injuries should be repaired primarily.
  - o Debride wound edges to normal, noncontused tissue.
  - o Perform two-layer closure or anastomosis.
- For **complex** injuries, **strongly consider colostomy/diversion**, especially when associated with:
  - o Massive blood transfusion requirement.
  - o On-going hypotension.
  - o Hypoxia (severe pulmonary injury).

    o Reperfusion injury (vascular injury).
    o Multiple other injuries.
    o High-velocity injuries.
    o Extensive local tissue damage.
- Potential breakdown of a repair or anastomosis is highest in the setting of concomitant pancreatic injury.
- Damage control technique: control contamination with ligation/stapling of bowel, delay creation of the stoma to the definitive reconstruction.
- Clearly document treatment for optimal follow-up throughout Levels of Care.
- At the time of formation, a colostomy should be matured.

Rectal Injuries

Rectal injuries can be difficult to diagnose unless very dramatic. Any question of an injury raised by proximity of another injury, rectal examination, or plain abdominal film radiography MANDATES proctoscopy. Gentle distal washout with dilute Betadine solution is usually required to be able to perform rigid proctoscopy. Findings can be dramatic disruptions of the rectal wall but more commonly are subtle punctuate hemorrhages of the mucosa. All abnormal findings should prompt corrective intervention.

- Consider the traditional 4 "Ds" of rectal injury: **D**iversion, **D**ebridement, **D**istal washout, and **D**rainage.
    o Of these, diversion is the most important.
        ♦ Transabdominal sigmoid colostomy is easiest.
        ♦ If the injury has not violated the peritoneum, exploration of the extraperitoneal rectum should NOT be done at laparotomy unless indicated for an associated nonbowel injury. This avoids contaminating the abdominal cavity with stool.
    o Debridement and closure of small- to medium-sized wounds is unnecessary in patients who have been diverted and drained. In any but the lowest of wounds, debridement and closure are difficult and troublesome.
    o Distal washout is usually necessary to assess the injury. Use gentle pressure when irrigating to minimize contamination of the perirectal space.

o Fecal contamination of the perirectal space mandates presacral drainage. Presacral drains should be placed any time the patient will leave your immediate care.

   ◆ Drains are placed through the perineum into the retrorectal space (Fig. 17-9).

● Peritonealized rectal injuries are easily accessed transabdominally and should be repaired and protected with diversion.

● Hematoma in the perirectal space should be drained either transluminally by leaving the injury open or by placing presacral and/or intraabdominal drains.

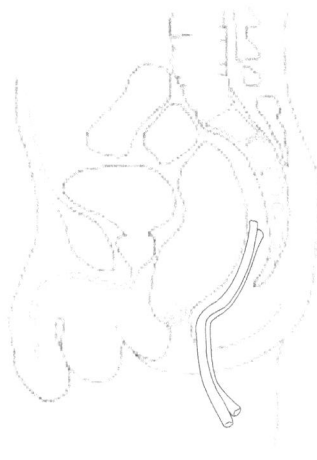

Fig. 17-9. Presacral drain.

Retroperitoneal Injuries

● Left medial visceral rotation moves the colon, pancreas, and small bowel to expose the aorta rapidly. Proximal aortic control can be rapidly obtained with compression or a clamp on the aorta at the hiatus, or through the left chest.

● Right medial visceral rotation (colon plus Kocher maneuver to elevate duodenum) exposes the subhepatic vena cava.

● Three zones of the retroperitoneum (Fig. 17-10).

   o **I-Central, supracolic:** explore for all injuries.
   o **II-Central, infracolic:** penetrating trauma, explore; blunt trauma, explore for expanding hematoma.
   o **III-Lateral:** blunt trauma, avoid exploration if possible because exploration increases the likelihood of opening a stable hematoma and, thus, precipitating nephrectomy. Explore for penetrating trauma.

● Gain proximal vascular control before entering the hematoma.

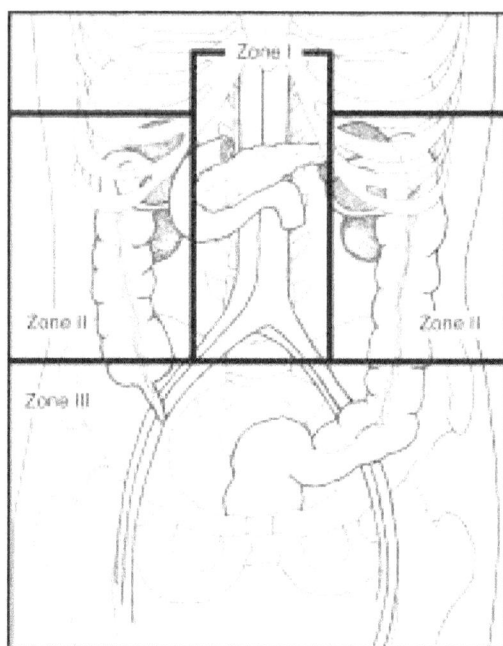

Fig. 17-10. Three zones of the retroperitoreum.

Abdominal Closure

- Close fascia if possible.
  - o Massive swelling associated with large amounts of blood loss and resuscitation and large injuries may necessitate temporary closures (see Chapter 12, Damage Control Surgery). Otherwise, closure is usually possible.
- A few penetrating battlefield wounds are isolated, small, and without visceral contamination, and it is perhaps safe to close the skin. **Most are not, and these patients will be passed quickly from one surgeon to the next, so the risk of missed and catastrophic infection is increased; the skin should not be closed.**
- Retention sutures are strongly recommended for the same reasons.

Chapter 18

Genitourinary Tract Injuries

Introduction

Genitourinary (GU) injuries constitute approximately 5% of the total injuries encountered in combat. Their treatment adheres to established surgical principles of hemostasis, debridement, and drainage. Proper radiographic evaluation prior to surgery may replace extensive retroperitoneal exploration at the time of laparotomy in the diagnosis of serious GU injuries.

> **GU wounds, aside from injuries of the external genitalia, are typically associated with serious visceral injury.**

Renal Injuries

- Most renal injuries, except for those of the renal pedicle, are not acutely life threatening. Undiagnosed or improperly treated injuries, however, may cause significant morbidity.
- While the vast majority of blunt renal injuries will heal uneventfully with observation and conservative therapy, a significant number of renal injuries in combat will come from penetrating wounds and require exploration.

> **The evaluation of a suspected renal injury is based on the type of injury, physical examination, and urinalysis.**

- Hematuria is usually present in patients with renal trauma, and gross hematuria in the adult patient is concerning for a significant injury. **The absence of hematuria, however, does not exclude renal trauma**. Renal injury must be suspected in patients who have sustained significant concurrent injuries such as multiple rib fractures, vertebral body or transverse process fractures, crushing injuries of the chest or thorax, or penetrating injury to the flank, chest, or upper abdomen.

- Adult patients who present with gross hematuria, microscopic hematuria with shock at any time following the injury, and significant concurrent injury require further evaluation of their kidneys. Computed tomography (CT) provides excellent staging of renal injuries and aids in the decision whether or not to explore the injured kidney.
- In the combat setting, many patients require rapid exploration before definitive radiographic staging can be completed. An intraoperative single-shot intravenous pyelogram (IVP) is useful in their evaluation.
  - o Procedure for one-shot IVP:
    - ♦ 2 cc/kg of high-dose contrast is injected in either the ED or OR setting.
    - ♦ A single standard KUB radiograph is obtained 10 minutes following the contrast injection.
  - o While high-osmolality contrast (Renografin, Hypaque, or Conray) is adequate, low-osmolality contrast (Omnipaque, Isovue, Optiray) is less likely to generate a reaction and is less toxic to the kidney.
- Major renal injuries usually appear as obscured renal shadows on IVP.
  - o Detailed anatomic information regarding the degree of renal injury or presence of urinary extravasation should not be expected on the trauma IVP. Delayed films, however, may improve detection of urinary extravasation.
  - o The study should confirm the presence and function of the **contralateral** kidney and may demonstrate congenital anomalies such as renal ectopia or fusion. Understanding the function of the contralateral kidney is imperative to sound intraoperative decision making during exploration and possible salvage of the injured kidney.
- Renal trauma is categorized by the extent of damage to the kidney.
  - o Minor injuries.
    - ♦ Consist of renal contusions or shallow cortical lacerations.
    - ♦ Most common after blunt trauma and usually resolve safely without renal exploration.
    - ♦ Hydration, antibiotics, and bed rest are the cornerstones of successful nonoperative management.

o Major injuries.
   ♦ Consist of deep cortical lacerations (with or without urinary extravasation), shattered kidneys, renal vascular pedicle injuries, or total avulsion of the renal pelvis.
   ♦ There is an 80% incidence of associated visceral injuries with major renal trauma. Most cases will require a laparotomy for evaluation and repair of concurrent intraperitoneal injuries.
   ♦ Operative intervention includes debridement of nonviable renal tissue (partial nephrectomy), closure of the collecting system, and drainage of the retroperitoneal area.
   ♦ Kidney preservation should be considered if at all possible, although total nephrectomy may be required for the severely damaged kidney or the unstable patient.

> **Vascular control of the renal pedicle can be obtained prior to opening the perirenal fascia when control of hemorrhage from the kidney requires exploration of the retroperitoneum.**

- **Operative Technique.**
  o Obtain vascular control from a periaortic approach to the renal vascular pedicle.
     ♦ The small intestine is retracted laterally and superiorly, and the posterior peritoneum is incised over the aorta.
     ♦ The left renal vein, crossing anterior to the aorta, must be mobilized to gain control of either renal artery.
     ♦ Atraumatic vascular clamps are used to occlude the appropriate artery.
  o While vascular control in this fashion may provide the safest approach against renal hemorrhage and reduce the likelihood of nephrectomy, it is not a commonly performed maneuver by either urologists or general surgeons. Direct reflection of the colon to expose the kidney is feasible (Fig. 18-1). A kidney pedicle clamp should be readily available for this approach.

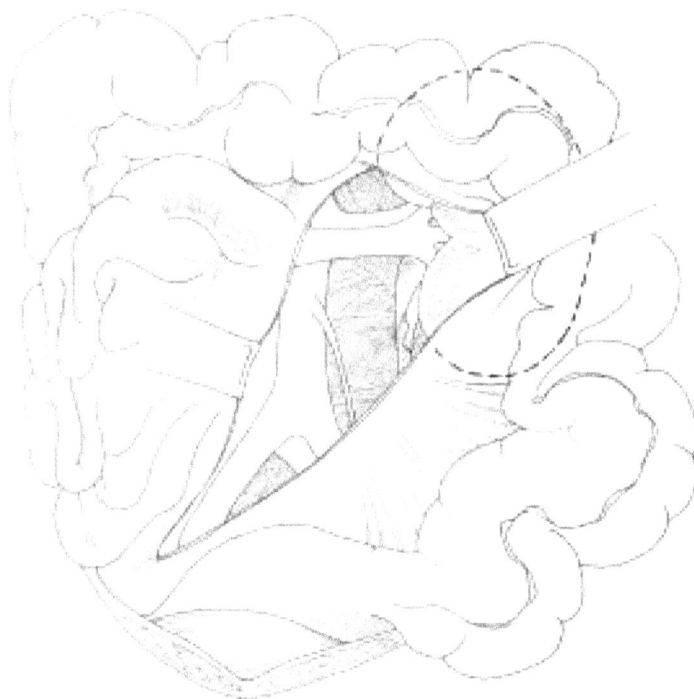

Fig. 18-1. Exposure of left renal hilum.

o Damaged renal parenchyma can be locally debrided (Fig. 18-2), excised in a partial nephrectomy (Fig. 18-3), or removed in a total nephrectomy depending on the degree of injury and the condition of the patient.

> **Nephrectomy may be the best solution for major renal injuries when associated life-threatening injuries are present.**

o Watertight closure of the collecting system with absorbable suture prevents the development of a urine leak.
  ♦ Urinary diversion is typically unnecessary if formal renal reconstruction is accomplished.

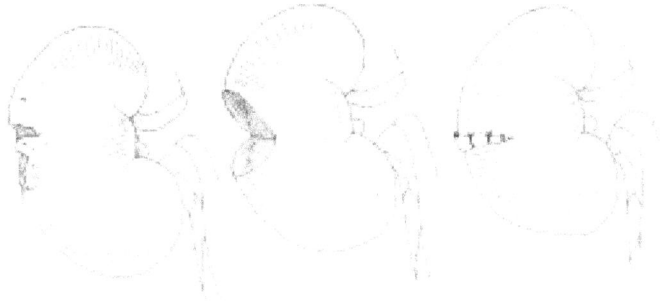

Fig. 18-2. Steps in renal debridement.

◊ For the sake of expedience or in the presence of associated injuries of the duodenum, pancreas, or large bowel, diversion may be required.
◊ Tube nephrostomy, ureteral stent, or ureterostomy may be utilized.
o The reconstructed kidney should be covered by perirenal fat, omentum, or fibrin sealant.
o A closed suction drain should be left in place.

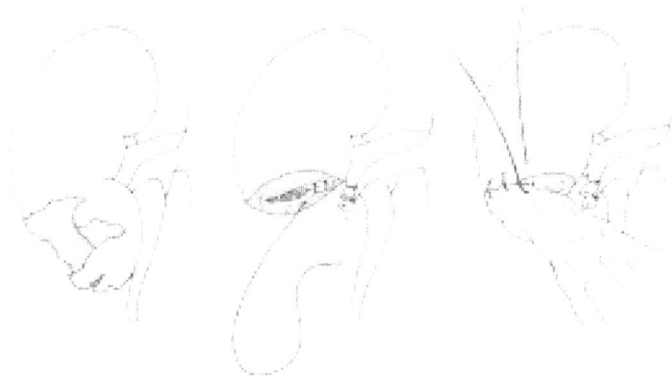

Fig. 18-3. Steps in partial nephrectomy.

Ureteral Injuries

> Ureteral injuries are rare but are frequently overlooked
> when not appropriately considered. They are more likely
> in cases of retroperitoneal hematoma and injuries of the
> fixed portions of the colon, duodenum, and spleen.

- Isolated ureteral injuries are rare and usually occur in conjunction with other significant injuries. They can represent a difficult diagnostic challenge in both the preoperative and intraoperative settings.
  - o Ureteral injuries are not reliably diagnosed by the preoperative IVP.
  - o Hematuria is frequently absent.
  - o Blast injury to the urethra may produce significant delayed complications even when the IVP is normal and the ureter appears visibly intact. Placement of an indwelling stent is reasonable when a high-velocity or blast injury occurs in proximity to the ureter.
  - o If a ureteral injury is initially missed and presents in a delayed fashion, urinary diversion with a nephrostomy tube and delayed repair at 3–6 months is a safe approach.

- Operative Technique.
  - o Intraoperative localization of the ureteral injury is facilitated by IV injection of indigo carmine or direct injection into the collecting system under pressure.
  - o Basic principles of repair.
    - ◆ Minimal debridement.
    - ◆ Primary tension free, 1 cm spatulated anastomosis using an interrupted single-layer absorbable suture (4–0 or 5–0) closure technique.
    - ◆ Internal (double J ureteral stent) and external drainage.
    - ◆ Lengthening maneuvers.
      - ◊ Ureteral mobilization.
      - ◊ Kidney mobilization.
      - ◊ Psoas hitch (Fig. 18-4).
      - ◊ Boare flap.

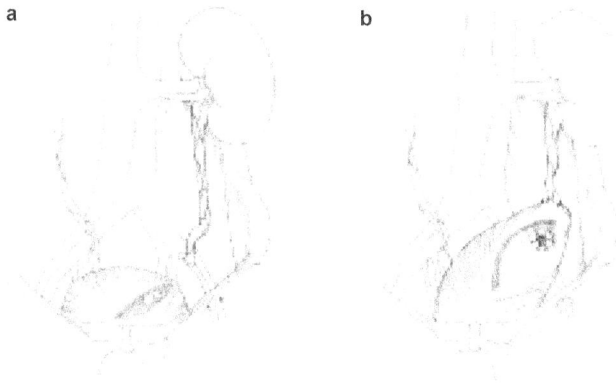

Fig. 18-4. The psoas hitch.

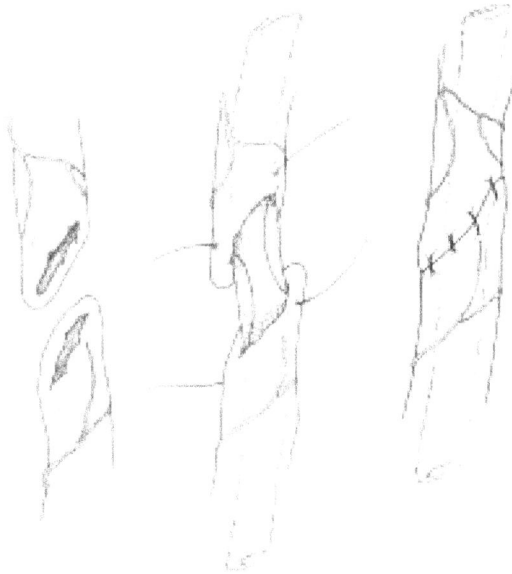

Fig. 18-5. Ureteroureterostomy.

- ♦ Isolate repairs with omentum or posterior peritoneum.
- o The type of repair is based on the following:
  - ♦ Anatomical segment of the traumatized ureter (upper, middle, and lower third).
  - ♦ Extent of segmental loss.
  - ♦ Other associated injuries.
  - ♦ Clinical stability of the patient.
- o Upper or Middle ureteral injuries:
  - ♦ Short segment loss/transection: Perform a primary ureteroureterostomy (Fig. 18-5).
  - ♦ Long segment loss: May require a temporizing tube/cutaneous ureterostomy with stent placement or ureteral ligation with tube nephrostomy.
- o Lower ureteral injuries.
  - ♦ When the injury occurs near the bladder, an ureteroneocystostomy should be performed (Fig. 18-6). This is typically completed by fixing the bladder to the fascial covering of the psoas muscle using permanent suture such as 2.0 or 3.0 Prolene. A transverse cystotomy assists in elongating the bladder to that location and facilitates the development of a submucosal tunnel for the reimplanted ureter.
  - ♦ When a distal ureteral injury is associated with a rectal injury, ureteral reimplantation is not recommended; temporary diversion should be performed.

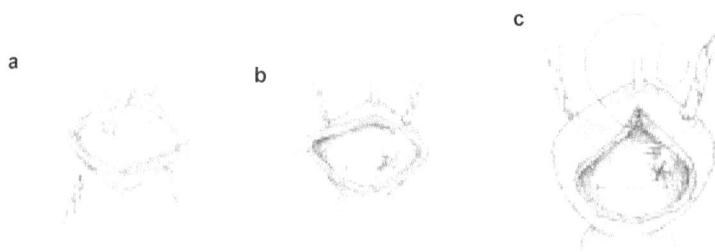

Fig. 18-6. Ureteroneocystostomy.

> Ureteral injuries in the combat setting may be best
> managed with temporary tube drainage with a small
> feeding tube or ureteral stent followed by delayed
> reconstruction.

Bladder Injuries

> Bladder wounds should be considered in patients with
> lower abdominal gunshot wounds, pelvic fractures with
> gross hematuria, or those patients unable to void
> following abdominal or pelvic trauma.

- Bladder disruptions can occur on the intraperitoneal or
  extraperitoneal surface of the bladder. The location may
  change the symptoms, complications, and management of
  this injury.
- After ensuring urethral integrity in appropriate cases (see
  Urethral Injuries, below), evaluation of the bladder is
  performed radiographically with a cystogram.
  - Cystography is performed using a 3-film technique: (1)
    scout or plain film KUB concentrating on the pelvis, (2)
    full-bladder radiograph after retrograde filling of the
    bladder with contrast, and (3) a postdrainage radiograph.
  - **Technique:** Fill the bladder by gravity with a urethral
    catheter using radiopaque contrast medium elevated 20–
    30 cm above the level of the abdomen. At least 300 cc (5–7
    cc/kg in children) are required for an adequate study. Take
    a full-bladder radiograph.
  - Drain the bladder using the catheter and take a postdrainage
    radiograph. Small extraperitoneal areas of extravasation
    may be apparent only on the postevacuation film.
- Operative Technique.
  - Intraperitoneal Injuries.
    - ◆ Cystography reveals contrast medium interspersed
      between loops of bowel.
    - ◆ Management consists of immediate exploration,
      multilayer repair of the injury with absorbable suture,
      suprapubic tube cystostomy, and drainage of the

perivesical extraperitoneal space.

o Extraperitoneal injuries.

♦ Bladder laceration is most often the result of laceration by bony fragments from a pelvic fracture.

♦ Cystography reveals a dense, flame-like extravasation of contrast medium in the pelvis on the postevacuation film.

♦ The bladder usually heals with 10–14 days of Foley catheter drainage without the need for primary repair. If the urine is clear, catheter drainage alone is preferred for treatment of most extraperitoneal ruptures.

♦ In cases of abdominal exploration for other injuries, primary repair and drainage are necessary if the extra-peritoneal space is entered. Repair can be completed from inside the bladder through a cystotomy to avoid disturbing any pelvic hematoma. Patients with concurrent rectal injuries should be managed more aggressively and may benefit from hematoma evacuation and primary bladder repair.

Urethral Injuries

> A urethral injury should be suspected in patients with a scrotal hematoma, blood at the meatus, or a floating/high-riding prostate. Catheterization is contraindicated until urethral integrity is confirmed by retrograde urethrography.

● Retrograde urethrography is performed to evaluate the anatomy of the urethra.

o Take oblique radiographs of the pelvis to avoid "end-on" imaging that obscures the bulbar urethra.

o Insert the end of a sterile catheter tip syringe (60 cc) into the urethral meatus while grasping the glans to prevent leakage. Alternately, insert an unlubricated Foley catheter into the fossa navicularis (approximately 3 cm) and inflate the balloon with 3 cc of water.

o Gently instill 15–20 cc of water-soluble contrast. The radiograph is taken during injection.

o Contrast must be seen flowing into the bladder to clear the proximal urethra of injury. Posterior urethral injuries seen in pelvic fractures may be missed otherwise.
o If no injury is identified, carefully place a Foley catheter.

If any difficulty in passing the catheter is encountered, the urethra should not be instrumented and a suprapubic tube cystostomy is performed.

- Operative Technique.
  o The urethra is divided into **anterior** and **posterior** (prostatic) segments by the urogenital diaphragm.
    ♦ Anterior urethral injuries may result from blunt trauma, such as results from falls when astride an object (straddle) or from penetrating injuries.
      ◊ Blunt trauma resulting in minor nondisruptive urethral injuries may be managed by gentle insertion of a 16 French Foley catheter for 7–10 days.
      ◊ Penetrating wounds should be managed by exploration and judicious debridement.
        ▪ Small, clean lacerations may be repaired primarily by reapproximation of the urethral edges using interrupted 4-0 chromic suture.
        ▪ Do not mobilize the entire urethra for a primary anastomosis, because the shortened urethral length in the pendulous urethra may produce ventral chordee and an anastomosis under tension.
        ▪ Instead, marsupialize the injured urethral segment by suturing the skin edges to the cut edges of the urethra. Marsupialization should be performed until healthy urethra is encountered both proximally and distally. Closure of the marsupialized urethra is subsequently performed at 6 months to reestablish urethral continuity.
    ♦ Posterior urethral disruption commonly occurs following pelvic fracture injuries.
      ◊ Rectal examination reveals the prostate to have been avulsed at the apex.

18.11

◊ Improved continence and potency rates are attained when suprapubic tube cystostomy is used as the initial management.

◊ Suprapubic urinary diversion is maintained for 10–14 days and urethral integrity is confirmed radiographically prior to removal of the suprapubic tube.

◊ With expectant observation, virtually all these injuries will heal with an obliterative prostatomembranous urethral stricture, which can be repaired secondarily in 3–6 months after reabsorption of the pelvic hematoma.

◊ Initial exploration of the pelvic hematoma is strictly reserved for patients with concomitant bladder neck or rectal injury.

External Genitalia Injuries

> **The management of wounds to the penis, scrotum, testes, or spermatic cord should be as conservative as possible and consists of hemorrhage control, debridement, and early repair to prevent deformity.**

- Injuries to the penis that disrupt Buck's fascia should be sutured to prevent further bleeding and avoid future penile curvature with erection. When extensive penile skin is lost, the penis may be placed in a scrotal tunnel until a plastic repair can be performed.
- The scrotum is highly vascularized, and extensive debridement is usually not necessary for scrotal wounds.
  - Most penetrating scrotal injuries should be explored to evaluate the testicle for injury and reduce the risk of hematoma formation.
  - Most partial scrotal avulsions are best treated by primary closure with absorbable 3-0 sutures in two layers.
  - Primary closure is selected for patients without associated life-threatening injuries who sustained injury less than 8 hours prior. A Penrose drain or small closed drain can be placed to reduce hematoma formation. The testes can be

placed in protective pockets in the medial thigh for complete scrotal avulsion.

- It is essential, when dealing with testicular wounds, to conserve as much tissue as possible.
  - o Herniated parenchymal tissues should be debrided, and the tunica albuginea closed by mattress sutures.
  - o The testicle is placed in the scrotum or in a protective pocket in the medial thigh.
  - o A testicle should never be resected unless it is hopelessly damaged and its blood supply destroyed.

Chapter 19

Gynecologic Trauma and Emergencies

Introduction
The current active duty population consists of 14% women, many of whom are subject to the same risks of combat injury as their male colleagues. This chapter deals with OB/GYN emergencies that may present to a deployed medical treatment facility (MTF), particularly in military operations other than war (MOOTW).

Gynecologic Trauma
Vulva
- Vulvar injuries include lacerations and hematomas.
  - o **Lacerations** that are superficial, clean, and less than 6 hours old can be primarily closed with absorbable suture. Debridement of obviously devitalized tissue is recommended.
    - ♦ Deep lacerations should be examined and explored to rule out urethral, anal, rectal mucosa, or periclitoral injuries.
    - ♦ Placing a urethral catheter will assist in determining injury. If found, single-layer closure with fine (4-0 or smaller), absorbable suture, leaving the catheter in place, is recommended. Rectal and periclitoral injuries are closed in a similar fashion.
    - ♦ Anal lacerations should be repaired by approximating the cut ends of the anal sphincter with size 0 or 1 absorbable suture.
    - ♦ Antibiotics (2nd generation cephalosporin) are recommended with contaminated wounds.

- Vulvar trauma may cause **infrafascial** (below the pelvic diaphragm) **hematoma.**
  - o Because the deeper layer of subcutaneous vulvar fascia is not attached anteriorly to the pubic rami, hematoma can spread freely into the anterior abdominal wall.
  - o **Most vulvar hematomas are treated conservatively.**
  - o **External compression** and ice packs should be applied until hemostasis is ensured by serial examination of the vulva, vagina, and rectum.
  - o **Signs of shock in association with a decreasing hematocrit should prompt consideration of extraperitoneal expansion.** Ultrasound or computed tomography is useful for detecting expansion not diagnosed by clinical exam.

A vulvar hematoma continuing to expand despite external pressure, or presenting acutely with a size greater than 10 cm, should be incised and evacuated, with ligation of bleeding vessels and packing placed to secure hemostasis.

Vagina
- Trauma to the vagina can cause **lacerations**, and less commonly, suprafascial (above the pelvic diaphragm) hematoma.
- Vaginal trauma has been reported in **approximately 3.5% of women with traumatic pelvic fractures. Concomitant urologic trauma, most often involving the bladder and/or urethra, has been described in about 30% of patients with vaginal trauma.**
- Thorough inspection and palpation of the vagina and rectovaginal exam are necessary for detection of vaginal trauma and to determine the need for further urologic evaluation/imaging. **Due to pelvic instability (in fracture cases) or pain, examination under sedation or anesthesia may be necessary.**
- Patients with vaginal lacerations typically present with bleeding, sometimes profusely, from the well-vascularized vagina.

- Lacerations are repaired using the guidelines given above for vulvar lacerations.
- Vaginal hematoma is usually accompanied by severe rectal pressure and is diagnosed by palpation of a firm, tender mass bulging into the lateral vagina. **Vaginal hematoma should be treated by incision, evacuation, ligation, and packing.**
- Unrecognized vaginal trauma can result in dyspareunia, pelvic abscess, and fistula formation.

Uterus/Cervix

- Trauma to the uterus and cervix is most commonly found in association with pregnancy, but may be seen as a result of penetrating vaginal or abdominal trauma.
- Noninfected simple cervical lacerations should be repaired to optimize restoration of normal anatomy (and possibly decrease the risk of cervical incompetence or stenosis with dysmenorrhea from poor healing). Absorbable 0 grade suture can be used.
- Acute penetrating trauma involving the uterine fundus usually causes little bleeding and can be managed expectantly without repair. Damage to the uterine wall with bleeding can be repaired with size 0 absorbable suture.
- **Trauma involving the lateral wall of the uterus may cause significant bleeding**, but can usually be controlled by successive ligation of the ascending and descending branches of the uterine artery as described below in the obstetrical section "uterine atony."

> **Hemorrhage not responding to ligation, or extensive mutilating damage to the cervix or uterus, is best treated by hysterectomy.**

- Prophylactic antibiotics should be given. **Adnexa should be retained unless there is an indication for removal** (see next page).

Basic steps for performing an emergent total abdominal hysterectomy.

- Ligate/cauterize round ligaments (Fig. 19-1).
- Incise anterior leaves of broad ligaments bilaterally, then continue across midline to incise vesicouterine fold.
- Mobilize bladder downward by blunt dissection (and sharp dissection if necessary) from lower uterine segment and cervix.[*]
- To **retain** adnexa, clamp/cut/ligate utero-ovarian ligaments and fallopian tubes near their connections to uterine fundus (Fig. 19-2).
- To **remove** adnexa with uterus, clamp/cut/ligate infundibulopelvic ligaments after making windows in posterior leaves of broad ligaments above ureters.
- Incise posterior peritoneum to mobilize adnexa either away from (if being retained) or toward (if being removed) uterus.
- Incise peritoneum overlying rectovaginal space, then mobilize rectum downward and away from posterior vagina by blunt dissection (Fig. 19-3).[*]
- Clamp/cut/ligate uterine arteries along lateral surface of uterus at uterocervical junction, staying within 1 cm of uterus to avoid damaging ureters.
- Clamp/cut/ ligate remainder of cardinal ligaments, paracervical tissue, and uterosacral ligaments by taking successive inferior bites until cervicovaginal junction is reached; each bite should be placed medial to previous bite to avoid injuring ureter and bladder.
- Crossclamp vagina below cervix.
- Transect vagina, removing uterus (and attached adnexa, if applicable).
- Suture vaginal cuff closed, ensuring bladder is not incorporated.

[*]In case of dense adhesions between cervix and bladder or rectum in emergent setting, or ongoing hemorrhage with poor visualization, supracervical hysterectomy can be performed. After mobilizing bladder and rectum from uterus and ligating uterine arteries, uterine fundus is transected from cervix with a knife. Cervix is then oversewn with a baseball stitch, staying medial to ligated uterine arteries.

Anterior View

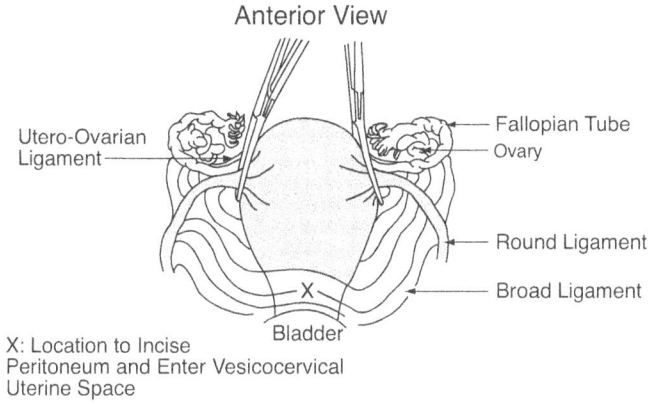

Utero-Ovarian Ligament

Fallopian Tube
Ovary

Round Ligament

Broad Ligament

X: Location to Incise Peritoneum and Enter Vesicocervical Uterine Space

Bladder

Fig. 19-1. Abdominal hysterectomy anterior view.

Adnexa
● **Fallopian Tubes.**
  o Damage to the wall of the fallopian tube by ruptured ectopic pregnancy or penetrating abdominal trauma should be treated by salpingectomy if there is significant damage to the tube, due to the risk of subsequent or recurrent ectopic pregnancy if left in situ. If the damage is

Adnexal View

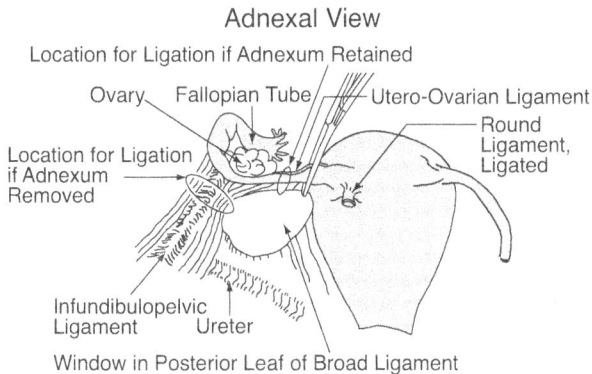

Location for Ligation if Adnexum Retained

Ovary Fallopian Tube Utero-Ovarian Ligament

Round Ligament, Ligated

Location for Ligation if Adnexum Removed

Infundibulopelvic Ligament   Ureter

Window in Posterior Leaf of Broad Ligament

Fig. 19-2. Abdominal hysterectomy adnexal view.

Posterior View

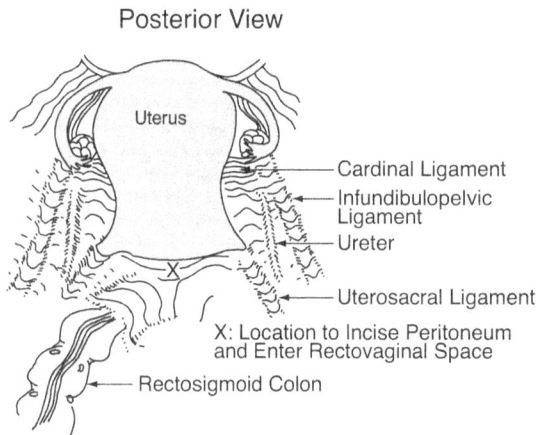

Fig. 19-3. Abdominal hysterectomy posterior view.

equivalent to a linear salpingotomy (see below), achieve hemostasis, then allow healing by secondary intention.
o The mesosalpinx is ligated or cauterized, then the tube ligated and cut at its connection with the uterine fundus.
o Unruptured ampullary/isthmic ectopic pregnancy can be treated by linear salpingotomy, with extraction of the ectopic gestation. The tubal incision is left open to heal by secondary intention.
o An unruptured or ruptured corneal/interstitial ectopic pregnancy requires wedge resection of the uterine cornuum with salpingectomy.
o An ectopic spontaneously aborted into the abdominal cavity through the end of the tube should be removed, but the tube may be left in situ if hemostasis is attained.

● **Ovaries.**
o A **ruptured ovarian cyst** should be treated via cystectomy by shelling the cyst wall out of the ovary, then cauterizing or ligating any bleeding vessels, usually at the base of the cyst.

o **Torsion of an ovarian mass** is first treated by assessing the ovary. Untwist the ovary and or fallopian tube. If it appears healthy with some continuing blood supply, it can be left in situ. If the ovary contains a large (> 4 cm) simple appearing cyst, the cyst can be drained and the cyst wall removed. Interrupted sutures using a fine monofilament or electrocautery can be used to obtain hemostasis. If the ovary appears dark and dusky after untwisting, perform a salpingo-oophorectomy by ligating the infundib-ulopelvic ligament first (after identifying the ureter), then the utero-ovarian ligament and fallopian tube.

o Hemorrhage from an infundibulopelvic ligament, as a result of penetrating abdominal trauma, is best treated by ligation with salpingo-oophorectomy.

Retroperitoneal Hematoma

- **Laceration of an arterial branch of the hypogastric artery can cause a retroperitoneal hematoma.**
- A large amount of blood may collect in the broad ligament with few symptoms. Dissection of the hematoma can extend up to the level of the renal vessels. The hematoma may be discovered during emergency surgery for trauma or during re-operation or post pelvic surgery, or can be prompted by signs of shock suggesting internal bleeding.
- Retroperitoneal hematoma can be treated by hypogastric artery ligation on the affected side. **Bilateral hypogastric artery ligation may be necessary for hemostasis.** The uterus, tubes and ovaries may be left in situ if viable and without other indication for removal.

Gynecologic/Obstetric Emergencies

- **Acute Vaginal Hemorrhage Unrelated to Trauma.**
  - o **Bright red vaginal bleeding filling more than one large perineal pad per hour is considered vaginal hemorrhage.** A pregnancy test and pelvic exam direct initial therapy.
    - ♦ **If the patient is not pregnant**, hormonal management with 25 mg IV Premarin or 50 mcg estrogen-containing oral birth control pills (OCPs) should be given every 6 hours.

◊ If the bleeding responds to hormonal management, OCPs should be continued qid for 5–7 days while more definitive diagnosis and management plans are made.

◊ If the bleeding has not decreased significantly within 24 hours, dilatation and curettage is reasonable. If the heavy bleeding continues, imaging studies and possibly coagulation studies will be needed to help direct further therapy.

♦ **In the pregnant patient,** heavy bleeding from the cervical os with uterine size < 20 weeks (fundus at/or below the level of patient's umbilicus) suggests spontaneous abortion. Dilatation and suction curettage should be performed.

◊ Ectopic pregnancy uncommonly presents with acute hemorrhage, but should be considered if the patient has an acute abdomen or if scant tissue is obtained on curettage.

◊ In a pregnant patient with uterine size consistent with a third trimester gestation (> 4 cm above the umbilicus in a singleton pregnancy), vaginal hemorrhage is usually an indication of placental abruption or placenta previa.

◊ Emergent cesarean section will be necessary if the uterine hemorrhage does not spontaneously resolve within several minutes.

◊ After delivery of the fetus and placenta, persistent hemorrhage unresponsive to more conservative measures may require hysterectomy (see **emergent cesarean** and **uterine atony** below).

◊ Pregnant patients (mothers) with acute vaginal hemorrhage who have Rh negative bloodtype, or if their Rh status is unknown, should be given RhoGAM 300 mcg IM.

o **A hemorrhaging mass in the vagina is most likely cervical cancer.** The vagina should be packed to tamponade the bleeding after placing a urethral catheter. Placing sutures is generally futile and may make the bleeding worse.

Precipitous Vaginal Delivery

- **Preparation.**
  - o Supplies needed for the delivery, include povidone-iodine sponges, a 10 cc syringe, lidocaine, 2 Kelly clamps, ring forceps, dry towels, a bulb syringe, and scissors.
  - o The mother should be placed on her left side for labor.
  - o The fetal heart rate should be determined every 15 minutes prior to pushing, and following each contraction during the pushing phase using a vascular Doppler. **Normal heart rate is between 120–160 bpm**. The heart rate often drops with the contraction, but should recover to normal prior to the next contraction.

> **If the heart rate drops below 100 and stays low for more than 2 minutes, a cesarean section should be considered.**

  - o When the patient presents, the cervix should be examined to determine dilation and fetal position. For the woman to begin pushing, the cervix should be completely dilated (10 cm) and no cervix should be felt on either side of the fetal head. If the baby's head is not presenting, move to cesarean section immediately. If there is any question, and ultrasound is available, it should be used to determine the presentation.
- **Delivery.**
  - o Once the patient begins pushing, flex the hips to optimally open the pelvis. The patient may be on her back, or tilted slightly to the left. Assistants should support the legs during pushing and relax them between contractions.
  - o Clean the perineum with sterile Betadine solution. If this is the patient's first delivery, the perineum should be anesthetized with lidocaine in case an episiotomy is needed. There is little support for prophylactic episiotomy, but may be necessary if the fetus is large, or tearing is anticipated.
  - o The fetal head delivers by extension. Pushing upward on the fetal chin through the perineum can assist this process.

Additionally, it is extremely important to control the rate of delivery of the head with the opposite hand.

o If an episiotomy is needed, it should be cut in the posterior midline from the vaginal opening approximately $1/2$ the length of the perineum, and extend about 2–3 cm into the vagina.

o After delivery of the head, the mouth and nose should be suctioned and the neck palpated for evidence of a nuchal cord. If present, this should be reduced by looping it over the fetal head, or by clamping twice and cutting if it will not reduce.

o Next, the operator's hands are placed along the parietal bones and the patient is asked to push again to allow delivery of the anterior shoulder. Gentle downward traction should allow the shoulder to clear the pubis, and the fetus should be directed anteriorly to allow delivery of the posterior shoulder. The remainder of the body will normally follow rapidly. Wrap infant in dry towels.

o Once the fetus delivers, the cord should be doubly clamped and cut. The placenta usually delivers within 15 minutes of delivery, but may take up to 60 minutes. Delivery of the placenta is heralded by uterine fundal elevation, lengthening of the cord, and a gush of blood. While waiting, gentle pressure may be placed on the cord, however, vigorous uterine massage and excessive traction can lead to complications.

o Following delivery of the placenta, the patient should be started on an infusion of lactated ringers with 20 units of oxytocin (Pitocin). Oxytocin can also be given IM if there is no IV access. If there is no oxytocin available, alternatives are methylergonovine maleate (Methergine) 0.2 mg intramuscular (IM) or allowing the patient to breastfeed. **The placenta should be inspected for evidence of fragmentation that can indicate retained products of conception.**

● **Inspection and repair.**

o Following delivery of the placenta, the vagina and cervix should be inspected for lacerations. Downward digital pressure on the posterior vagina and fundal pressure (by an assistant, if available) will facilitate visualization of the cervix. A ring forceps is then used to grasp and visualize the entire cervix.

o The vagina should be inspected with special attention to the posterior fornix. The perineum and periurethral areas should also be inspected. Vaginal and cervical lacerations may be repaired with 3-0 vicryl or an equivalent suture in running or interrupted layers.

o If the anal sphincter is lacerated, it should be reapproximated with 2-0 absorbable interrupted single or figure-of-eight sutures.

o If the patient has torn into the rectum, the rectal-vaginal septum should be repaired with interrupted sutures of 3-0 vicryl. A second layer imbricating the underlying tissue will decrease the risk of breakdown. Care should be taken to preserve aseptic technique. If a large tear is noted, a saddle block or spinal anesthetic may be necessary.

o Patients with a periurethral tear may require urethral catheterization. In addition to lacerations, hematoma in the vulva, vagina, or retroperitoneum may occur. See above gynecologic trauma for management.

Emergency Cesarean Section
- Indications.
  o Fetal heart rate drops below 100 and stays down for more than 2 minutes.
  o Acute uterine hemorrhage persisting for more than a few minutes (suggestive of placental abruption or previa).
  o Breech or transverse fetal presentation.
- The patient should be placed in the left tilt position with an IV bag or towel displacing the uterus to the left. She should undergo a quick prep from just below the breasts to the mid thigh. A major abdominal equipment set should have most of the instruments that you will need.
- **Basic steps to performing an emergency C-section** (Fig. 19-4 a,b,c,d).
  o Enter the abdomen through lower midline.

Uterine Incision

a

Uterus

Incision in Lower
Uterine Segment

Bladder Retracted After
Incising Vesicouterine Fold

b   **Delivery of Fetus**

Fundal Pressure
Exerted

Placenta

Operator's Hand
in Position to
Deliver Fetal Head

c   **Delivered Infant on Abdomen**

Nose and Mouth Suctioned

Umbilical Cord Doubly Clamped,
Then Cut

Uterine Fundus Exteriorized

d

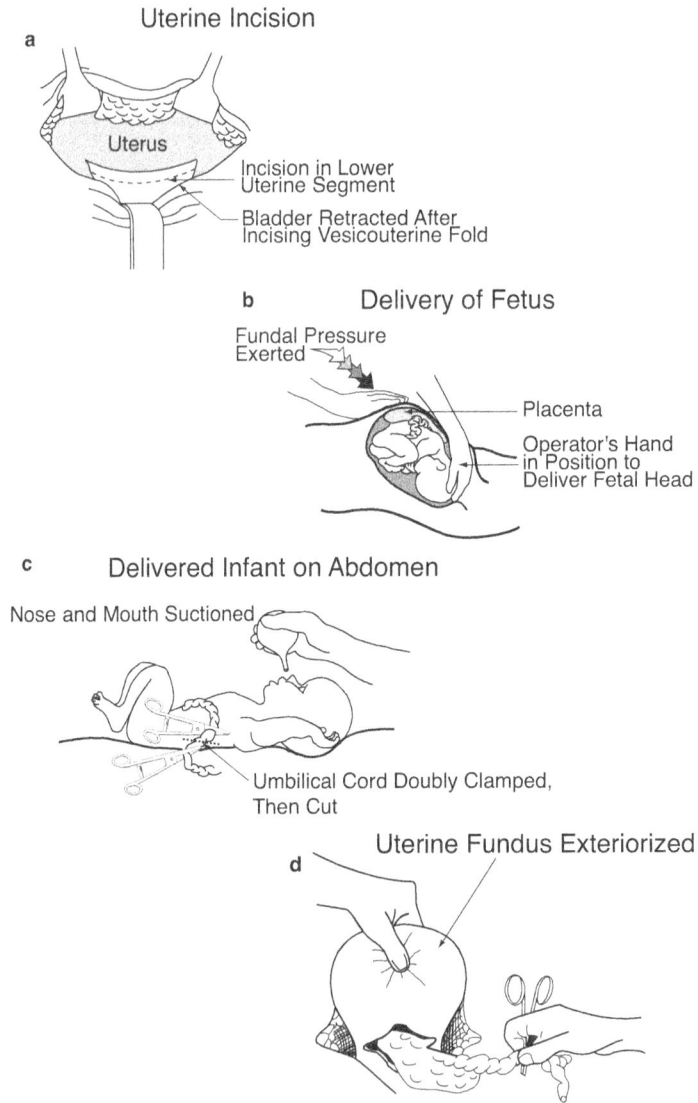

Fig. 19-4. Emergency C-Section.

o Identify and incise the peritoneal reflection of the bladder transversely, and create a bladder flap to retract the bladder out of the field.

o Using a scalpel, carefully incise the uterus transversely across the lower uterine segment (where the uterine wall thins).

o Once the amniotic membranes are visible or opened, extend the incision laterally, either bluntly or by **carefully** using bandage scissors. **Avoid the uterine vessels laterally.** If necessary, the incision can be extended at one or both of its lateral margins in a J-fashion by vertical incision.

o Elevate the presenting fetal part into the incision, with an assistant providing fundal pressure.

o Upon delivery of the fetus, suction the nose and mouth and clamp and cut the cord. Hand the infant off for care (see below).

o Direct anesthetist to administer 2 grams of cefazolin (Ancef) once the cord is clamped.

o Allow the placenta to deliver by providing gentle traction on the cord and performing uterine massage.

o Begin oxytocin, if available as above.

o Using a sponge, clean the inside of the uterus, and vigorously massage the fundus to help the uterus contract.

o Quickly close the incision with 0-vicryl. A single layer (running, locking) is adequate, if hemostatic, for transverse incisions. Take care to avoid the lateral vessels. If the incision has a vertical extension, close it in 2 or 3 layers.

o Once hemostasis is assured, close the fascia and abdomen in the usual fashion.

o In the rare case of continued uterine hemorrhage, evaluate and treat as outlined in the section below.

Uterine Atony

● The majority of postpartum hemorrhage is secondary to uterine atony (failure of uterine contracture).

> **When the uterus fails to contract following delivery of the placenta, bleeding may be torrential and fatal.**

- Initial management should include manual uterine exploration for retained placenta. Without anesthesia, this procedure is painful. An opened sponge is placed around the examiner's fingers. Place the opposite hand on the patient's uterine fundus and apply downward pressure. Gently guide your fingers through the open cervix and palpate for retained placenta. The inside of the uterus should feel smooth, and retained placenta will feel like a soft mass of tissue. This may be removed manually or by using a large curette if available.
- If no tissue is encountered, use both hands to apply vigorous uterine massage to improve the uterine tone.
- Medications should also be used if available. Oxytocin may be given by IV bolus using 40 units in 1000 cc, or up to 10 units IM, but never by IV push. Although unlikely to be available, other medications that can be considered are Methergine, dinoprostone (Prostin), and misoprostol (Cytotec).
- If no medication is available, the patient should be encouraged to breast feed or do nipple stimulation to increase endogenous oxytocin release.

> **If conservative measures fail to arrest the postpartum hemorrhage, laparotomy (if the hemorrhage is occurring post vaginal delivery), should be performed.**

- Intraoperative massage of the uterine fundus may be tried.
- **If the massage fails to improve uterine tone, the uterine arteries should be ligated in a stepwise fashion.** Begin with the ascending branch at the junction of the upper and lower uterine segment. Using 0 or No. 1 chromic, place a stitch through the myometrium medial to the artery from front to back. The stitch is then brought out through the adjacent broad ligament and tied. If bilateral ligation of the ascending branch does not control bleeding, the descending branch should be ligated at the level of the uterosacral ligament. **If this fails, consider bilateral hypogastric artery ligation (see above). If this fails, proceed to hysterectomy** as outlined in the gynecologic portion of this chapter.

Neonatal Resuscitation
- **Immediately following delivery, every infant should be assessed for need for resuscitation.** Equipment that may be needed includes warm towels, bulb syringe, stethoscope, flow-inflating or self-inflating bag with oxygen source, laryngoscope and blade, suction catheter, and endotracheal tube. The two medications that may be needed are epinephrine 1:10,000 and naloxone (Narcan) 0.4 mg/ml.
- Nearly 90% of term babies are delivered without risk factors and with clear fluid, requiring only to be dried, suctioned and observed. **If the baby is less than 36 weeks, or if there is meconium in the fluid at delivery, the baby will need to be observed more closely.**
  - In the first 30 seconds after delivery, dry and stimulate the baby, position it in order to open the airway, and give free flow oxygen if the color is poor.
  - At 30 seconds, evaluate the heart rate. **If it is < 100 begin to provide positive pressure ventilation.** After 30 seconds of ventilation, recheck the heart rate. **If it is < 60, then chest compressions should be started.** After 30 seconds of chest compressions, again re-evaluate. If the heart rate remains < 60 you should administer epinephrine. Epinephrine can be given either through the umbilical vein or the endotracheal tube. The level of experience of the team present should dictate which route should be used. The dose is 0.1–0.3 ml/kg of the 1:10,000 solution.
  - If heart rate rises over 100, stop the positive pressure ventilations, but continue to provide free flow oxygen. If the mother has been given a dose of narcotics in the 4 hours prior to delivery, and positive pressure ventilation has resulted in a normal heart rate and color but poor respiratory effort, then naloxene is indicated. Administer naloxene by IV, IM, or endotracheal route at a dosage of 0.1 mg/kg.
- If at any time during resuscitation the heart rate goes above 100, with good respiratory effort, tone and color, the baby may be moved to an observation status.

Chapter 20

Wounds and Injuries of the Spinal Column and Cord

Introduction
Combat injuries of the spinal column, with or without associated spinal cord injury, differ from those encountered in civilian practice. These injuries are often open, contaminated, and usually associated with other organ injuries.

Following the ABCs of advanced trauma life support (ATLS), management principles include:
- Initial spine stabilization to prevent neurologic deterioration.
- Diagnosis.
- Definitive spinal stabilization.
- Functional recovery.

> In complete injuries, the likelihood of neurological recovery is minimal and is not influenced by emergent surgical intervention. However, incomplete injuries with neurological deterioration may benefit from emergent surgical decompression. Emergent, life-saving, soft tissue exploration, and debridement may still be required, particularly with colorectal involvement.

Classification
Four discriminators must be considered in the classification and treatment of spinal injuries.
- Is injury open or closed?
- Neurologic status: complete vs incomplete vs intact.
  - o Complete injury demonstrates no neurologic function **below the level of injury** after the period of spinal shock

(usually 24–48 h, evidenced by return of the bulbocavern-osus reflex).
- Location of the injury: cervical, thoracic, lumbar, or sacral.
- Degree of bony and ligamentous disruption: stable vs unstable.

Pathophysiology of the Injury to the Spinal Cord
- Injury to the spinal cord is the result of both primary and secondary mechanisms.
  - o Primary: the initial mechanical injury due to local deformation and energy transmission.
    - ◆ High-velocity missile wounds in the paravertebral area can cause injuries even without direct trauma. Stretching of the tissue around the missile's path during formation of the temporary cavity, or fragmentation of the projectile and bone resulting in secondary missiles, cause injury without any direct destruction of the spinal column.

> **The destructive nature of high-velocity wounds explains the futility of decompressive laminectomy in the management of these wounds.**

  - o Secondary: the cascade of biochemical and cellular processes initiated by the primary process that causes cellular damage and even cell death.

> **The critical care of spinal cord injury patients includes attempts to minimize secondary injury from hypoxia, hypotension, hyperthermia, and edema.**

Mechanical integrity of the vertebral column
The vertebral column is composed of three structural columns (Table 20-1).

Table 20-1. Support of the Spinal Column.

Column	Bony Elements	Soft-Tissue Elements
Anterior	Anterior two-thirds of vertebral body	Anterior longitudinal ligament Anterior annulus fibrosus
Middle	Posterior one-third of vertebral body Pedicles	Posterior longitudinal ligament Posterior annulus fibrosus
Posterior	Lamina Spinous processes Facet joints	Ligamentum flavum Interspinous ligaments

- Injuries occur by either direct penetrating forces or a combination of flexion, axial loading, rotation, and distraction forces.
- Loss of integrity of two of the three columns results in instability of the spine.
- **Instability is common following blunt injury of the vertebral column, but is not usually the case with gunshot or fragment wounds of the vertebral column.**
- Cervical instability by lateral radiograph (must include C-7/T-1 junction) is defined by:
  - o 3.5 mm or greater sagittal displacement or translation.
  - o Angulation of 11° or more on the lateral view.
  - o Should questions exist regarding cervical stability, flexion and extension lateral radiographs can be obtained in the awake, cooperative patient.
- Thoracic and lumbar spine instability:
  - o 5 mm of sagittal translation.
  - o 20°–30° of sagittal angulation.
  - o 50% loss of vertebral body height.
  - o Widened pedicles on anterior-posterior (AP) radiographs.

Computed tomography (CT) is very effective in demonstrating spinal instability and has become available in some field environments.

Instability must be presumed (and the spine stabilized) in any patient with:
- Complaints of a sense of instability (holds his head in his hands).
- Vertebral column pain.
- Tenderness in the midline over the spinous processes.
- Neurologic deficit.
- Altered mental status.
- SUSPECTED, but NOT PROVEN injury.

Patient Transport

On the battlefield, preservation of the life of the casualty and medic are of paramount importance. In these circumstances, EVACUATION TO A MORE SECURE AREA TAKES PRECEDENCE OVER SPINE IMMOBILIZATION. Data do not support the use of cervical collars and spine boards for PENETRATING spine injuries on the battlefield.

Extrication
- Cervical spine.
  o **The neck should never be hyperextended.**
  o If an airway is needed.
    ♦ If appropriate, attempt endotracheal intubation with in-line neck stabilization.
    ♦ Cricothyroidotomy is necessary if intubation fails.
  o The head should be maintained in alignment with the body.
    ♦ Requires several people, including one just to stabilize the neck.
    ♦ Log roll with the most experienced person stabilizing the neck.
  o A stiff cervical collar and sandbags provide stabilization of the neck during the transport. The head and body should be secured to the extrication device.
- Thoracic and lumbar spine.

o Use log roll or two-man carry as demonstrated in Fig. 20-1.
  ♦ The two-man carry alone does not protect the cervical spine.
  ♦ The cradle-drop drag may also be used.
o In the absence of a spine board, makeshift litters can be fashioned from local materials.

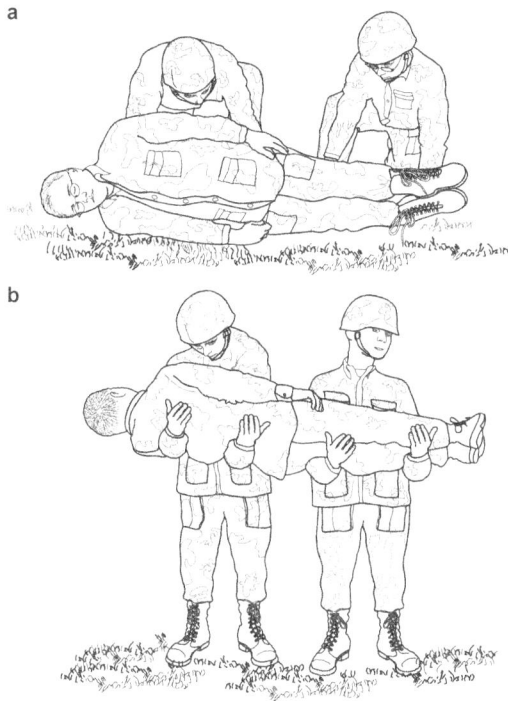

Fig. 20-1. (**a**) Log roll (**b**) two-man carry.

Anatomical Considerations
Cervical Spine
All potentially unstable cervical spine injuries should be immobilized in a rigid collar, unless halo immobilization is required.
● Indications for halo use:

o The role of halo immobilization in the acute combat setting is quite limited. In nonpenetrating trauma to the cervical spine, immobilization with a cervical hard collar or sand bags is preferable until arrival at a definitive treatment site

o Should traction be indicated for cervical spine injuries (eg, facet joint dislocations or burst fractures with a tenuous neurologic status), the Gardner-Wells tongs should be applied and sufficient weight (generally 2–10 kg) placed in line of the spine (Fig. 20-2, Table 20-2). It is paramount to remember that injuries to occiptocervical articulation should not be treated with traction-in effect, putting these injuries in traction "pulls the head off". If traction is applied, radiographs must be obtained to be certain that no undiagnosed ligamentous injury has been exacerbated by the weight.

o The role of collar immobilization in penetrating injuries to the cervical spine is less well established. Soft-tissue care is compromised by the collar's position and, in general, penetrating injuries coupled with osseous instability should be managed in Gardner-Wells traction.

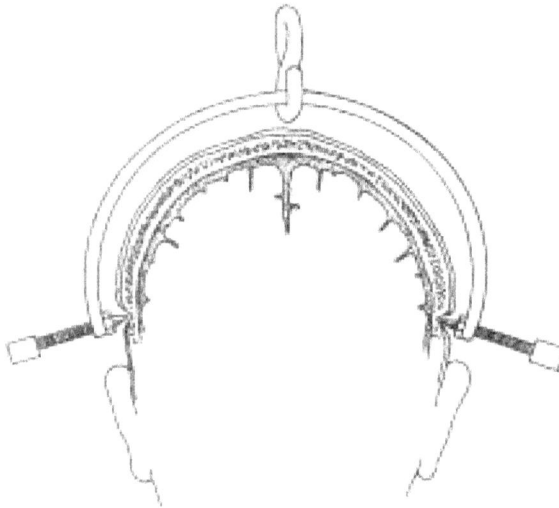

Fig. 20-2. Gardner-Wells tongs.

Table 20-2. Application of Gardner-Wells Tongs.

Step	Procedure	Comment
1	**Inspect Insertion Site:** Select a point just above apex of each ear.	Rule out depressed skull fracture in this area.
2	**Shave and Prep Pin Insertion Site.**	
3	**Inject Local Anesthetic:** Inject 2–3 cc of 1% Xylocaine or equivalent agent 1 cm above each ear in line with the external auditory meatus.	May omit if patient is unconscious.
4	**Advance Gardner-Wells Tong Pins:** Insert pins into skull by symmetrically tightening the knobs.	A spring-loaded device in one of the two pins will protrude when the pins are appropriately seated. (A data plate on the tongs provides additional information.)
5	**Apply Skeletal Traction:** Use a pulley fixed to the head of the litter or frame to direct horizontal traction to the tongs.	Use 5 lb rule (ie, 5 lb of weight for each level of injury). High cervical fractures usually require minimal traction to reduce. Monitor with series radiographs. The tong-pin site requires anterior or posterior positioning to adjust for cervical spine flexing or extension as indicated.
6	**Elevate Head of Litter:** Use blocks in order to provide body-weight counter traction.	The knot in the cord should not be permitted to drift up against the pulley. Should this occur, traction is no longer being applied.
7	**Decrease Traction Weight:** When radiographs confirm that reduction is adequate, decrease traction to 5–15 lb.	Unreducible or unstable fractures should be maintained in moderate traction until surgical intervention. If neurological deterioration occurs, immediate surgical intervention must be considered.
8	**Daily Pin Care.**	Cleanse tracts with saline and apply antibiotic ointment to the pin sites. Maintain pin force (see Step 4) by tightening as necessary to keep spring-loaded device in the protruded position.

| 9 | **Turn Patient Appropriately:** Use Stryker, Foster, or similar frame and turn patient every 4 h. | When initially proned, obtain radiographs to ensure that the reduction is maintained. If reduction is not maintained when the patient is proned, rotate the patient only between the 30° right and left quarter positions. The use of a circle electric bed is contraindicated with injuries of the spinal cord or column. |
| 10 | **If Satisfactory Alignment Cannot Be Obtained, Further Workup Is Necessary.** | Consider myelogram, CT scan, tomograms, and neurosurgical /orthopedic consultations. |

Thoracic and Lumbar Spine

- Although the thoracic rib cage contributes considerable rotatory stability, it does not protect completely against injuries.
- The vascular supply of the spinal cord is most vulnerable between T-4 and T-6 where the canal is most narrow. Even minor deformity may result in cord injury.
- The most common place for compression injuries is at the thoracolumbar junction between T-10 and L-2.
- Most burst fractures result from an axial load, and occur at the thoracolumbar junction. These fractures are associated with compromise of the spinal canal and progressive angular deformity. They are often associated with significant neurologic injury.
- Evaluation for surgical stabilization and spinal cord decompression should be done with advanced imaging such as CT and/or magnetic resonance imaging (MRI).

> **When complex wounds involving the head, thorax, abdomen, or extremities coexist with vertebral column injuries, lifesaving measures take precedence over the definitive diagnosis and management of spinal column and cord problems. During these interventions, further injury to the unstable spine must be prevented by appropriate protective measures.**

Emergent Surgery

> **Emergent spine surgery for penetrating or closed injuries of the spinal cord is indicated only in the presence of neurological deterioration.**

- Penetrating Spine Injuries.
  - o Injuries associated with a hollow-viscus should undergo appropriate treatment of the viscus injury without **extensive** debridement of the spinal injury, followed by appropriate broad-spectrum antibiotics for 1–2 weeks. Inadequate debridement and irrigation may lead to meningitis.
  - o Removal of a fragment from the spinal canal is indicated for patients with neurologic deterioration.
  - o In neurologically stable patients with fragments in the cervical canal, delaying surgery for 7–10 days reduces problems with dural leak and makes dural repair considerably easier.
  - o Casualties not requiring immediate surgery may be observed with spine immobilization and treated with 3 days of IV antibiotics. Surgical stabilization can be performed following evacuation.

Pharmacologic Treatment
- **Penetrating injuries of the spine should NOT receive corticosteroid treatment.**
- **Closed** spinal cord injuries may be treated with an IV corticosteroid if started within 8 hours of injury.
  - o 30 mg/kg bolus of methylprednisolone initially.
  - o 5.4 mg/kg/h of methylprednisolone for the next 24–48 hours.
    - ♦ If therapy is started within 3 hours of injury, continue treatment for 24 hours.
    - ♦ If therapy is started within 3–8 hours after injury, then treat for 48 hours.

General Management Considerations

Neurogenic shock
- Traumatically induced sympathectomy with spinal cord injury.
- Symptoms include bradycardia and hypotension.
- Treatment:
  - o Volume resuscitation to maintain systolic BP > 90 mm Hg.
  - o May use phenylephrine (50–300 µg/min) or dopamine (2–10 µg/kg/min) to maintain BP.

Gastrointestinal tract
- Ileus is common and requires use of a nasogastric tube.
- Stress ulcer prevention using medical prophylaxis.
- Bowel training includes a schedule of suppositories and may be initiated within one week of injury.

Deep vein thrombosis
- Start mechanical prophylaxis immediately.
- Initiate chemical prophylaxis after acute bleeding has stopped (See Chapter 11, ICU Care).

Bladder Dysfunction
- Failure to decompress the bladder may lead to autonomic dysreflexia and a hypertensive crisis.
- The bladder is emptied by intermittent or indwelling catheterization.
- Antibiotic prophylaxis for the urinary tract is not advised.

Decubitus ulcers
- Skin breakdown begins within 30 minutes in the immobilized hypotensive patient.
- **For prolonged transport, the casualty should be removed from the hard spine board and placed on a litter.**
- Frequent turning and padding of prominences and diligence on the part of caretakers are essential to protect the insensate limbs.
- All bony prominences are inspected daily.
- Physical therapy is started early to maintain range of motion in all joints to make seating and perineal care easier.

Chapter 21

Pelvic Injuries

Introduction
- Injuries of the pelvis are an uncommon battlefield injury.
- **Blunt injuries** may be associated with major hemorrhage and early mortality.
- **Penetrating injuries** to the skeletal pelvis are usually associated with abdominopelvic organ injury.

Blunt Injuries
- Patterns and mechanisms are the same as those seen in civilian blunt trauma.
  - o Lateral compression injuries are marked by internal rotation or midline displacement of the hemipelvis.
  - o Anterior posterior injuries demonstrate external rotation of the hemipelvis.
  - o Vertical shear injuries have cephalad displacement of the hemipelvis.
- Increasing degrees of displacement in any direction are associated with greater risk of hemorrhage.
  - o Anterior posterior injuries with complete disruption of all sacroiliac ligaments represent an internal hemipelvectomy and have the greatest potential for hemorrhage.

> **Early pelvic stabilization can control hemorrhage and reduce mortality.** This is particularly true in an austere environment with limited blood replacement products and other treatment resources.

- Open injuries require early recognition and prompt treatment to prevent high mortality due to early hemorrhage and late sepsis.

- Diagnosis.
  - o Physical examination demonstrates instability of the pelvis when manual pressure is applied to the iliac crests.
  - o Leg length difference, scrotal or labial swelling/ecchymosis, or abrasions over the pelvis raise suspicion for pelvic ring injury.
  - o **Perineum, rectum, and vaginal vault must be evaluated for lacerations to rule out an open injury.**
  - o Radiograph (AP pelvis, and when possible, inlet and outlet views) confirm the diagnosis. Computed tomography (CT) defines the location of injury more accurately.
  - o Bladder and urethral injuries are suspected when blood is present at the meatus or in the urine, or when a Foley catheter cannot be passed. Retrograde urethrogram and cystography confirm the diagnosis.
- Treatment.
  - o Hemorrhage control.
    - ◆ Mechanical stabilization.
      - ◊ Tying a sheet or placing a binder around the pelvis at the level of the greater trochanters.
      - ◊ Bean bags or sand bags.
      - ◊ Lateral decubitus positioning with the affected side dependent.

> **External fixator placement in the iliac crests allows for the most direct control of the pelvis.**

  - ◆ Angiography is a useful adjunct, but is not usually available in the deployed environment.
  - ◆ As a last resort, retroperitoneal packing may be attempted, but will expend tremendous resources and is often unsuccessful.
  - o Open blunt injuries require:
    - ◆ Immediate hemorrhage control by packing.
    - ◆ Aggressive and thorough debridement.
    - ◆ Pelvic stabilization.
    - ◆ Diverting colostomy in the presence of wounds at risk for fecal soilage.

o Definitive internal pelvic stabilization (plates, screws, among others) is done outside of the combat zone.

> **Missile and fragmentation wounds can cause fracture of the pelvis.**
> - **The pelvis usually remains stable.**
> - **The colon, small intestine, rectum, and the genitourinary tracts must all be assessed for associated injury.**
> - **Major hemorrhage can result from injury to the iliac vessels.**

Penetrating Injuries
- Evaluation.
    o Diagnosis of associated injuries may require exploratory laparotomy.
    o Fractures should be assessed with radiographs and CT scans, when available, to **rule out extension into the hip and acetabulum**.
- Treatment.
    o Control hemorrhage.
    o Control hollow visceral injury.
    o Debride wounds and fractures.

> **For combined hollow-viscus and acetabulum /hip joint injuries, the joint is contaminated and must be explored and treated as described in Chapter 24, Open Joint Injuries.**

- Technique of pelvic external fixator placement (Fig. 21-1).
    o Prep the iliac crests.
    o Place a 2-cm horizontal incision over the iliac crest, 2 fingerbreadths proximal or medial ventral to the anterior superior iliac crest.
    o Bluntly dissect to the iliac crest.
    o To determine the angle of the pelvis, first slide a guide pin between the muscle and the bone along the inner table of the iliac wing, no deeper than 3–4 cm.

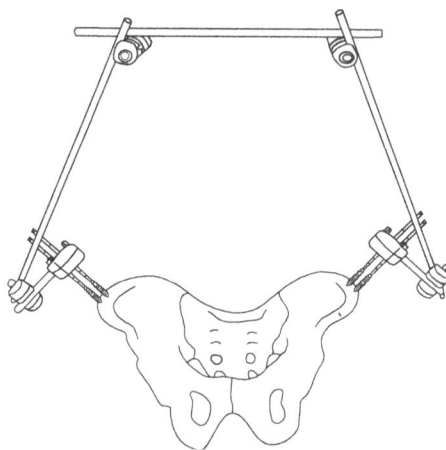

Fig. 21-1. Pelvic external fixator placement.

> **Failure to properly determine the angle of the iliac wing leads to inadequate fixation and may cause significant complications.**

- o Locate the junction of the middle and medial thirds of the thickness of the iliac crest with the tip of a 5-mm external fixator pin.
- o Paralleling the guide pin, begin drilling the pin into the crest.
- o Drill between the inner and outer tables to a depth of about 4 cm, aiming generally towards the greater trochanter. **Only gentle pressure should be applied once the pin threads have engaged, to allow for the pin to guide itself between the tables.**
- o A second pin is inserted 1–2 cm more posteriorly on the crest.
- o Check the stability of each pin. If unsatisfactory, attempt reinsertion by aiming between the tables.
- o Place pins in the contralateral iliac crest in the same manner.
- o Reduce the pelvis by applying pressure on the pelvis (**not the pins!**) and connect the extreme fixator pins with bar(s) across the abdomen and pelvis to maintain reduction.

Chapter 22

Soft-Tissue Injuries

> **All war wounds are contaminated and should not be closed primarily.**

The goal in treatment of soft-tissue wounds is to save lives, preserve function, minimize morbidity and prevent infections through early and aggressive surgical wound care far forward on the battlefield.

Presurgical Care
- Prevent infection.
  - o Antibiotics:
    - ◆ **Antibiotics are not a replacement for surgical treatment.**
    - ◆ Antibiotics are therapeutic, not prophylactic, in war wounds.
    - ◆ Give antibiotics for **all** penetrating wounds as soon as possible.
  - o Sterile dressing.
    - ◆ Place a sterile field dressing as soon as possible.
    - ◆ Leave dressing undisturbed until surgery. **A one-look** soft-tissue examination may be performed on initial presentation. Infection rate increases with multiple examinations prior to surgery. Initial wound cultures unnecessary.

Surgical Wound Management Priorities
- Life-saving procedures before limb and soft-tissue wound care.
- Save limbs.
  - o Vascular repair.
  - o Compartment release.

- Prevent infection.
  - o Wound surgery within 6 hours of wounding.
  - o Antibiotics.
  - o Sterile dressing.
  - o Fracture immobilization.
- **Superficial penetrating fragment (single or multiple) injuries usually do not require surgical exploration.** Simply cleanse the wounds with antiseptic and scrub brush. Nonetheless, depending on location and clinical presentation, maintain high suspicion for vascular injury or intraabdominal penetration.
  - o Avoid "Swiss cheese" surgery (in an attempt to excise all wounds and retrieve fragments).

Wound Care

> **Primary Surgical Wound Care**
> - **Limited longitudinal incisions.**
> - **Excision of foreign material and devitalized tissue.**
> - **Irrigation.**
> - **LEAVE WOUND OPEN—NO PRIMARY CLOSURE.**
> - **Antibiotics and tetanus prophylaxis.**
> - **Splint for transport** (improves pain control).

- Longitudinal incisions.
  - o Wounds are extended with incisions parallel to the long axis of the extremity, to expose the entire deep zone of injury. At the flexion side of joints, the incisions are made obliquely to the long axis to prevent the development of flexion contractures.
  - o The use of longitudinal incisions, rather than transverse ones, allows for proximal and distal extension, as needed, for more thorough visualization and debridement.
- Wound excision (current use of the term **debridement**).
  - o Skin.
    - ♦ Conservative excision of 1–2 mm of damaged skin edges (Fig. 22-1a).
    - ♦ Excessive skin excision is avoided; questionable areas can be assessed at the next debridement.

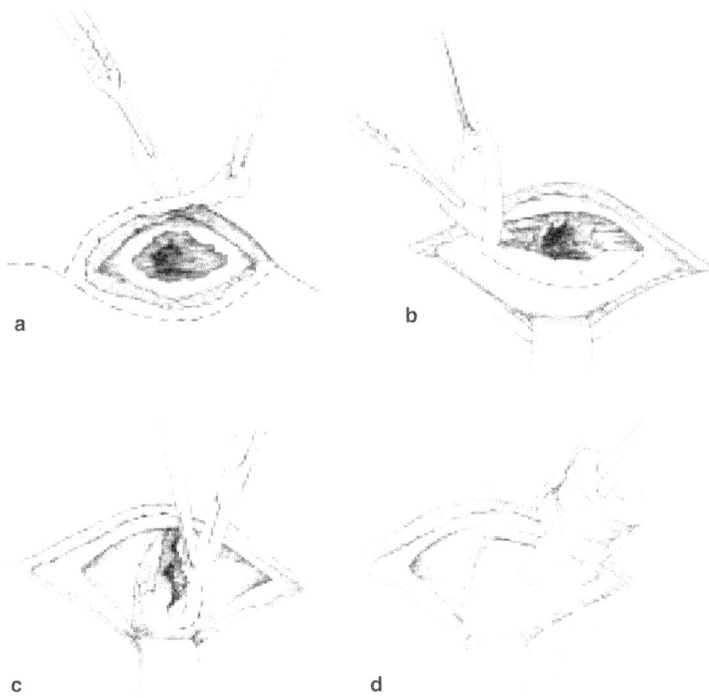

Fig. 22-1. (**a**) Skin excision, (**b**) removal of fascia, (**c**) removal of avascular tissue, (**d**) irrigation.

- o Fat.
    - ◆ Damaged, contaminated fat should be generously excised.
- o Fascia.
    - ◆ Damage to the fascia is often minimal relative to the magnitude of destruction beneath it (Fig 22-1b).
    - ◆ Shredded, torn portions of fascia are excised, and the fascia is widely opened through longitudinal incision to expose the entire zone of injury beneath.
    - ◆ Complete fasciotomy is often required as discussed below.
- o Muscle.

> **Removal of dead muscle is important to prevent infection.** ACCURATE INITIAL ASSESSMENT OF MUSCLE VIABILITY IS DIFFICULT. **Tissue sparing debridement is acceptable if follow-on wound surgery will occur within 24 hours. More aggressive debridement is required if subsequent surgery will be delayed for more than 24 hours.**

- ♦ Sharply excise all nonviable, severely damaged, avascular muscle (Fig. 22-1c).
- ♦ The "4 Cs" may be **unreliable** for initial assessment of muscle viability (**color, contraction, consistency, circulation**).
  - ◊ Color is the least reliable sign of muscle injury. Surface muscle may be discolored due to blood under the myomesium, contusion, or local vasoconstriction.
  - ◊ Contraction is assessed by observing the retraction of the muscle with the gentle pinch of a forceps.
  - ◊ Consistency of the muscle may be the best predictor of viability. In general, viable muscle will rebound to its original shape when grasped by a forceps, while muscle that retains the mark has questionable viability.
  - ◊ Circulation is assessed via bleeding tissue from a fresh wound. Transient vasospasm, common with war wounds, may not allow for otherwise healthy tissue to bleed.
- o Bone.
  - ♦ Fragments of bone with soft-tissue attachments and large free articular fragments are preserved.
  - ♦ Remove all devitalized, avascular pieces of bone smaller than thumbnail size that have no soft-tissue attachment.
  - ♦ Deliver each of the bone ends of any fracture independently, clean the surface and clean out the ends of the medullary canal.
- o Nerves and tendons.
  - ♦ Do not require debridement, except for trimming frayed edges and grossly destroyed portions.
  - ♦ **Primary repair is not performed**. To prevent desiccation, use soft-tissue or moist dressings for coverage.

o Vessels.
  ♦ Only minimal debridement of vessel is required for a successful repair.
o Irrigation.
  ♦ Following surgical removal of debris and nonviable tissue, irrigation is performed until clean (Fig. 22-1d).
  ♦ While sterile physiologic fluid is preferred, do not deplete resuscitation fluid resources. May use potable water as an alternative. The last liter of irrigant should be a sterile solution with antibiotics.
o Local soft-tissue coverage.
  ♦ The development and rotation of flaps for this purpose should not be done during primary surgical wound care.
  ♦ Local soft-tissue coverage through the gentle mobilization of adjacent healthy tissue to prevent drying, necrosis, and infection is recommended. Saline-soaked gauze is an alternative.

No Primary Closure of War Wounds.

---

o Dressing.
  ♦ **Do not plug the wound** with packing as this prevents wound drainage. Leaving the wound open allows the egress of fluids, avoids ischemia, allows for unrestricted edema, and avoids the creation of an anaerobic environment.
  ♦ Place a nonconstricting, nonocclusive dry dressing over the wound.

Wound Management After Initial Surgery
● The wound undergoes a planned second debridement and irrigation in 24–72 hours, and subsequent procedures until a clean wound is achieved.
● Between procedures there may be better demarcation of nonviable tissue or the development of local infection.
● Early soft-tissue coverage is desirable within 3–5 days, when the wound is clean, to prevent secondary infection.

- Delayed primary closure (3–5 days) requires a clean wound that can be closed without undo tension. This state may be difficult to achieve in war wounds.
- Soft-tissue war wounds heal well without significant loss of function through secondary intention. This is especially true of simple soft-tissue wounds.
- Definitive closure with skin grafts and muscle flaps should not be done in theater when evacuation is possible. These techniques may be required, however, for injured civilians or prisoners of war.

Crush Syndrome
- When a victim is crushed or trapped with compression on the extremities for a prolonged time, there is the possibility for the crush syndrome (CS), characterized by ischemia and muscle damage or death (rhabdomyolysis).
  - o With rhabdomyolysis there is an efflux of potassium, nephrotoxic metabolites, myoglobin, purines, and phosphorous into the circulation, resulting in cardiac and renal dysfunction.
  - o Reperfusion injury can cause up to 10 L of third-space fluid loss per limb that can precipitate hypovolemic shock.
  - o Acute renal failure (ARF) can result from the combination of nephrotoxic substances from muscle death (myoglobin, uric acid) and hypovolemia resulting in renal low-flow state.
- Recognition.
  - o History.
    - ♦ Suspect in patients in whom there is a history of being trapped (eg, urban operations, mountain operations, earthquakes, or bombings) for a prolonged period (from hours to days).
    - ♦ Clear history is not always available in combat, and the syndrome may appear insidiously in patients who initially appear well.
  - o Physical findings.
    A thorough examination must be done with attention to extremities, trunk, and buttocks. The physical findings depend on the duration of entrapment, treatment rendered, and time since the victim's release.

- ◆ Extremities.
  - ◊ May initially appear normal just after extrication.
  - ◊ Edema develops and the extremity becomes swollen, cool, and tense.
  - ◊ May have severe pain out of proportion to examination.
  - ◊ Anesthesia and paralysis of the extremities, which can mimic a spinal cord injury with flaccid paralysis, but there will be normal bowel and bladder function.
- ◆ Trunk/buttocks: may have severe pain out of proportion to examination in tense compartments.
- o Laboratory findings.
  - ◆ Creatinine phosphokinase (CK) is elevated with values usually > 100,000 IU/mL.
  - ◆ The urine may initially appear concentrated and later change color to a typical reddish–brown color, so called "port wine" or "iced tea" urine. The urine output decreases in volume over time.
  - ◆ Due to myoglobin, urine dipstick is positive for blood, but microscopy will not demonstrate red blood cells (RBCs). The urine may be sent to check for myoglobin, but results take days and should not delay therapy.
  - ◆ Hematocrit/hemoglobin (H/H) can vary depending on blood loss, but in isolated crush syndrome H/H is elevated due to hemoconcentration from third spacing fluid losses.
  - ◆ With progression, serum potassium and CK increase further with a worsening metabolic acidosis. Creatinine and BUN will rise as renal failure ensues. Hyperkalemia is typically the ultimate cause of death from cardiac arrhythmia.
- • Therapy.
  - o On scene while still trapped.
    - ◆ The primary goal of therapy is to prevent acute renal failure in crush syndrome. Suspect, recognize, and treat rhabdomyolysis early in victims of entrapment.
    - ◆ Therapy should be initiated as soon as possible, preferably in the field, while the casualty is still trapped. Ideally it is recommended to establish IV access in a free arm or leg vein.

◊ Avoid potassium and lactate containing IV solutions.
◊ At least 1 L should be given prior to extrication and up to 1 L/h (for short extrication times) to a maximum of 6–10 L/d in prolonged entrapments.
♦ As a last resort, amputation **may** be necessary for rescue of entrapped casualties (ketamine 2 mg/kg IV for anesthesia and use of proximal tourniquet).
o Hospital care.
  ♦ Other injuries and electrolyte anomalies must be treated while continuing fluid resuscitation, as given above, to protect renal function.
  ♦ Foley catheter for urine output monitoring.
  ♦ Establish and maintain urine output > 100 cc/h until pigments have cleared from the urine. If necessary, also
    ◊ Add sodium bicarbonate to the IV fluid (1 amp/L D5W) to alkalinize the urine above a pH of 6.5.
      ▪ If unable to monitor urine pH, put 1 amp in every other IV liter.
    ◊ Administer mannitol, 20% solution 1–2 g/kg over 4 hours (up to 200 g/d), in addition to the IV fluids.
  ♦ Central venous monitoring may be needed with the larger volumes (may exceed 12 L/d to achieve necessary urine output) of fluid given.
  ♦ Electrolyte abnormalities.
    ◊ Hyperkalemia, hyperphosphatemia, hypocalcemia, hyperuricemia must be addressed.
  ♦ Dialysis.
    ◊ ARF requiring dialysis occurs in 50%–100% of those with severe rhabdomyolysis.
  ♦ Surgical management centers on diagnosis and treatment of **compartment syndrome**—remember to check torso and buttocks as well.
    ◊ Amputation: consider in casualties with irreversible muscle necrosis/necrotic extremity.
  ♦ Hyperbaric oxygen therapy: may be useful after surgical therapy to improve limb survival.

Compartment Syndrome (see Chapter 27, Vascular Injuries)
- Compartment syndrome may occur with an injury to any fascial compartment.
- The fascial defect caused by the injury is not adequate to fully decompress the compartment, and compartment syndrome may still occur.
- Mechanisms of injuries associated with compartment syndrome.
  o Open fractures.
  o Closed fractures.
  o Penetrating wounds.
  o Crush injuries.
  o Vascular injuries.
  o Reperfusion following vascular repairs.
- Early clinical diagnosis of compartment syndrome.
  o Pain out of proportion.
  o Pain with passive stretch.
  o Tense, swollen compartment.
- Late clinical diagnosis.
  o Paresthesia.
  o Pulselessness and pallor.
  o Paralysis.
- Measurement of compartment pressures: **Not recommended, just do the fasciotomy**.
  o The diagnosis of a compartment syndrome is made on clinical grounds.
  o Measurement of compartment pressures is not recommended in the combat zone.
- Consider **prophylactic fasciotomy.**
  o High-energy wounds.
  o Intubated, comatose, sedated.
  o Closed-head injuries.
  o Circumferential dressings or casts.
  o Vascular repair.
  o Prolonged transport.
  o High index of suspicion.

Fasciotomy Technique
- Upper extremity.
  - o Arm: The arm has two compartments:
    The **anterior flexors** (biceps, brachialis) and the **posterior extensors** (triceps).
    - ◆ Lateral skin incision from the deltoid insertion to the lateral epicondyle.
    - ◆ Spare the larger cutaneous nerves.
    - ◆ At the fascial level the intermuscular septum between the anterior and posterior compartment is identified, and the fascia overlying each compartment is released with longitudinal incisions.
    - ◆ Protect the radial nerve as it passes through the intermuscular septum from the posterior compartment to the anterior compartment just below the fascia.
    - ◆ Compartment syndrome in the hand is discussed in Chapter 26, Injuries to the Hands and Feet.
  - o Forearm: The forearm has three compartments:
    The **mobile wad** proximally, the **volar** compartment, and the **dorsal** compartment (Fig 22-2).
    - ◆ A palmar incision is made between the thenar and hypothenar musculature in the palm, releasing the carpal tunnel as needed.
    - ◆ This incision is extended transversely across the wrist flexion crease to the ulnar side of the wrist, and then arched across the volar forearm back to the ulnar side at the elbow.
    - ◆ At the elbow, just radial to the medial epicondyle, the incision is curved across the elbow flexion crease. The deep fascia is then released.
    - ◆ At the antecubital fossa, the fibrous band of the lacertus fibrosus overlying the brachial artery and median nerve is carefully released.
    - ◆ This incision allows for soft-tissue coverage of the neurovascular structures at the wrist and elbows, and prevents soft-tissue contractures from developing at the flexion creases.
    - ◆ A second straight dorsal incision can be made to release the dorsal compartment, reaching proximally to release the mobile wad if necessary.

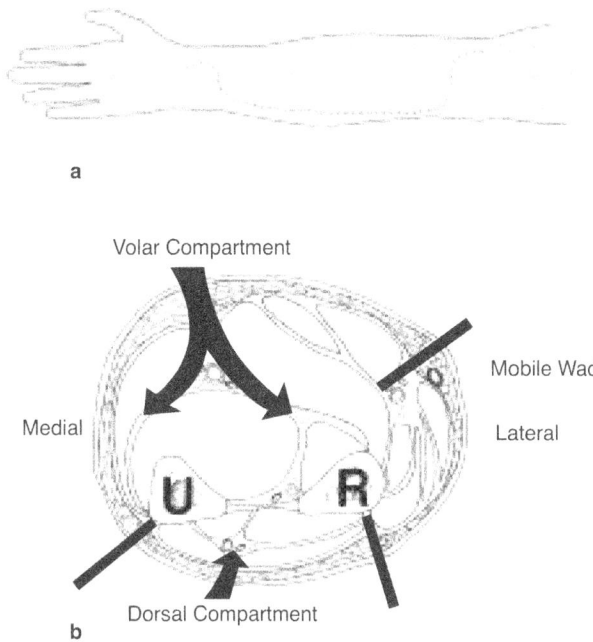

Fig. 22-2. Forearm compartments.

- Lower extremity.
  - o Thigh: The thigh has three compartments:
    The **anterior** (quadriceps), the **medial** compartment (adductors), and the **posterior** compartment (hamstrings).
    - ◆ A lateral incision is made from greater trochanter to lateral condyle of the femur.
    - ◆ Then iliotibial band is incised, and the vastus lateralis is reflected off the intermuscular septum bluntly, releasing the anterior compartment.
    - ◆ The intermuscular septum is then incised the length of the incision, releasing the posterior compartment.
    - ◆ This release of the intermuscular septum should not be made close to the femur, because there are a series of perforating arteries passing through the septum from posterior to anterior near the bone.
    - ◆ The medial adductor compartment is released through

a separate anteromedial incision.

o Calf: The calf has four compartments:

The **lateral** compartment, containing peroneal brevis and longus; the **anterior** compartment, containing extensor hallucis longus, extensor digitorum communis, tibialis anterior, and peroneus tertius; the **superficial posterior** compartment, containing gastrocnemius and soleus; and the **deep posterior** compartment, containing the flexor hallucis longus, flexor digitorum longus, and the tibialis posterior (Fig. 22-3).

♦ Two-incision technique.

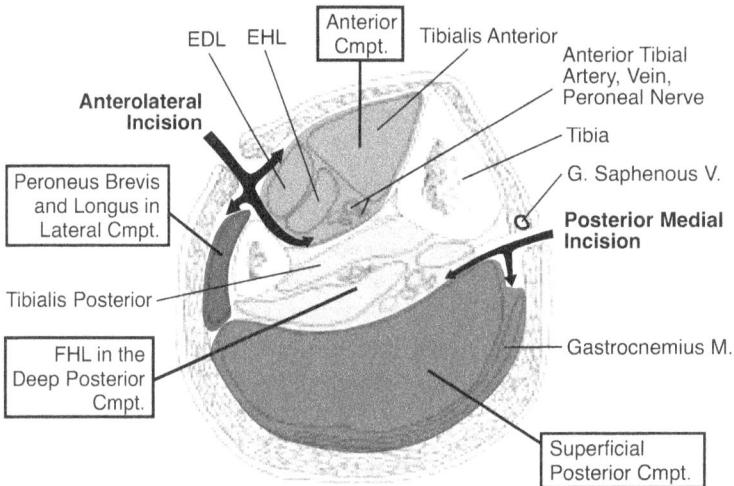

Fig. 22-3. Calf compartments.

◊ Incisions must extend the entire length of the calf to release all of the compressing fascia and skin (Fig. 22-4).

◊ A lateral incision is made centered between the fibula and anterior tibial crest.

◊ The lateral intermuscular septum and superficial peroneal nerve are identified, and the anterior compartment is released in line with tibialis anterior

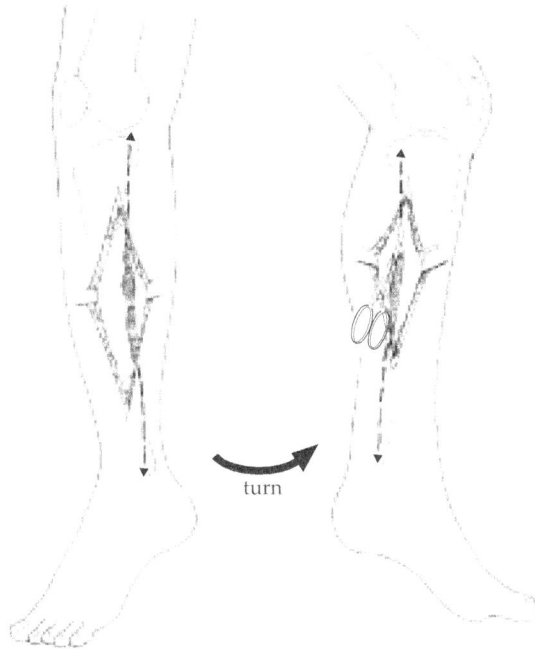

Fig. 22-4. Anteromedial incision of the calf.

   muscle, proximally toward the tibial tubercle, and distally toward anterior ankle.

◊ The lateral compartment is then released through this incision in line with the fibular shaft, proximally toward the fibular head, distally toward the lateral malleolus.

◊ A second incision is made medially at least 2 cm medial to the medial-posterior palpable edge of the tibia.

◊ A medial incision over or near the subcutaneous surface of the tibia is avoided, preventing exposure of the tibia when the tissues retract.

◊ The saphenous vein and nerve are retracted anteriorly.

◊ The superficial compartment is released through its length, and then the deep posterior compartment over the FDL is released. Then identify the tibialis posterior and release its fascia.

22.13

- o Foot: See Chapter 26, Injuries to Hands and Feet.
- Fasciotomy wound management.
    - o Following the fasciotomy, the fasciotomy wound undergoes primary surgical wound management, removing all devitalized tissue.
    - o As with all war wounds, the fasciotomy is left open, and covered with sterile dressings.

The treatment of soft tissue injury is the most common denominator in the management of war wounds. This chapter summarizes some principles of this mangement.

Chapter 23

Extremity Fractures

Introduction
This chapter discusses two techniques for safe transportation of a wounded soldier with a long bone fracture: **transportation casts** and **temporary external fixation**. Both of these methods are acceptable for initial treatment of a patient who will be evacuated out of theater. Precise indications for external fixator use versus casting have not been established.

In general, good indications for external fixator use include when the soft tissues need to be evaluated while en route, such as with a vascular injury; when other injuries make use of casting impractical, such as with a femur fracture and abdominal injury; or when the patients have extensive burns. **Advantages of external fixation** are that it allows for soft tissue access, can be used for polytrauma patients, and has a minimal physiologic impact on the patient. **Disadvantages** are the potential for pin site sepsis or colonization and less soft tissue support than casts.

Advantages of transportation casts are that they preserve the maximum number of options for the receiving surgeon; the soft tissues are well supported, and the casts are relatively low tech. **Disadvantages** are that casts cover soft tissues, may not be suitable for polytrauma patients, and are more labor-intensive than external fixators.

Both transportation casts and external fixators are equally acceptable methods for the initial management of long bone fractures. In the end, the choice of initial fracture stabilization must be made on a case-by-case basis by the treating surgeon. That decision should be based on the surgeon's experience, his/her assessment of the evacuation process, the materials available, the nature of the patient's wounds and the patient's overall condition.

> Though standard in civilian trauma centers, intramedullary nailing of major long bone fractures is **contraindicated** in combat zone hospitals because of a variety of logistical and physiologic constraints. This method may be used once a patient reaches an echelon above corps (EAC) or other site where more definitive care can be provided.

In this chapter, the term **casting material** is used in place of describing either plaster or fiberglass for constructing casts. Both are acceptable materials for application of transportation casts.

General Considerations of Wound Management

- Initial management.
  - o Treat by irrigation and debridement as soon as feasible to prevent infection.
  - o Femur fractures are at high risk for infection (about 40%, historically).
  - o Biplanar radiographs should be obtained.
  - o Neurovascular status of the extremity should be documented and checked repeatedly.
  - o Internal fixation is contraindicated.
  - o Begin IV antibiotics as soon as possible and maintain throughout the evacuation chain. Use a broad spectrum cephalosporin (cefazolin 1 g q 8 h). An aminoglycoside may be harmful for someone in shock or dehydrated. The two most harmful bacteria—clostridia and strep—are covered by a 1st generation cephalosporin.

- Wound incision/excision.
  - o Guidelines as per soft tissue injury section.
  - o Longitudinal incisions to obtain exposure.
  - o Fascia incised longitudinally to expose underlying structures and **compartment release.**
  - o All foreign material in the operative field must be removed (Fig. 23-1a, b, c).

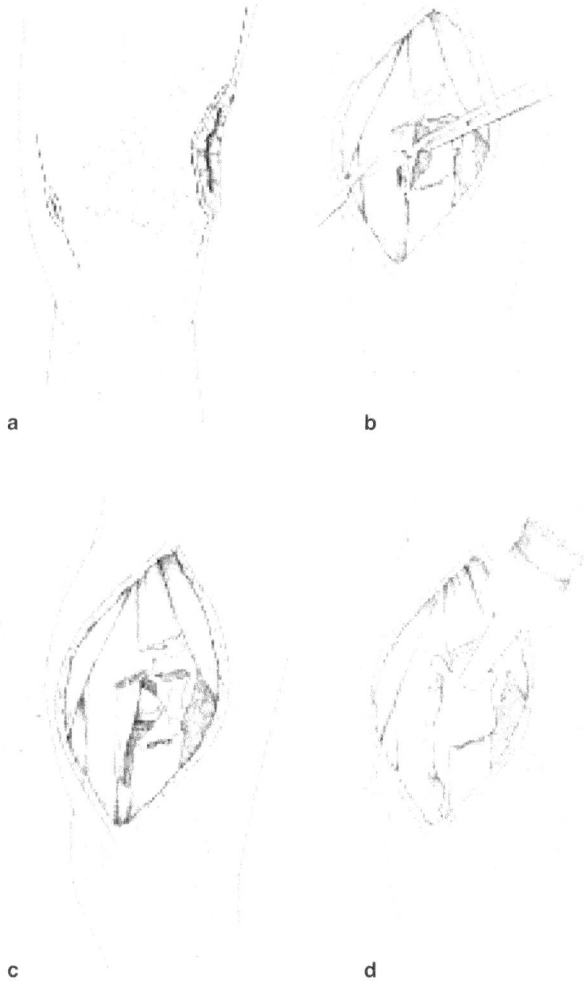

Fig. 23-1. Wound incision/excision.

o Bone fragments should be retained if they have a soft tissue attachment.

23.3

o Detached bone fragments smaller than a thumbnail are discarded.
o Larger fragments that contribute to the structural integrity of the long bone should be retained.
o Irrigation is essential (Fig. 23-1d).

● Closure of wounds.
o Primary closure is never indicated. Loose approximation of tissues with one or two retention sutures is appropriate to cover nerves, vessels, and tendons, but there must be a provision for substantial free drainage.
o Skin grafts, local flaps, and relaxing incisions are contraindicated in the initial management.
o Delayed primary closure may be attempted as described in the section on soft tissue wounds. This should be accomplished in a stable environment.

Transportation Casts
● Introduction.
o A transportation cast is a well-padded cast that is unique to the treatment of combat casualties. It is used to transport patients between hospitals and not intended as a means of definitive care.
o Definitive reduction is not required with the initial surgical procedure.
o The goal of transportation casts is to immobilize a fracture along the evacuation chain. The cast must meet the dimensions of the standard NATO litter (FM 8-10-6).
o Transportation casts are applied prior to evacuation.
o All casts must be bivalved prior to evacuation. (Hip spica — univalved.)
o If a patient is expected to have multiple procedures at the same hospital, balanced skeletal traction should be utilized until the last procedure prior to transportation. The traction pin may be incorporated into the transportation cast.
o Slab splinting may not be adequate for transportation, particularly for severely unstable fractures Splinting is appropriate for stable fractures, particularly in the hand, wrist, forearm, foot, ankle and lower leg.

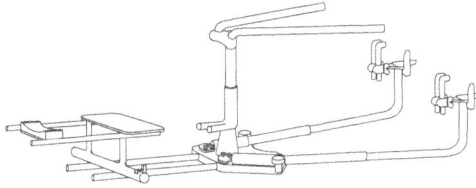

Fig. 23-2. Portable fracture table.

o Portable skeletal traction should not be used for transportation of a patient.
o Tobruk splint (a Thomas splint with circular plaster) should not be used.

● **Hip, femur, and knee, and some proximal tibia fractures.**
  o Low hip spica transportation cast.
  o Disadvantages: Limited soft tissue access. Not suitable in polytrauma.
  o Technique.
    ♦ Adequate anesthesia is given, and patient is placed on fracture table (Fig. 23-2).
    ♦ Irrigation and debridement as indicated above.
    ♦ Precise reduction not necessary, but usually requires two assistants.
    ♦ Stockinette over abdomen, distal thigh of uninvolved side, and foot of the involved side (Fig. 23-3).

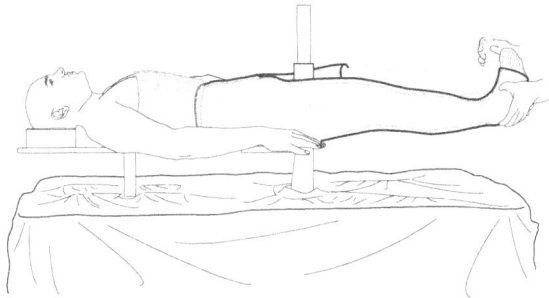

Fig. 23-3. Patient position on fracture table.

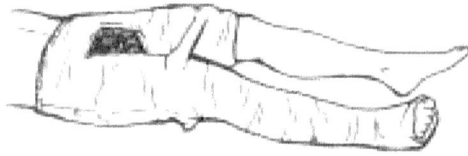

Fig. 23-4. Hip spica transportation cast.

♦ Felt padding is placed over sacrum and anterior superior iliac spine (ASIS) and other bony prominences.
♦ Towel is placed over abdomen to allow breathing space.
♦ Six-inch Webril or similar cotton batting is wrapped, 2-4 layers.
♦ Six-inch casting material is then rolled over the Webril from ASIS to the foot on the affected side to the distal thigh on the unaffected side (Fig. 23-4). Splints are applied over the posterior, lateral, or groin areas to reinforce the groin (Fig. 23-5). Use a finishing roll after turning down the edges of the stockinette to give a neat appearance.
♦ An adequate perineal space must be left for hygiene.
♦ Use a $1/2$" dowel or similar material to make anterior/posterior crossbars.
♦ Affected knee bent about 20°.
♦ Space between feet must not exceed standard litter, although this makes perineal access difficult.
♦ Towel is removed, cast is bivalved, and a circular area over the abdomen is cut out.

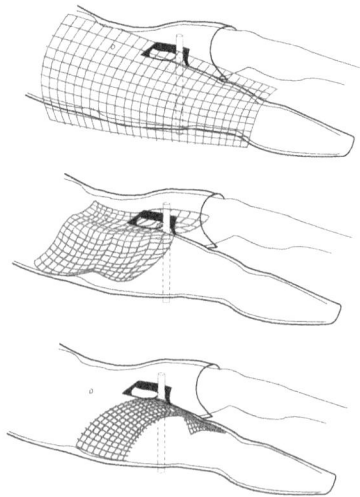

Fig. 23-5. Reinforce cast at hip with splints.

♦ Use an indelible marker to draw the fracture configuration, and note the dates of surgery and wounding on the cast.
♦ Support the cast with towels, blankets, or pillows to relieve pressure on the cast, especially the back edge.

● Proximal/**mid/distal tibia and ankle fractures**.
  o Long Leg Cast (Fig. 23-6).

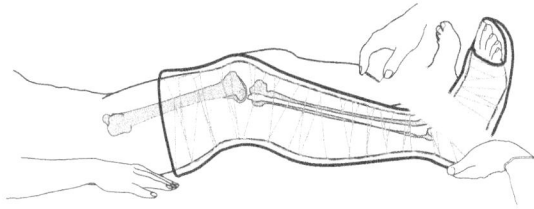

Fig. 23-6. Long leg cast.

  o Technique.
    ♦ The foot, leg, and thigh are placed in a stockinette at the conclusion of the operation for the open wounds.
    ♦ Two people are needed to maintain the reduction and apply the cast. Hold the knee flexed about 20°.
    ♦ Webril applied from the toes to the groin.
    ♦ Six-inch wide casting material is then rolled over this region, with a turn down of the stockinette prior to the final layer, to make a neat edge.
    ♦ Reinforce the knee to strengthen the cast.
    ♦ Make a supracondylar mold to provide support (Fig. 23-7).

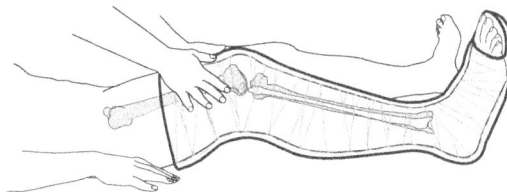

Fig. 23-7. Supracondylar mold of long leg cast.

- ◆ Bivalve the cast.
- ◆ Label the cast with the dates of injury and surgery, and draw the fracture on outside of the cast.
- ◆ Elevate the leg so the tibia is parallel to the litter or bed.

- ● **Shoulder and humeral shaft fractures**.
  - o Velpeau technique. (External fixator is an acceptable alternative, however without direct visualization there is a high risk of iatrogenic injury to the radial nerve and vascular structures. Review anatomy carefully.)
    - ◆ At the conclusion of open wound treatment, the extremity is manipulated on the fracture table to obtain the best alignment.
    - ◆ Large cotton pads are placed under the axilla and arm (Fig. 23-8a).
    - ◆ The Webril is wrapped around the torso and affected extremity to the wrist (Fig. 23-8b).
    - ◆ Six-inch wide casting material is then wrapped over the extremity and the torso. The first wrap should start around the trunk, go over the shoulder posteriorly, down the arm anteriorly, around the elbow, and then up the posterior aspect of the arm (Fig. 23-8c).
    - ◆ The trunk and the extremity should be wrapped in plaster to stabilize the cast.
    - ◆ Four layers should be sufficient (Fig. 23-8d).
    - ◆ Bivalve this cast, and wrap with elastic bandages. There are no cast saws available on the aircraft. If a patient in a Velpeau cast developed any respiratory problems, emergency measures could not be taken if the cast couldn't be removed.

- ● **Elbow/forearm.**
  - o Long arm cast.
  - o Technique.
    - ◆ After treatment of open wounds, the extremity is wrapped in stockinette from the fingers to the axilla.
    - ◆ Gross alignment of fractures is the goal. Precise reduction is not necessary.
    - ◆ Four-inch wide Webril is wrapped from metacarpal heads to axilla.

♦ Four-inch wide casting material is applied from metacarpal heads to axilla.
♦ Fold the stockinette before finishing layer for a neat edge.
♦ Bivalve cast after drying.
♦ Reassess neurovascular status.

Bivalving Casts

When a cast is bivalved, it is completely split longitudinally along opposing sides of the cast. Splitting the cast into anterior and posterior halves is preferred. The purpose of bivalving is to allow room for soft tissue swelling, thus lessening the chance

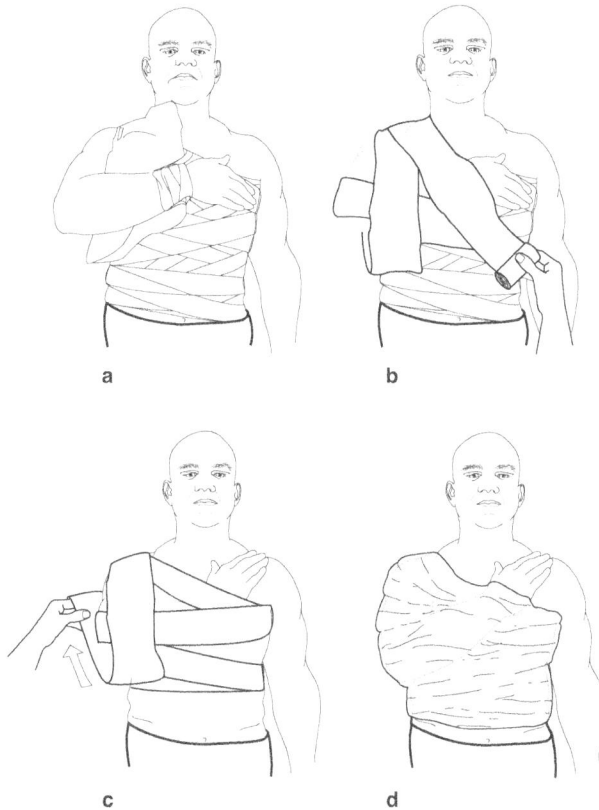

Fig. 23-8a. Padding Velpeau.
Fig. 23-8b–c. Webril application for Velpeau cast.
Fig. 23-8d. Completed Velpeau cast.

of postcasting compartment syndrome. It is important that the underlying cast padding also be completely split underneath the cast cuts; otherwise, the cast padding can restrict swelling and a compartment syndrome could still develop.

External Fixation

- General technique: The surgeon should be familiar with four types of standard constructs of external fixation for use in the initial care of battle casualties: femur, tibia, knee, and ankle. External fixation can also be applied for humerus and ulna fractures as needed.
  - o A thorough understanding of the anatomy of the lower extremity is essential for application of the pins in a safe corridor.
  - o The external fixator for military purposes should be modular and allow for building up or down as healing progresses.
  - o Application of the external fixator may be done without the use of plain films or fluoroscopy.
  - o Pins can be inserted by hand using a brace without power instruments.
  - o Enough pins should be used to adequately stabilize the fracture for transport. This is usually two per clamp, but three may occasionally be required.
  - o The present external fixation system (Hoffmann II) allows for the use of either single pin clamps or multipin clamps. Both clamps are acceptable to use in standard constructs.
  - o Multipin clamps provide geater stability and are the current fixators fielded. Dual pin placement (with multipin clamps) is described here. The technique for single pin placement is similar.

- **Femur diaphyseal fracture technique.**
  - o The entire limb is prepared for surgery, from the ASIS to the toes.
  - o A standard OR table or portable fracture table may be used.
  - o An assistant should apply counter pressure while pins are inserted.
  - o Precise reduction is not necessary. A padded "bump" under the thigh will help reduce the fracture (Fig. 23-9).

o The position of the proximal femur should be identified by palpation. A 1-cm longitudinal stab incision is made over the midaxis, or midlateral axis, of the femur (Fig. 23-10). The pin closest to the fracture should be outside of the fracture hematoma, and at least three fingerbreadths from the fracture (Fig. 23-11).
o Bluntly spread with a clamp down to bone. Put the pin down on the bone, and determine the midportion of the bone by moving the pin back and forth across the width of the femur. You do not want to plunge to one or the other side. Your assistant should provide stability and counter

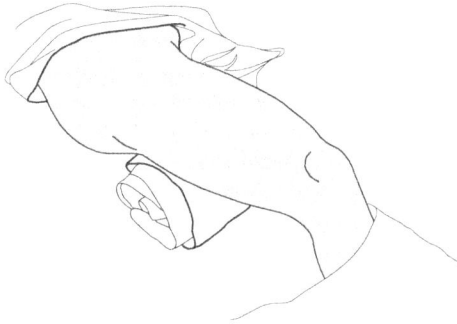

Fig. 23-9. Placing a towel underneath the thigh helps to reproduce the bow of the femur.

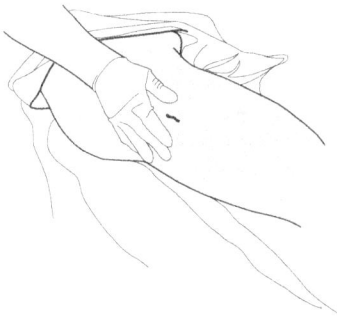

Fig. 23-10. A 1-cm or so incision directly over the middle of the bone, cut in a longitudinal direction.

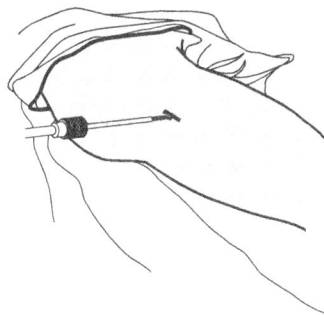

Fig. 23-11. Femur pin placement.

pressure. Two taps on the end of the bit brace should provide an indent in the bone and allow you to start insertion. Apex pins are placed by hand. There is no predrill nor power insertion. 5-mm half-pins should be used. Insert the pin in the midportion of the bone through both the near and far cortex of the bone (Fig. 23-12). The pin will move easier as it enters the inter-medullary canal, and then get more difficult to drive as it enters the far cortex.

o Place a multipin clamp over the inserted pin (Fig. 23-13). Ideally, the pin should occupy one of the end positions (eg, position 1, Fig. 23-14).

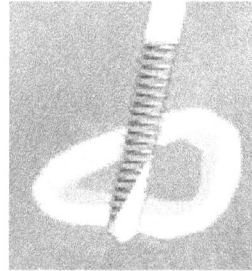

Fig. 23-12. Bicortical placement of 5-mm half-pin.

o Using the clamp as a guide, insert a second pin through the clamp. An assistant should hold the clamp. Ensure that the clamp is aligned to the bone and that bicortical purchase is obtained with the second pin. The second pin must be parallel to the first (Fig. 23-15). Use the pin sites that are the farthest apart on the clamp as possible for biomechanical stability (clamp positions 1 and

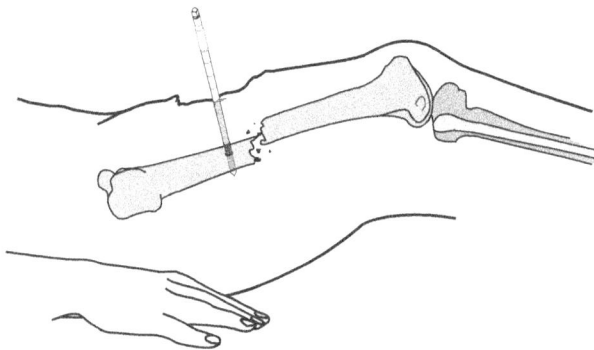

Fig. 23-13.

5 are best, see Fig. 23-14). A third pin may be inserted if needed for additional clamp stability.

o Apply a second multipin clamp and pins in the same manner to the distal femoral fracture fragment.

o Connect the two clamps with elbows, bar-to-bar clamps, and two longitudinal bars placed parallel to each other (Fig. 23-16).

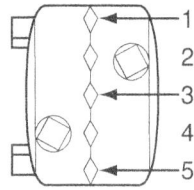

Fig. 23-14. Multipin clamp showing pin positions 1-5.

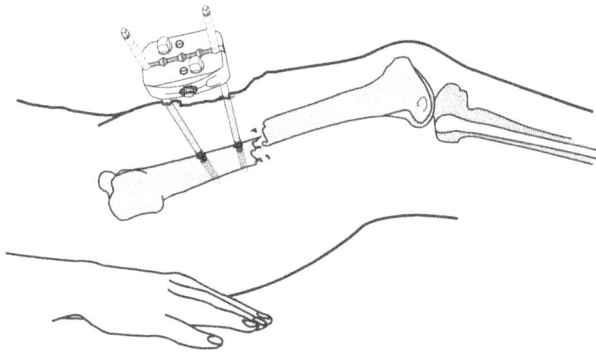

Fig. 23-15.

o Reduce the fracture with longitudinal traction. Manipulating the fracture fragments using the clamps may be helpful. Once adequate reduction is achieved, tighten all the connections. Precise reduction is not necessary.

● **Tibia shaft fracture technique.**
   o Palpate the anterior-medial border of the tibia. Place a 1-cm longitudinal incision over the midportion of the surface (Fig. 23-17). The pin closest to the fracture site should be outside the hematoma and at least three fingerbreadths away from the fracture site (Fig. 23-18).

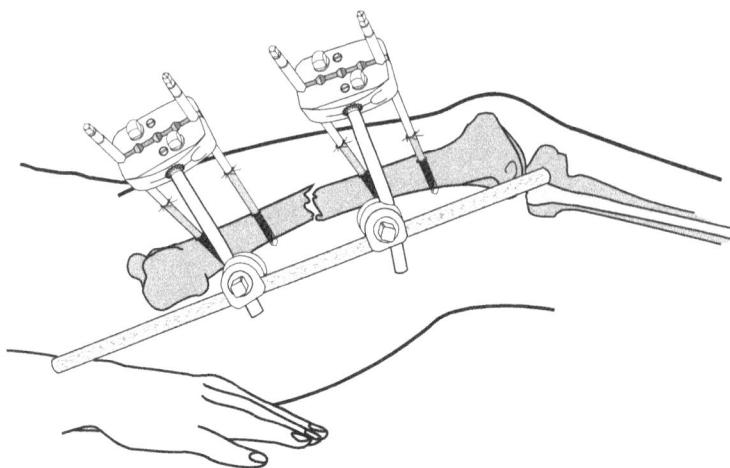

Fig. 23-16.

 o Insert one pin into either the proximal or distal fragment, engaging both cortices. This pin should be placed perpendicular to the subcutaneous border of the tibia, and centered across the width of the tibia (Fig. 23-19).

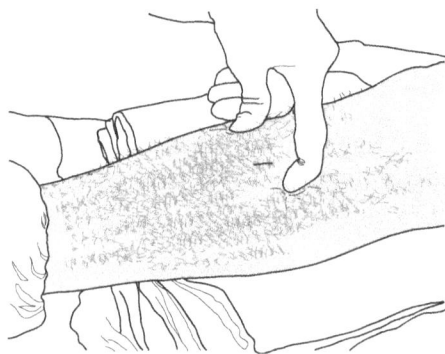

Fig. 23-17. Palpation of the anterior and posterior margins of the medial face of the tibia where a 1 cm incision has been made midway between these two points.

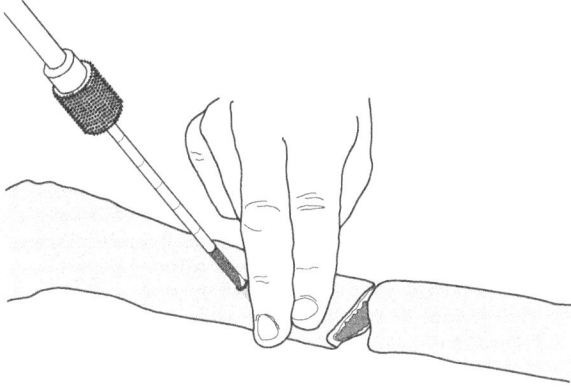

Fig. 23-18. The anteriomedial surface is the safest way to introduce pins to the tibia. The pin should be a minimum of two or three fingerbreadths from the fracture site.

    o Using the clamp as a guide, insert a second pin through the clamp. An assistant should hold the clamp. Ensure that the clamp is aligned to the bone and that bicortical purchase is obtained with the second pin. The second pin

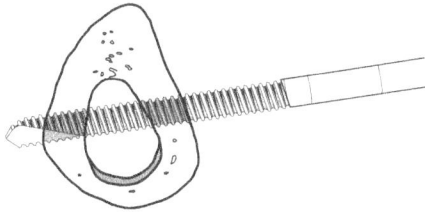

Fig. 23-19. This is the ideal bicortical placement for a pin in the tibia.

must be parallel to the first. Use the pin sites as far apart on the clamp as possible for biomechanical stability (Figure 23-20 and positions 1 and 5 in Fig. 23-14). The second pin should be through the clamp farthest away from the fracture site (Fig. 23-20).

23.15

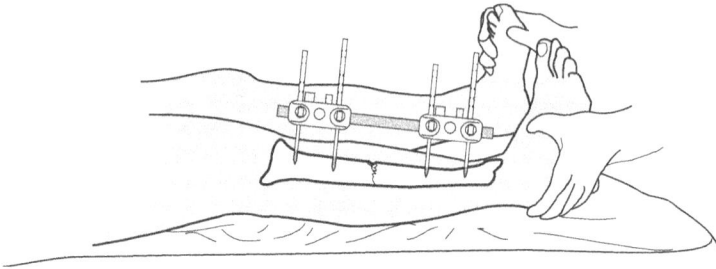

Fig. 23-20. Application of tibia external fixation with multipin clamps.

o Apply a second multipin clamp and two pins in the same
  manner to the other main fracture fragment (Fig. 23-21).
  Connect the two clamps via two elbows, bar–bar clamps,
  and a single bar (Fig. 23-22).
o Most battle caused fractures are comminuted; therefore, a
  second bar should be added to the construct (Fig. 23-23).
  Use a single bar for stable fractures only.
o Check the reduction.

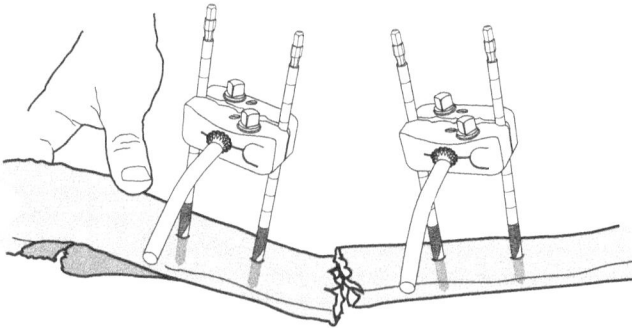

Fig. 23-21. Application of the second multipin clamp and two pins.
Repeat those steps with the other major fracture fragment so that
you have two sets of multipin clamps as shown here. You will then
add the 30 degree elbows as shown here, pointing them in a
direction that allows for the best access. At this point you should
have gross alignment of the fracture.

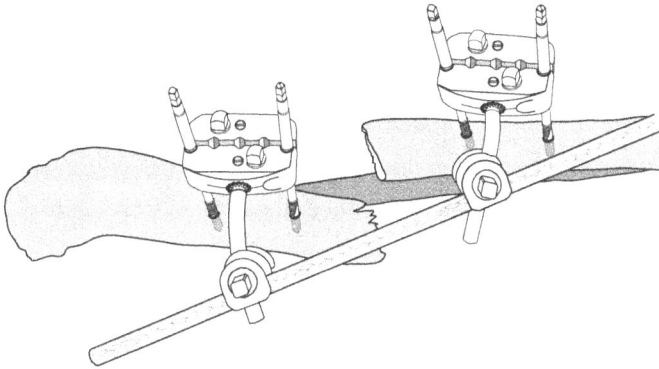

Fig. 23-22. Addition of the cross bar and two bar-to-bar clamps. Have your assistant apply longitudinal traction to reduce the frame, and then tighten the frame in alignment.

● **Technique to span knee.**
  o Indications are proximal tibia fractures, distal femur fractures, or extensive knee injuries, or vascular repairs in the popliteal fossa.

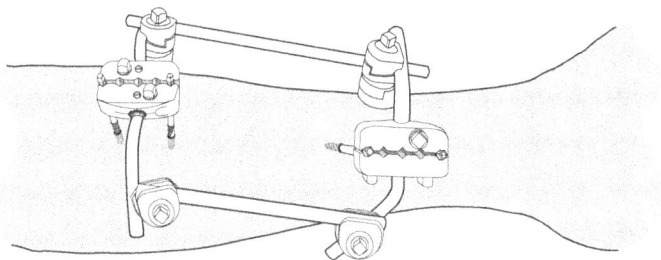

Fig. 23-23. Two-bar apparatus. As the majority of tibia fractures are unstable, it creates a more stable construct by adding a second bar. This requires the use of two of the kits but makes little difference when you are using the tub container at the CSH or equivalent hospitals.

o Check the distal vascular status of the limb prior to and after the procedure. If there is a vascular injury, refer to Chapter 27, Vascular Injuries.

o An assistant will be required to help apply the frame.

o General reduction maneuver should be longitudinal traction with slight (10°–15°) flexion at the knee.

o Pins are placed anterior medial on the proximal tibia and antero-lateral on the distal femur. Pin placement should be outside of the zone of injury, at least three fingerbreadths from a fracture site, and outside of the knee joint. At the distal femur, a longitudinal stab incision is made over the antero-lateral aspect of the bone, so that the pin may be inserted into the center of the bone at about a 45° angle from the horizontal. Depending on the fracture configuration, it may also be placed directly anteriorly, though it is generally better to avoid the quadriceps tendon.

o Blunt dissection is used to create a corridor to the bone.

o A single pin is inserted by hand through both cortices of the bone fragment.

o A multipin clamp is used as a guide for a second pin. The second pin **must** be parallel to the first and also bicortical — care should be taken to maintain pin alignment. The proximal tibia should be palpated on the anterior medial surface and the anterior and posterior border should be identified. Midway anterior/posterior, a 1-cm longitudinal stab incision should be made and a blunt soft tissue dissection made to bone.

o A multipin clamp should be used as a guide to insert a second pin in the proximal tibia.

o The two pin clusters (femur and tibia) should be connected via two elbows, two bar-bar clamps, and a single bar. The knee should be aligned.

o A second bar should be added in the manner described above.

● **Technique to span ankle.**
o An assistant will be required to help apply the frame and reduce the ankle.

o General indications are for open distal tibia fractures and open ankle wounds.

o Pins should be inserted on the anterior medial surface of the tibia and the medial aspect of the calcaneus.

o Check the distal vascular status prior to and after the procedure. Mark where the posterior tibial and dorsalis pedis artery pulses can be felt.

o Palpate the anterior medial border of the tibia. Make a 1-cm longitudinal incision midway between the anterior and posterior border of the tibia. Insert the most distal pin on the tibia outside the zone of injury, at least three fingerbreadths from the fracture site.

o Using a multipin clamp as a guide, insert a second pin in the tibia more proximal to the first. The pin **must** be parallel and be aligned in the longitudinal axis to the first.

o Palpate the medial border of the calcaneus. Make a longitudinal incision over the calcaneus **away from the posterior neurovascular structures**: dissect to the bone with a clamp and insert the pin.

o Using a multipin clamp as a guide, insert a second pin in the calcaneus.

o Connect the two clamps via two elbows, two bar–bar clamps, and a single bar.

- **Skeletal traction.**
    o Skeletal traction provides a quick means to immobilize a large number of fracture cases with a minimum of technical support.
    o Indications.
        ♦ Patients who are expected to have more than one procedure in the same forward hospital prior to evacuation.
        ♦ Large casualty load.
    o Technique.
        ♦ Large threaded Steinman pins are used to obtain skeletal traction of a femur or tibia.
        ♦ Aseptic preparation of a pin site is necessary prior to placement.
        ♦ Apply local anesthetic to pin site.

- ◆ Incise skin and dissect to bone bluntly.
- ◆ For femur fractures, incision is made 2 cm posterior and lateral to the tibial tuberosity (directly under, as in Fig. 23-24). Place pin from lateral to medial through and through the proximal tibia.
- ◆ Apply a Thomas splint with Pierson device, with weight applied midthigh (10–20 lb), to the leg (10–20 lb), and to the traction pin (20–40 lb) to obtain balanced skeletal traction as shown in Fig. 23-25.
- ◆ For tibia fractures, incise medially 2 cm anterior and 2 cm cephalad from the tip of the heel. Place the pin from medial to lateral through and through the calcaneus. Place the leg on a Bohler-Braun frame and apply traction to the calcaneal pin (10–20 lb).
- ◆ Wait at least $^1/_2$ hour after applying traction to obtain radiographs.

- **Care in the evacuation chain.**
  - o **Patients do not improve in the evacuation system.**

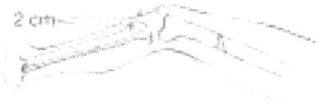

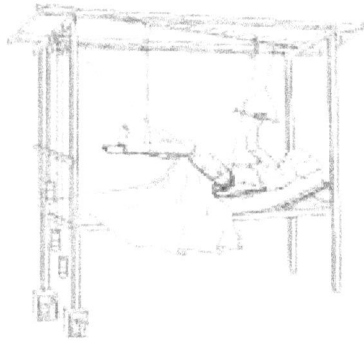

Fig. 23-24. Thomas splint with Pierson device.

Fig. 23-25. Bohler-Braun frame with traction.

Consider patient safety during evacuation when planning procedures.
- o Medications should be arranged prior to departure. **Ensure adequate pain control.**
- o Skeletal traction should **not** be used for transportation.

o Casts should be bivalved. Follow neurovascular status during transport because **casts may act as tourniquets due to tissue swelling**.
o All documentation, including radiographs, should accompany the patient.

Chapter 24

Open-Joint Injuries

Introduction

Open injuries to the joints are rarely immediately life threatening. They are frequently quite dramatic in appearance and draw the inexperienced caregiver's attention away from the truly life threatening, associated injuries. **Neurovascular structures are in close proximity to the major joints, and may require vascular management and repair.** Open joints have long-term morbidity and some secondary mortality from infection due to missed injury or inadequate treatment.

> **All open-joint injuries must be explored and treated within 6 hours to prevent infection and joint destruction.**

With rare exceptions, **closed**-joint injuries should be treated nonoperatively in the combat zone. Definitive intervention and rehabilitation usually require months before complete recovery. Thus, patients with closed injuries to major joints should be evacuated from the theater for definitive surgical intervention and rehabilitation.

> **The key to treating open-joint injures is <u>recognition</u>. Once identified, goals are prevention of infection and preservation/restoration of normal joint function.**

- Signs of possible open-joint injury are a wound associated with the following:
  o Proximity to a joint.
  o Periarticular fracture.
  o Exposed joint.
  o Effusion.

    o Loss of joint motion.
    o Intra-articular air or foreign body on biplanar radiographs.
    o Abnormal joint aspiration demonstrating hemarthrosis.
    o Extravasation from joint on diagnostic injection.

Open-joint injuries always require surgery. Joint aspiration/injection may be performed to confirm a suspected open joint. If in doubt, treat as an open-joint injury to prevent missed injury sequelae.

- The technique for aspiration / injection involves:
  - Sterile prep.
  - 18-gauge needle, 30-cc syringe.
  - Enter suspected joint, avoiding neurovascular structures.
  - Attempt aspiration — if blood is aspirated a hemarthrosis is present.
  - If no hemarthrosis, inject with normal saline (methylene blue if available) until joint is fully distended — the joint is damaged if extravasation is detected.
  - If there is no extravasation, open joint injury may still be present.
- Approaches for aspiration are shown for the shoulder, elbow (Lateral), knee (Medial parapatellar), and ankle (Antero-lateral) (Fig. 24-1a,b,c,d).

Treatment of All Open-Joint Injury
- IV antibiotics should be started ASAP after wounding, and continued postop for 48 hours.
- Tourniquet control of operative bleeding is essential.
- Standard arthrotomy incisions are utilized (Fig. 24-2a,b,c). (Wound margins are incorporated if possible, provided they do not compromise exposure or create non-viable flaps).
- The extremity must be draped free to allow full range of motion during surgery.
- All intra-articular foreign material, loose cartilage (including flaps), blood clots, and detached bony fragments without major articular surface must be removed.

Shoulder

Elbow

b

a

Ankle

Knee

d

c

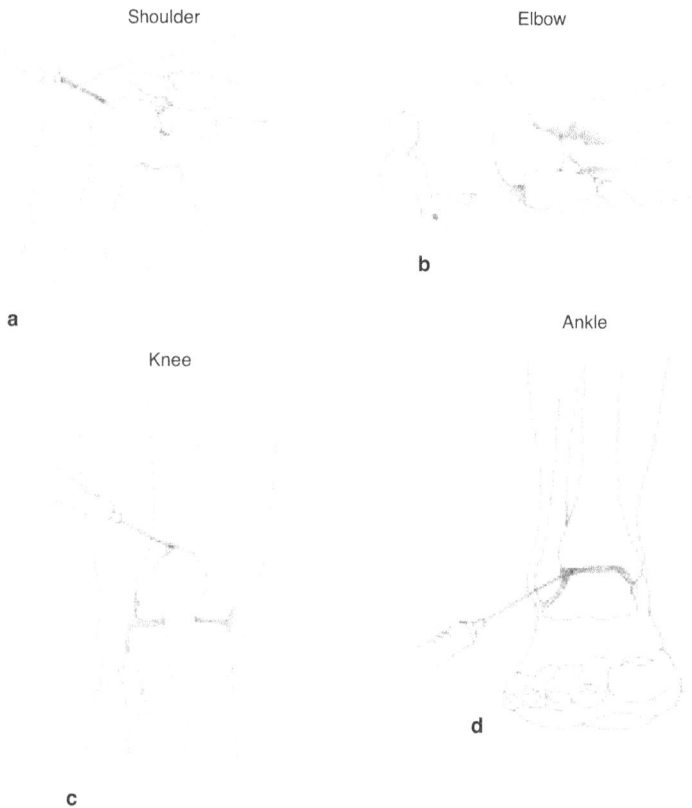

Fig. 24-1a,b,c,d. Aspiration/injection approaches to the shoulder, elbow, knee, and ankle.

- All recesses must be explored and all damaged tissue must be removed.
- The joint must be thoroughly irrigated with normal saline (pulse lavage and 6 to 9 L is recommended).
- Internal fixation is **contraindicated** with the **exception of large articular fragments** that may be stabilized with Kirscher wire (K-wire) or Steinmann pins.

Ankle   Elbow

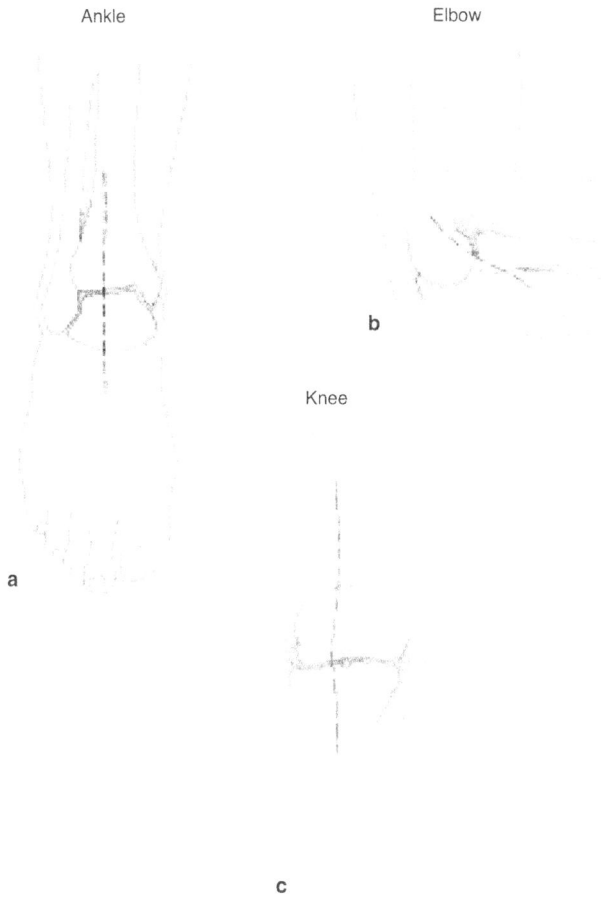

b

Knee

a

c

Fig. 24-2a,b,c. Surgical approaches to the ankle, elbow, and knee.

- Close synovium if possible without tension and without surgical tissue advancement. **The remainder of the wound should <u>never</u> be closed at the initial surgical exploration.**
- If synovial closure is not possible, the joint should be dressed open with moist fine mesh gauze occlusive dressing.
- The wound should be reexplored in 48–72 hours.
- A bivalved cast or splints can be used to stabilize the joint.

- If there are delays in evacuation or inability to move the patient, the following steps can be taken:
  - o Delayed primary closure (DPC) can be undertaken in 4–7 days if there are no signs of infection.
  - o If there is extensive soft-tissue loss, split-thickness skin grafts may be applied to granulating synovium.
- After DPC, gentle range-of-motion therapy is begun, based on consideration of any associated fractures or neurovascular injuries.

> **Any time joint infection is suspected, the joint should be <u>immediately</u> explored/re-explored.**

Signs of Joint Sepsis
- Persistent swelling.
- Marked pain.
- Local warmth.
- Fever.
- **Intense pain with restriction of the range of motion.**

Special Considerations for Hip Wounds
- Open injuries of the hip joint are problematic for several reasons.
  - o Difficulty in diagnosis.
  - o Highly virulent organisms leading to mortality or long-term morbidity.
- Violations of the hollow viscus organs associated with fractures that extend into the acetabulum or femoral neck uniformly contaminate the joint.
  - o Ruling out joint involvement is difficult in the field environment due to poor radiographic support and difficulty in reliable joint aspiration/injection. Therefore, a high index of suspicion with a low threshold for joint exploration is essential for preventing devastating complications.
- Presacral drainage is highly encouraged in rectal injury with joint extension.

Hip Exploration Technique

- Semilateral or lateral decubitus position, with the abdomen, pelvis, and full lower extremity prepped and draped free.
- A tibial traction pin to suspend the leg from the ceiling is advantageous.
- Anterior iliofemoral (Fig. 24-3a,b,c) approach gives the most extensive exposure to the hip, acetabulum, and ilium. (If the incision was extended superior and posterior, closure of the

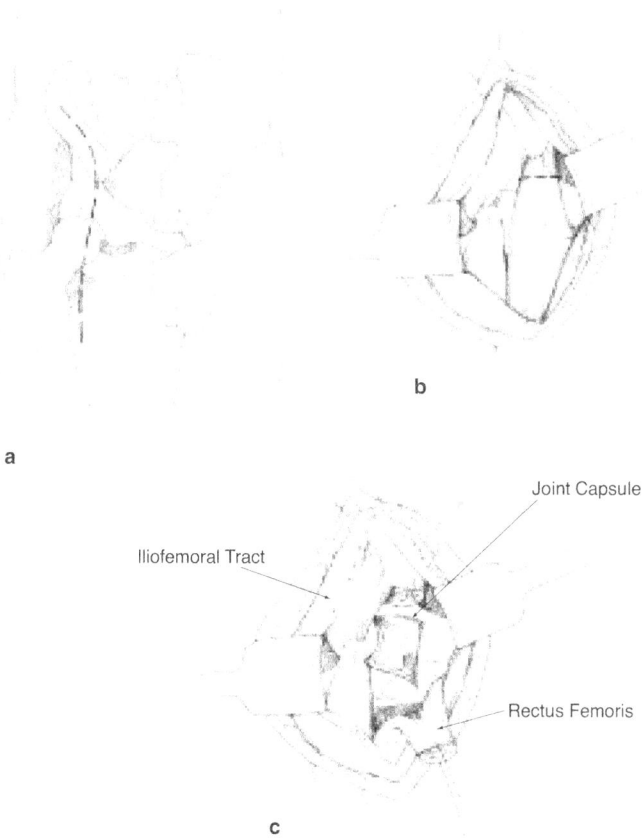

a

b

Joint Capsule

Iliofemoral Tract

Rectus Femoris

c

Fig. 24-3a,b,c. Anterior iliofemoral approach to the hip.

superior/posterior aspect of the incision only over the iliac crest is necessary at the initial surgery to prevent muscle retraction and subsequent inability to close the wound.)

- A posterior or Kocher approach (Fig. 24-4a,b) allows for posterior exposure and allows for posterior drainage. It may be used in conjunction with the iliofemoral approach or in select cases alone for debridement. In an echeloned care/delayed evacuation scenario, dependent posterior drainage may be more critical than currently practiced in the civilian environment.

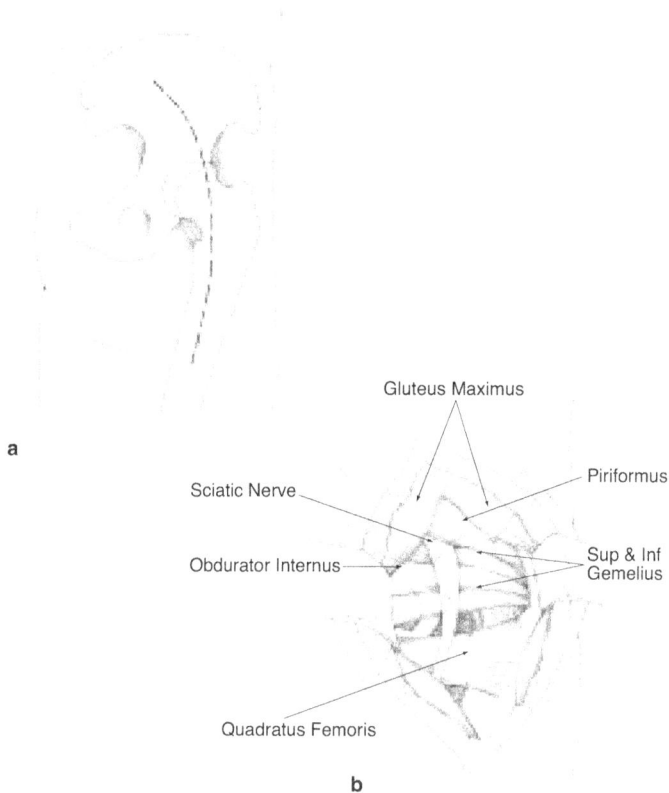

Fig. 24-4a,b. Posterior approach to the hip.

- Complete fractures of the femoral neck/head should be resected due to nearly uniform complications of sepsis and avascular necrosis.
- Except as described above, the surgical incision is not closed. Dressing of the wound is as previously described. The patient may be placed in a spanning external fixator from the iliac crest to the distal femur, or placed in a one and one-half hip spica cast. (See Chapter 23, Extremity Fractures, for diagram.)

Special Considerations for the Shoulder
- Often associated with life-threatening thoracic or vascular injuries. See Chapter 27, Vascular Injuries, for approaches to the axillary and subclavian arteries.
- Technique for shoulder exploration:
  - Semilateral position will allow both anterior and posterior approaches to the glenohumeral joint.
  - Anterior deltopectoral approach is recommended (Fig. 24-5a,b,c,d). (Detachment of the short biceps, coracobrachialis, and pectoralis minor off the coracoid may be needed for adequate exposure.) The subscapularis is detached and the joint capsule is trimmed of devitalized tissue. All attempts are made to preserve the supraspinatus attachment.
  - Loose fragments or a completely devitalized humeral head are resected to prevent infection. In an echeloned care/delayed evacuation scenario, dependent posterior shoulder drainage may be more critical than currently practiced in the civilian environment.
  - At the time of the DPC, 4–7 days later, the infraspinatus and teres minor are reattached if previously detached.
  - A Velpeau dressing is utilized for the wounds.
  - For transport, the shoulder can be wrapped in plaster, suspending the cast from the opposite shoulder for comfort. If this is not feasible, a sling and swath, immobilizing the arm against the chest wall, may be used. These patients will require litter transport.

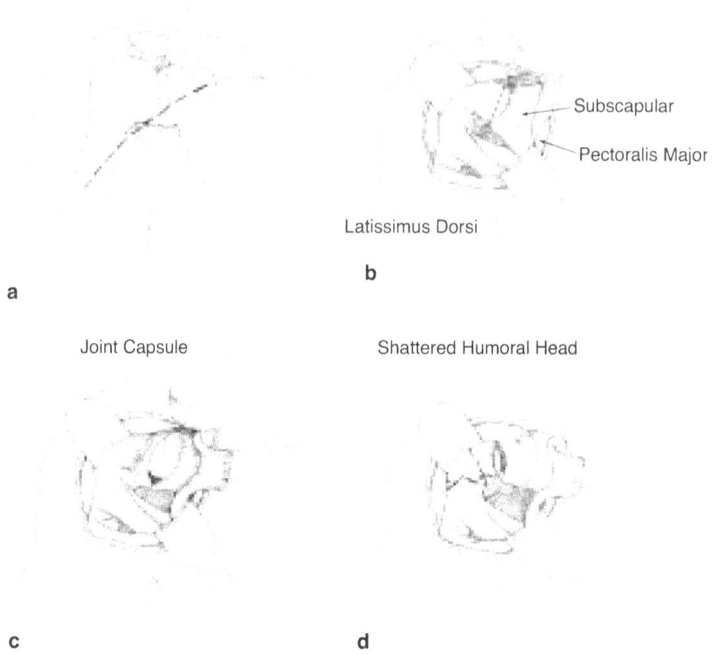

a

b

Subscapular

Pectoralis Major

Latissimus Dorsi

Joint Capsule

Shattered Humoral Head

c

d

Fig. 24-5a,b,c,d. Anterior deltopectoral approach to the shoulder.

The key to success in dealing with open joints is a high index of suspicion. If the joint is open, then aggressive surgical management is imperative.

Chapter 25

Amputations

Introduction
Battle casualties who sustain amputations have the most severe extremity injuries.

- Historically, one in three patients with a major amputation (proximal to the wrist or ankle) will die, usually of exsanguination.
- Though amputations are visually dramatic, attention must be focused on the frequently associated life-threatening injuries.

Goals for initial care are to preserve life, prepare the patient for evacuation, and leave the maximum number of options for definitive treatment.

- The following are indications for amputation.
    - o Partial or complete traumatic amputation.
    - o Irreparable vascular injury or failed vascular repair with an ischemic limb.
    - o Life-threatening sepsis due to severe local infection, including clostridial myonecrosis.
    - o Severe soft-tissue and bony injury to the extremity precluding functional recovery.

The surgeon must balance the realistic likelihood of ultimate reconstruction of a functional extremity against the risk of death associated with attempts to preserve a limb. It is always desirable to secure the opinion of a second surgeon before amputating. The tactical situation may require amputation in cases where the limb might otherwise have been preserved.

- Battlefield amputations are unique.
  - Most commonly due to explosive munitions, with penetration and blast effects (see Chapter 1, Weapons Effects and Parachute Injuries).
  - Involve a large zone of injury with a high degree of contamination, which may affect the level of amputation and/or surgical intervention.
  - Require staged treatment with evacuation out of the combat zone prior to definitive closure.

Amputations should be performed at the <u>lowest viable level of soft tissues</u>, in contrast to traditional anatomic amputation levels (eg, classic above knee (AK), below knee (BK), and so forth), to preserve as much limb as possible. A longer stump is desirable for final prosthetic fitting.

- The Open **Length Preserving Amputation** (formerly Open Circular Amputation) procedure has two stages.
  - **Initial**. Complete the amputation at lowest possible level of bone and prepare the patient for evacuation to the next level of care.
  - **Reconstructive**. Involves final healing of the limb to obtain the optimal prosthetic stump.
  - **Final level of amputation and definitive treatment of the residual limb should occur in the stable environment of a CONUS hospital, <u>not in the combat zone hospital</u>**.

  - All viable skin and soft tissues distal to the indicated level of bone amputation should be preserved for use in subsequent closure of the amputation stump. These tissues may be considered "Flaps of Opportunity" and can add length to the stump. This is especially true for amputations below the knee. Short tibial stumps can be saved with posteriorly based flaps because the gastrocsoleus is frequently preserved following landmine injury. To save length, any shape or form of a viable muscle or skin flap should be preserved. The lowest level may be an oblique or irregular wound, creating an oblique or irregular residual limb.

Technique of Amputation

- Surgical preparation of the **entire** limb, because planes of injury may be much higher than initially evident.
- Tourniquet control is mandatory. If a tourniquet was placed in the prehospital setting for hemorrhage control, it is prepped entirely within the surgical field.
- Excise nonviable tissue.
  - o Necrotic skin and subcutaneous tissue or skin without vascular support.
  - o Muscle that is friable, shredded, grossly contaminated, or noncontractile. (This muscle is usually at the level of the retracted skin.)
  - o Bone that is grossly contaminated or devoid of soft tissue support. Bone is transected at a level at which it has the potential for coverage. (This is usually at the level of the retracted muscle.)
- Identify and securely ligate major arteries and veins to prevent hemorrhage in transport.
- Identify nerves, apply gentle traction, and resect proximally to allow for retraction under soft tissue. Ligate the major nerves.
- Preserved muscle flaps should not be sutured, but should be held in their intended position by the dressing.
- Flaps should not be constructed at the initial surgery, to facilitate later closure.

In blast injuries, particularly landmine injuries, the blast forces drive debris proximally along fascial planes. It may be necessary to extend incisions proximally parallel to the axis of the extremity to ensure adequate surgical decontamination of the wound.

The stump is never closed primarily.

- **Special considerations**.
  - o Primary Symes (ankle disarticulation) has a high failure rate due to heel pad necrosis during transport. The wound should simply be debrided, retaining the clean hindfoot (talus and calcaneus).
  - o Primary knee disarticulation is problematic due to skin and tendon retraction necessitating reamputation at a higher less functional level. It is preferable to leave even a very short (1–2 cm) clean transtibial stump, even though nonfunctional, to prevent retraction.
  - o Fractures, when present proximal to the mangled segment, should not determine amputation level, but must be treated appropriately (cast, external fixator) to preserve maximal length.
  - o Plan the initial amputation solely on the qualities of the wound and surrounding tissues, never on the hope of achieving a particular level or flap pattern as a final result. The combat surgeon's goal is a thorough and complete debridement. Trying to preserve marginal tissue in the hope that a better stump can be constructed may lead to subsequent infection and a higher amputation level.

Dressings and Prevention of Skin Retraction

Since amputations must be left open, skin retraction is likely, causing the loss of usable limb length by making definitive closure difficult. This is particularly true of a patient who is the evacuation chain. Because of this, patients who will be evacuated should be placed in skin traction in order to leave the wound open and prevent skin retraction. Surgeons working for the International Committee of the Red Cross (ICRC) in a stable environment have successfully treated refugees by delayed primary closure. However, ICRC surgeons work in a relatively stable environment where evacuation is not a consideration for the refugee population. This situation does not apply to those in the air evacuation system.

Skin Traction

Ideally, skin traction should be maintained throughout the course of treatment. If evacuation times are reliably very short

(1–3 days), skin traction may be omitted. If there is the possibility of any delay, use skin traction to preserve limb length. When tactical conditions or resources are not available for application of casts, skin traction may be applied through weights off the end of the bed before and after transport.

o Dry fine mesh gauze is loosely placed over the open wound. Preserved flaps are not suspended freely, but are held in their intended position by the dressing (Fig. 25-1).

o Absorbent dressing is placed over the stump.

o Tincture of benzoin is applied proximally on the skin up to 2 cm from the wound edge, but not including the preserved flap.

o A stockinette for skin traction is applied.

o Wrap stockinette with a figure-of-8 elastic wrap.

o Two to six pounds of traction is applied through the stockinette/wrap. This may simply involve a weight attached via parachute cord to the stockinette. However, during transport, hanging weights are problematic

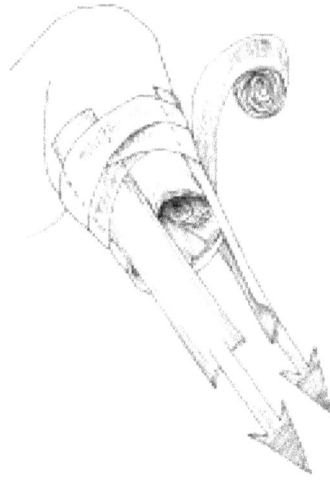

Fig. 25-1. Skin Tractions

and may be substituted with a light elastic such as surgical tubing or elastic exercise tubing applied through a transportation cast described below.

o A transportation cast should be applied to prevent contracture and allow for continuous traction (Fig. 25-2).

Postoperative Management
● Prevention of contracture.
  o BK amputations are at risk for knee flexion contractures. These contractures are preventable by using a long leg cast.

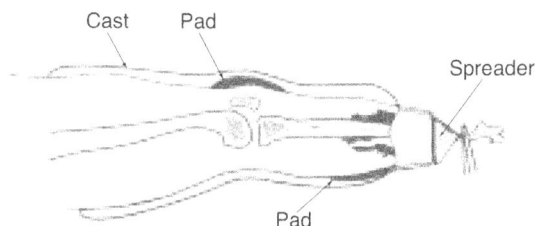

Fig. 25-2. Transportation cast allows for continuous traction.

Splinting in extension requires closer monitoring. Pillows should never support the knee, because of the increased risk of flexion contractures.

o AK amputations are at risk for hip-flexion contractures. Prone positioning and active hip extension exercises will avoid this complication. When the casualty is supine, sandbags may be applied to the anterior distal thigh as well.

● Prevention of hemorrhage: A tourniquet should be readily available at the bedside or during transport for the first week following injury.

● Pain control: Patient comfort is paramount following amputation, particularly if dressing changes are required. Adequate analgesia should be available and the patient should be counseled regarding phantom limb pain.

Transportation Casts
Prior to evacuation, transportation casts should be applied to maintain traction of the residual limb and support the soft tissues. The transportation cast is a well-padded cast that has integral skin traction maintained by use of an outrigger.

Cast Application Techniques
Low Hip Spica cast
● Indications: Transfemoral amputation.
● Technique.
   o Adequate anesthesia is administered and the patient is placed on the fracture table.

o Nonviable tissue is excised, as indicated above.
o Stockinette or Webril is applied over lower abdomen and thigh on side of amputation. Stockinette should already be applied for skin traction.
o Felt padding is placed over sacrum and anterior superior iliac spine (ASIS).
o Towel is placed over abdomen to allow breathing space.
o Six-inch Webril or similar cotton batting is wrapped in 1–2 layers (Fig. 25-3).
o Six-inch plaster is then rolled over the Webril from the ASIS to the end of the residual limb on the affected side. Splints are applied over the posterior, lateral, and groin areas. Use a finishing roll after turning down the edges of the stockinette to give it a neat appearance.
o Prior to the last roll, a Cramer wire splint should be attached over the distal end of the cast to provide skin traction via the stockinette.
o An adequate perineal space must be left for hygiene.
o The towel should be removed, the cast bivalved, and a circular area over the abdomen should be cut out.
o Use an indelible marker to label the cast with the date of injury and surgery(ies).

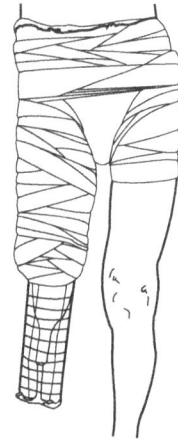

Fig. 25-3. Low hip spica cast.

- Indications: Transtibial amputations.
- Technique.
  o Adequate anesthesia is provided. The wound is evaluated, nonviable is tissue excised, and the wound is irrigated.
  o Stockinette is applied to the distal end of the residual limb with tincture of Benzoin to maintain skin traction.
  o Two to three layers of Webril are applied from the amputation to the proximal thigh.
  o A six-inch plaster is then rolled over the thigh and leg.
  o Prior to application of the last layer, a Cramer wire splint should be incorporated over the distal end of the residual limb. Apply skin traction when the cast is dry.

    o Bivalve the cast.
    o Label the cast with dates of injury and surgery(ies).

Shoulder Spica Cast
- Indications: Transhumeral amputation.
- Technique.
  - o Administer adequate anesthesia.
  - o Irrigate wound and excise nonviable tissue.
  - o Apply stockinette to axilla for skin traction applied with tincture of Benzoin.
  - o Wrap Webril over chest wall and around to edge of residual limb.
  - o Apply 4–6 in. plaster over the Webril.
  - o A Cramer wire splint outrigger should be applied with the last roll to allow for connection of the stockinette and application of skin traction.
  - o Label the cast with dates of injury and surgery(ies).

Long Arm Cast
- Indications: Transradial amputation.
- Technique.
  - o Administer adequate anesthesia.
  - o After treatment of open wounds and application of a dressing, apply a stockinette over the distal edge of the residual limb.
  - o Apply 4-inch Webril from the residual limb to the axilla.
  - o Apply 4-inch plaster from the residual limb to the axilla.
  - o Use plaster to incorporate a Cramer wire splint over the distal edge of the residual limb to be able to in order to apply skin traction.
  - o Bivalve the cast.
  - o Label the cast with dates of injury and surgery(ies).

Chapter 26

Injuries to the Hands and Feet

Introduction

Combat injuries to the hands and feet differ from those of the arms and legs in terms of mortality and morbidity. Death is rare, but a minor wound, causing no lasting impairment if inflicted, for example, on the thigh, can result in life-long disability when it occurs in a hand or foot. The hands and feet have an important commonality: an intricate combination of many small structures that must function smoothly together.

Types of Injury

- Nonbattle injuries resulting in laceration of the hands and crush injuries involving either the hands or feet are common. Such crush injuries may result in compartment syndrome.
- Missile and blast injuries involving the hands and feet are common in combat and may result in mutilating injuries with a permanent loss of function.

The Hand

> Even apparently minor wounds distal to the wrist crease may violate tendon sheaths and joints, resulting in a serious deep space infection. Such wounds require a high index of suspicion for injury and a low threshold for operative exploration.

Evaluation and Initial Management

- The casualty's upper extremities should be exposed.
- Rings, watches, and other constrictive material must be removed immediately.

- A preliminary neurologic exam should be performed and documented.
- Vascular status of the hand should include an assessment of radial and ulnar arteries (Allen test, Doppler, among others).

Treatment of Hand Compartment Syndrome
- The hand has 10 separate fascial compartments (4 dorsal interossei, 3 volar interossei, the thenar muscles, the hypothenar muscles, and the adductor pollicis [Fig. 26-1]).

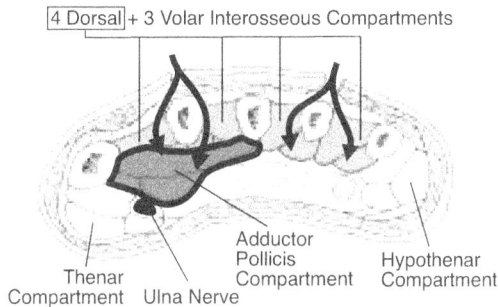

Fig. 26-1. Compartments of the hand.

- A complete hand fasciotomy consists of four incisions (shown in Fig. 26-2).
- One incision on the radial side of the thumb metacarpal releases the thenar compartment.
- A dorsal incision over the index finger metacarpal is used to release the 1st and 2nd dorsal interossei, and to reach ulnar-to-index finger metacarpal and to release the volar interossei and adductor pollicis.

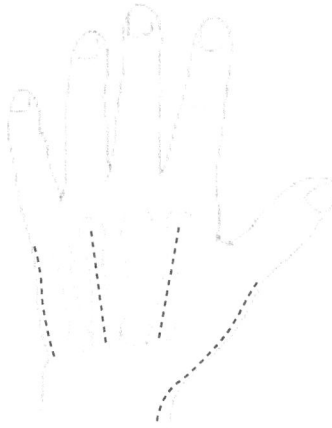

Fig. 26-2. Hand fasciotomy incisions.

26.2

- A dorsal incision over the ring finger metacarpal is used to release the 3rd and 4th dorsal interossei, and to reach down along the radial aspect of the ring finger and small finger metatarsal to release the volar interossei.
- An incision is placed at the ulnar aspect of the small finger to release the hypothenar muscles.
- Although compartments are not well defined in the fingers, grossly edematous fingers may require release of dermal and fascial constriction; care should be taken to place the skin incision away from the neurovascular bundles (Fig. 26-3).

Fig. 26-3. Incisions for finger fasciotomy.

Surgical Technique

Do not blindly clamp bleeding tissues because nearby nerves may be injured. If unable to control the bleeding with pressure, isolate the vessel under tourniquet control and tie off or clamp under direct vision.

- General or regional (block) anesthetic is required; local infiltration of anesthetic is inadequate. Epinephrine is never injected into the hands or fingers.
- Although either the radial or ulnar artery may be ligated, both should not.
- Thorough exploration under tourniquet down to normal tissue is mandatory to define the extent of the injury.
- Debridement removes buried foreign matter and deep devitalized tissue.
  - o Dead tissue is removed.
  - o Tissue, including skin, with marginal or questionable viability is left for subsequent evaluation to improve chances for optimal outcome.
- The fingers are not amputated unless irretrievably mangled.

- Viable tissue, even though nonfunctional, is retained and stabilized for later reconstruction.
- Provisional stabilization of fractures with Kirscher wires (K-wires) may enhance patient comfort and later management.

Specific Tissue Management

- **Bone:** Unless extruding from the body or severely contaminated, fragments should be left in place. At forward hospitals, only small K-wires should be used for internal fixation.
- **Tendon:** Minimal excision of tendons should occur. No attempt at repair should be made in the field.
- **Nerve:** Do not excise nerve tissue. No attempt at repair should be made in the field.
- The ends of lacerated nerves and tendons may be tagged with 4-0 suture so that they may be more easily identified later during definitive reconstruction and repair.

> Closure of wounds is delayed; however, exposed tendon, bone, and joint should be covered with viable skin, if possible, to prevent desiccation.

Dressing and Splinting

> Splint the hand in the safe position (Fig. 26-4). The wrist is extended 20°, the metacarpalphangeal joints are flexed 70°–90° and the fingers (proximal and distal interphangeal joints) are in full extension.

- Fine mesh gauze is first laid on the wounds and covered with a generous layer of fluffed gauze.
- The entire wound should be covered but the fingertips left exposed, if possible, to evaluate perfusion.

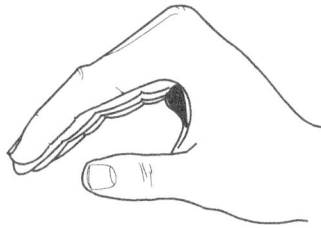

Fig. 26-4. Hand splint position.

- A splint is applied, immobilizing all injured parts and extending one bone or joint beyond. A palmar plaster slab is routine, but a dorsal one may be added for additional stability.

The Foot

Penetrating injuries of the foot frequently result in prolonged morbidity and disability. Crush injuries and injuries from blast are more likely to result in an unsatisfactory result than are wounds made by low-velocity bullets or isolated fragments. This is especially true when there is loss of the heel-pad, significant neurovascular injury or when the deep plantar space has been contaminated. The ultimate goal of treatment of these injuries is a relatively pain free, plantigrade foot with intact plantar sensation.

Evaluation and Initial Management

- The zone of injury with both open and closed injuries of the foot is often more extensive than is apparent with the initial inspection.
- The vascular status of the foot should be assessed by palpation of the dorsalis pedis and posterior tibial pulses. An assessment of capillary refill in the toes should also be made as a compartment syndrome of the foot can coexist with intact pulses.
- Anesthesia of the plantar aspect of the foot indicates an injury to the posterior tibial nerve or one of its major branches and portends a poor prognosis for a satisfactory outcome.
- Compartment syndrome of the foot can occur even in the presence of an open foot injury, and when identified, requires emergency treatment.
- At the time of debridement, small, contaminated bone fragments without soft tissue attachment should be removed.
- High-volume irrigation for all open wounds is mandatory.

> **All wounds should be left open.**

Injuries to the Hindfoot
- Severely comminuted, open fractures of the talus may require talectomy, but this decision should be left to higher levels of care.
- The talus is best debrided through an anterolateral approach to the ankle extended to the base of the 4th metatarsal.
- Penetrating wounds into the plantar aspect of the heel pad can be approached through a heel-splitting incision to avoid excessive undermining of this specialized skin.
- Transverse gunshot wounds of the hindfoot are best managed by medial and lateral incisions with the majority of surgery performed laterally to avoid medial neurovascular structure.

Injuries to the Midfoot
- Tarsal and metatarsals are best approached through dorsal longitudinal incisions. In addition, compartment release can be adequately performed through longitudinal incisions medial to the 2nd metatarsal and lateral to the 4th metatarsal in order to leave a wide skin bridge.
- Contamination of the deep plantar compartments of the foot is best managed through a plantar medial incision that begins 1 inch proximal and 1 inch posterior to the medial malleolus and extends across the medial arch ending on the plantar surface between the 2nd and 3rd metatarsal heads. The medial neurovascular structures must be identified during this approach. A full compartment release can also be performed through this incision.

Injuries to the Toes
- Even effort should be made to preserve the great toe.
- Amputation of the lateral toes is generally well-tolerated.

Foot Compartment Syndrome
- There are 5 compartments in the foot.
  o The interosseous compartment is bounded by the lateral 1st metatarsal medially, metatarsals and dorsal interossous fascia dorsally, and the plantar interosseous fascia plantarly.

o The lateral compartment is bounded by the 5th metatarsal shaft dorsally, the plantar aponeurosis laterally, and the intermuscular septum medially.

o The central compartment is bounded by the intramuscular septum laterally and medially, the interosseous fascia dorsally, and the plantar aponeurosis plantarly.

o The medial compartment is bounded by the inferior surface of the 1st metatarsal dorsally, the plantar aponeurosis extension medially, and the intramuscular septum laterally.

o The calcaneal compartment contains the quadratus plantae muscle.

- The foot may be released through a double dorsal incision.
- One incision placed slightly medial to the 2nd metatarsal, reaching between the 1st and 2nd metatarsals into the medial compartment, and between the 2nd and 3rd metatarsals, into the central compartment (Fig. 26-5).
- A second dorsal incision is made just lateral to 4th metatarsal, reaching between 4th and 5th metatarsals into the lateral compartment.
- To spare the dorsal soft tissue, a single incision medial fasciotomy may be used.

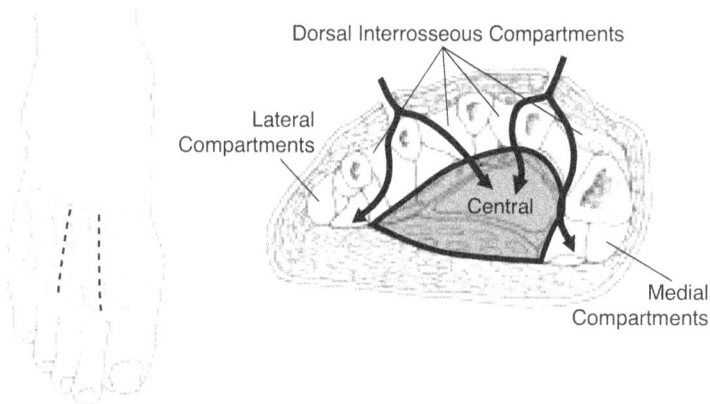

Dorsal Interrosseous Compartments

Lateral Compartments

Central

Medial Compartments

Fig. 26-5. Interosseous compartment releases through two dorsal incisions.

- A medial approach to the foot is made through the medial compartment, reaching across the central compartment into the interosseous compartment dorsally and lateral compartment releasing all the away across the foot (see description in this chapter's Injuries to the Midfoot and Fig. 26-6).
- Fasciotomy wound management.
  - o Following the fasciotomy, the fasciotomy wound undergoes primary surgical wound management; all devitalized tissue is removed.
  - o As with all battle wounds, the fasciotomy is left open and is covered with a sterile dressing.

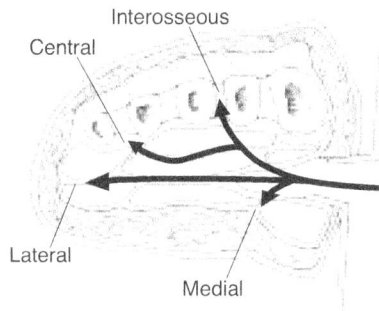

Fig. 26-6. Central compartment releases through medial approach.

Stabilization
- K-wires can be utilized for temporary stabilization.
- A bivalved cast or splint is adequate for transport to a site of more definitive care.

Chapter 27

Vascular Injuries

Introduction
- History.
  - o World War II: Popliteal artery injuries were routinely ligated with a 73% amputation rate.
  - o Korean War: Formal repair of peripheral arterial injuries instituted.
  - o Vietnam War: Further refinements in arterial repair; amputation rate for popliteal artery injuries is reduced to 32%.
- There are various types of wounds seen in combat.
  - o Low-velocity missile damages a blood vessel lying directly in its path.
  - o High-velocity missile blast effect causes fragmentation of the missile or bone and widespread destruction, including vascular injury at a distance.
  - o Blunt trauma, often resulting from sudden deceleration in motor vehicle accidents, falls, rail and air disasters.
  - o Popliteal artery injury associated with posterior knee dislocations.

Evaluation and Diagnosis
- Physical examination — detailed examination is paramount.
  - o **Hard signs of arterial injury** (pulsatile external bleeding, enlarging hematoma, absent distal pulses, a thrill/bruit, or ischemic limb) should lead to **immediate surgical exploration, without further preoperative studies**.
    - ♦ The 6 Ps of acute ischemia are: pain, pallor, pulselessness, poikilothermia, paresthesia, and paralysis.
    - ♦ Degree of injury and adequacy of collateral flow will determine the severity of distal ischemia. **Remember: Warm ischemia of striated muscle for > 4–6 hours will likely lead to myonecrosis and major amputation**.

- ◆ Falsely attributing loss of pulse, diminished pulse, or asymmetry of pulses to arterial spasm may cause delay in detection/repair of limb-threatening arterial injury.
- ◆ Distal pulses may be intact in up to 20% of patients with arterial injuries.
  - o **Soft signs** of arterial injury that require additional diagnostic evaluation include proximity of wound to major vessels, history of hemorrhage/shock, nonexpanding hematoma, diminished pulse, and anatomically related nerve injury.
- Doppler examination.
  - o A patient with penetrating or blunt trauma who has a normal distal pulse exam and ankle-brachial index (ABI) ≥ 1.0 does not require arteriography.
  - o In the patient without a palpable pulse distal to the injury, perform a Doppler examination and an ABI. ABI < 0.9 or a difference in ABI between extremities of > 0.1 indicate an arterial injury until proven otherwise. Because of extensive collateral flow, injuries to the deep femoral or deep brachial artery are not ruled out by this technique.
- Duplex ultrasound (US).
  - o Color flow duplex ultrasonography has demonstrated high sensitivity and specificity for detecting arterial injuries. It is noninvasive, portable, and painless, and repeated exams are easily performed.
  - o Duplex is highly operator-dependent and may fail to detect all arterial injuries (eg, deep femoral or tibial injuries).
- Contrast angiography.
  - o Precise localization of vascular injury is useful in patients with multiple pellet wounds (eg, shotgun blast), fractures, and penetrating injuries to the neck and thoracic outlet.
  - o Consider with high-velocity wounds, where arterial injury may occur outside the path of the missile, or in the presence of soft signs of arterial injury.
  - o Consider as routine for knee dislocations where occult arterial injuries may occur, and undetected delayed popliteal artery thrombosis may lead to major amputation.

Management Aspects
- Initial management.
    - o **Control external bleeding immediately!** Blind or imprecise placement of vascular clamps in a bloody field is discouraged. Direct pressure to the bleeding wound is preferable; **temporary tourniquet (BP cuff)** placed proximal to the injury site and inflated above systolic blood pressure may be useful.
    - o Administer IV antibiotics, tetanus toxoid, and analgesia.
    - o **In most long-bone fractures**, resuscitation and fracture alignment will restore distal flow.
    - o **Indications for operation for a suspected vascular injury:**
        - ◆ Hard signs as discussed above.
        - ◆ Soft signs confirmed by duplex US and/or angiography.
- Operative management.
    - o Preparation and draping of injured extremity as well as contralateral uninjured lower or upper extremity in case repair requires autogenous vein graft.
    - o Surgical approaches to the femoral popliteal, and brachial arteries are shown in Figures 27-1–Figure 27-5.

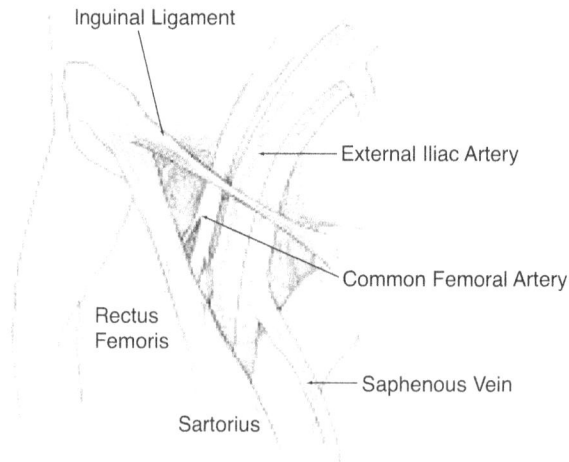

Fig. 27-1. Inguinal anatomy.

a

b

Vastus Medialis

Adductor Magnus

Medial Head
Gastrocnemius

Sartorius

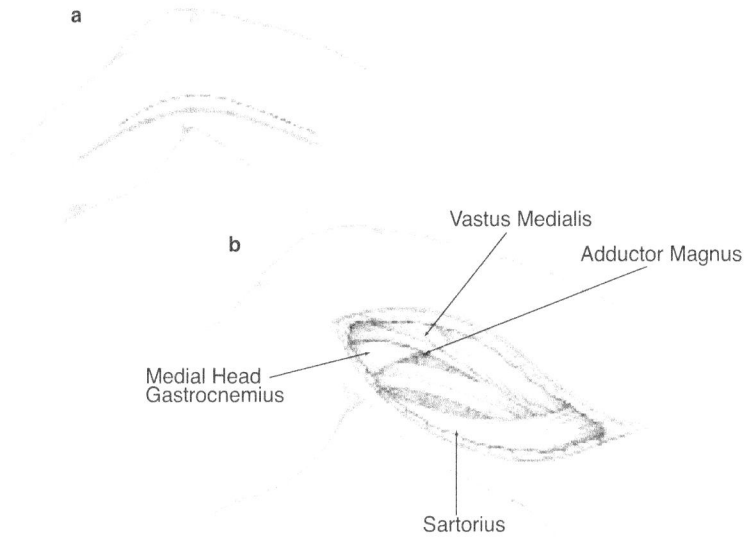

Fig. 27-2. Exposure of distal femoral and popliteal vessels.

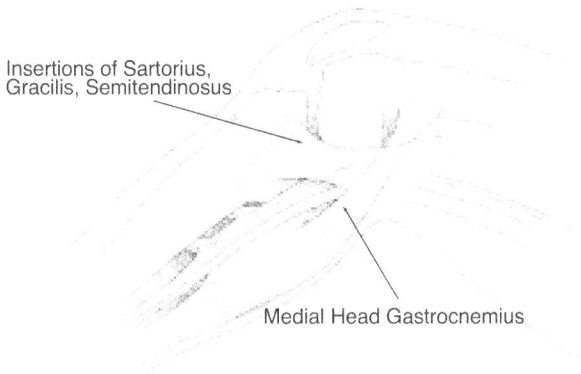

Insertions of Sartorius,
Gracilis, Semitendinosus

Medial Head Gastrocnemius

Fig. 27-3. Medial approach to popliteal vessels.

27.4

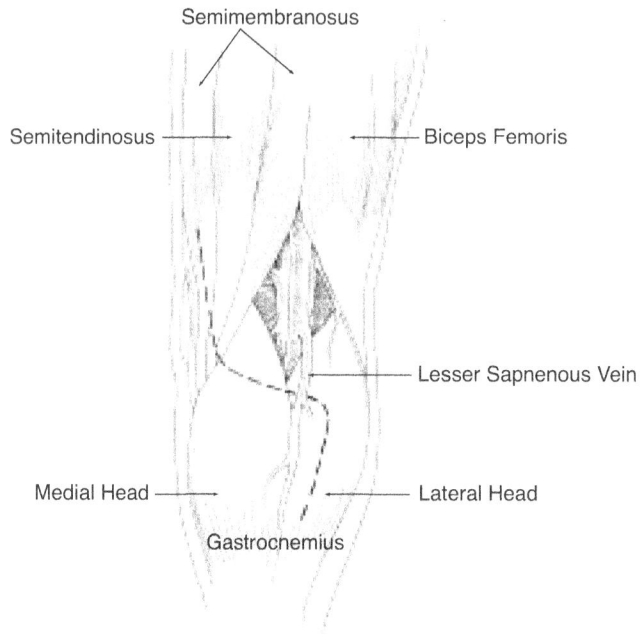

Fig. 27-4. Posterior approach to popliteal vessels.

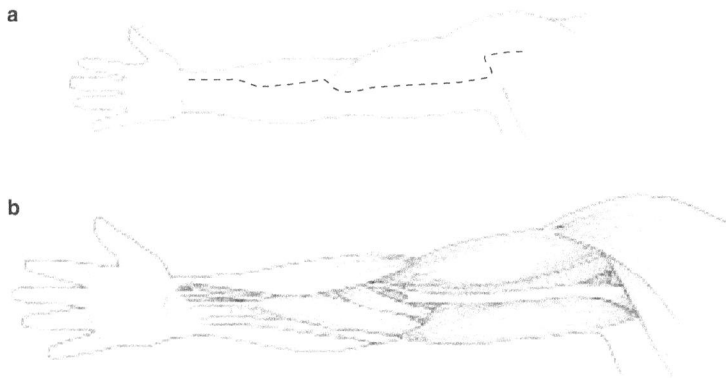

Fig. 27-5. Exposure of brachial and radial arteries.

o Longitudinal incisions usually directly over injured vessel followed by **proximal and distal control**. A tourniquet (eg, blood pressure cuff) may occasionally be useful to obtain proximal control or to improve intraoperative visualization.
o **Once control is obtained, perform the following steps:**
  ♦ Debride injured vessels to macroscopically normal wall.
  ♦ Pass balloon catheters proximal and distal to remove any residual thrombus.
  ♦ Flush both directions with heparinized saline.
o Consider temporary intraluminal shunting.
  ♦ Successful shunt placement allows ample time for wound debridement and copious irrigation, identification of nerve injuries, and careful consideration of reconstruction vs primary amputation.
- **Shunt placement technique.**
  o Proximal and distal vessel control with Silastic vessel loops or Rumel tourniquet.
  o Release proximal control to flush clot and place Argyle shunt.
  o Distal thrombectomy (Fogarty catheter) until no clot is returned.
  o Instill heparinized saline (20 U/mL) into distal vessel.
  o Place shunt into distal end and secure.
  o Check for distal pulse/perfusion.
- In injuries to **both artery and vein** in which no shunt is used, **repair artery first** to minimize ischemic time, followed by venous repair.
- **Suture:** 5-0 or 6-0 Prolene; 7-0 Prolene for small arteries. All completed repairs must be tension free.
- Upon completion, forward and back bleed repaired segment until clear of air and debris prior to final closure.
- **Type of repair** will depend on the extent of injury.
  o **Lateral suture repair**: Required for minimal injuries that, when repaired, will not compromise the lumen > 25%, result in a thrill, nor decrease pulse or Doppler signal.
  o **Patch angioplasty:** Needed for larger, tangential wounds; to prevent stenosis.
  o **End-to-end anastomosis:** Excise extensively damaged segments and perform anastomosis if able to mobilize ends (generally, < 2 cm gap) without tension. An oblique anastomosis is less likely to stenose.

o **Interposition graft:** Required if the vessel cannot be primarily repaired without undue tension.

♦ **Autogenous vein** grafts preferred, usually the contralateral greater saphenous vein (GSV).

◊ Harvest vein from the contralateral limb, if possible. The reason for this is in the injured limb, superficial veins may be an important source of venous outflow if deep veins are injured.

◊ Order of preference vein harvest for arterial conduit is contralateral GSV, ipsilateral GSV (if no concomitant deep venous injury), contralateral lesser saphenous vein (LSV), ipsilateral LSV (if no deep venous injury), cephalic vein, and basilic vein.

♦ **Prosthetic** grafts may be required when autogenous vein is inadequate or unavailable, expeditious repair is indicated, or for large vessels (aortoiliac system) for which there is a large size discrepancy.

◊ Polytetrafluoroethylene (PTFE) grafts are more resistant to infection than Dacron and have acceptable patency rates when used in the above-knee position.

◊ **The use of prosthetic grafts can hasten the completion of a procedure in patients whose physiology requires expeditious surgery.**

◊ **Prosthetics can also be used in areas of extensive soft-tissue debridement as a "prolonged shunt" where planned revision days to weeks later, out of theatre, will be expected.**

● **Graft coverage:** Exposed vein grafts will dessicate, leading to graft blow-out and potential exsanguination. They must be covered by soft tissue or muscle; superficial muscles such as sartorius or gracilis in the thigh may be mobilized to cover a graft. If coverage is not possible, an alternate subcutaneous or subfascial route through uncontaminated viable tissue must be chosen.

● **Prolonged shunting**: If the above techniques are unsuccessful or precluded by patient physiology or the tactical environment, shunting (as outlined above) with the following modifications can be used for up to 72 hours.

o Replace silastic loops with suture, and **secure firmly**.

o Systemic heparinization is not required.
o Monitor distal perfusion hourly.
o Re-evaluate/evacuate early for definitive repair.
- **Ligation of artery:** If the above options for repair are unsuccessful or unavailable, vessels can be ligated in light of known rates of morbidity. **Emphasis is Save Life Over Limb**.
- **Intraoperative completion angiogram** or duplex US (if available) should be done to evaluate the technical adequacy of the repair, visualize the runoff, and detect any missed distal clot.
  o Full strength contrast 30–60 cc.
  o 20 gauge Angiocath.
  o Inflow occlusion.
- **Venous repair:** Options are similar to arterial repairs outlined above.
  o **Ligation** of major veins is acceptable in life-threatening situations, although in a stable patient and time permitting, venous repair should be performed and may enhance arterial repair patency.
- **Compartment syndrome:** Muscle compartments of the forearm and palm in the upper extremity and anterior compartments of the lower leg are particularly susceptible.
  o Indications for fasciotomy:
    ♦ 4–6 hour delay after vessel injury.
    ♦ Combined vein and artery injury.
    ♦ Arterial ligation.
    ♦ Concomitant fracture/crush, severe soft-tissue injury, muscle edema or patchy necrosis.
    ♦ Tense compartment/compartment pressures exceeding 40 mm Hg.
    ♦ Prophylactic for patients with prolonged transport times or long periods without observation (no surgical care available enroute).
  o A standard two-incision, four-compartment approach for the calf is simple and effective (see Chapter 22, Soft-Tissue Injury).
  o Arm fasciotomy will consist of a longitudinal centrally placed incision over the extensor compartment and a curvilinear incision on the flexor aspect beginning at the antecubital fossa.

- **Post-op care.**
  - o Palpable pulses obtained in the operating room (OR) should remain palpable post-op.
    - ◆ Pulse changes, even if Doppler signals remain, may indicate graft thrombosis and should be investigated.
  - o Consider low-dose heparin as deep vein thrombosis (DVT) prophylaxis.
    - ◆ Use with caution in multiply injured and head-injured patients.
  - o Slight elevation of injured extremity improves post-op edema.

Chapter 28

Burn Injuries

Introduction

Burns constitute between 5% and 20% of combat casualties during conventional warfare, and are particularly common during war at sea and combat involving armored fighting vehicles. Even relatively small burns can be incapacitating, and can strain the logistical and manpower resources of military medical units. Optimal treatment currently results in salvage of approximately 50% of young adults whose burns involve 80% of the total body surface area (TBSA) or greater. Thus, in a battlefield triage scenario, expectant care should be considered for patients with burns that exceed 80%. Care can be delayed for those patients with burns of 20% or less who are otherwise stable.

Point-of-Injury Care

The following are key steps in the first aid of burn patients:

- **Stop the burning process.** Extinguish and remove burning clothing, and remove the patient from a burning vehicle or building. In an electrical injury, remove the patient from the power source, while avoiding rescuer injury. Wash chemical agents from the skin surface with copious water lavage.
- **Ensure airway patency, control hemorrhage, and splint fractures.**
- **Remove all constricting articles**, such as rings, bracelets, wristwatches, belts, and boots. However, do not undress the patient unless the injury has been caused by a chemical agent, in which case remove all contaminated clothing.
- **Cover the patient** with a clean sheet and a blanket, if appropriate, to maintain body temperature and to prevent gross contamination during transport to a treatment facility; special burn dressings are not required. Hypothermia is a complication of large surface area burns.
- **Establish intravenous access** through unburned skin if possible, and through burned skin if necessary. Intraosseous access is also acceptable.

- **Begin resuscitation** with lactated Ringer's solution (LR) or similar solution, and continue during evacuation.
- Dress white phosphorus-injured patients with saline-soaked dressings to prevent reignition of the phosphorus by contact with the air.

Primary Survey

> **Do not be distracted by the burn! The priorities of management for burn casualties are the same as those for other injured patients, with the addition of burn pathophysiology.**

- The primary survey includes airway management (with cervical spine control, if appropriate given the mechanism of injury), diagnosis and management of any breathing condition, rapid circulatory assessment, and hemorrhage control. **In the burn patient, special attention to exposure, removal of clothing that continues to burn the victim, and prevention of hypothermia are important.**
- Airway.

> - **Inhalation injury may be manifested by stridor, hoarseness, cough, carbonaceous sputum, dyspnea, and so forth. It may cause airway obstruction at any time during the first 2 days postburn.**
> - **Patients who may have sustained inhalation injury should be closely observed in an intensive care unit, and may be monitored without intubation if minimally symptomatic.**
> - **Prior to transport, prophylactically intubate patients having/or who have symptomatic inhalation injury.**
> - **Tubes, such as the orotracheal tube, should be definitively secured with cloth ties (eg, umbilical tape). Avoid adhesive tape.**

- o Cervical spine injury is uncommon in burn patients, except in those injured in explosions, high-speed vehicular accidents, and falls, or by contact with high-voltage electricity.

    o Burns are a "distracting injury," pain secondary to burns, and the treatment of pain with narcotics, may make the clinical diagnosis of spinal injury difficult.
- Breathing.
    o Inhalation injury is more common in patients with extensive cutaneous burns, a history of injury in a closed space (eg, building or vehicle), facial burns, and at the extremes of age.
    o Patients with major burns and/or inhalation injury require supplemental oxygen, pulse oximetry, chest radiograph and arterial blood gas measurement.
    o Circumferential burns of the chest may prevent effective chest motion. If this occurs, **perform immediate thoracic escharotomy as a life-saving procedure to permit adequate chest excursion** (see Fig. 28-1).
    o Definitive diagnosis of lower airway injury requires fiberoptic bronchoscopy.

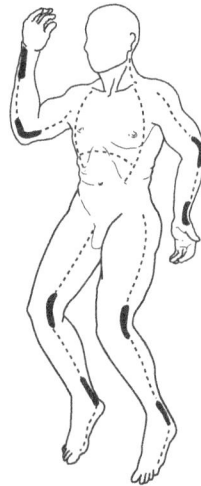

Fig. 28-1. The dashed lines indicate the preferred sites for escharotomy incisions. The bold lines in the figure indicate the importance of extending the incision over involved major joints. Incisions are made through the burned skin into the underlying subcutaneous fat using a scalpel or electrocautery. For a thoracic escharotomy, begin incision in the midclavicular lines. Continue the incision along the anterior axillary lines down to the level of the costal margin. Extend the incision across the epigastrium as needed. For an extremity escharotomy, make the incision through the eschar along the mid-medial or mid-lateral joint line.

    o Carbon monoxide (CO) poisoning causes cardiac and neurologic symptoms. Patients with CO poisoning require 100% oxygen for at least 3 hours or until symptoms resolve.
- Circulation.
    o Secure all cannulae (peripheral and central) with suture, because tape will not adhere well.

o Cuff blood pressure (BP) measurements may be inaccurate in patients with burned or edematous extremities. Arterial BP is preferred.

Estimation of Fluid Resuscitation Needs

> **Initiate resuscitation with LR based on the patient's weight and the burn size. Then, use the urine output as the primary index of adequacy of resuscitation (see below). It is equally important to avoid both over-resuscitation and under-resuscitation.**

- **Determine the burn size** based on the Rule of Nines (Fig. 28-2). A patient's hand (palm and fingers) is approximately 1% of the total body surface area (TBSA). Only 2nd and 3rd degree burns are included in burn size calculations.
  o Overestimation is common and may lead to over-resuscitation and over-evacuation.
- **Estimate crystalloid needs for the first 24 hours**, using the following formula:

    Total Volume = (2 mL) • (% burn) • (kg weight).

- **Half of this total volume is programmed for the first 8 hours postburn,** and half for the second 16 hours postburn:
  o Hourly rate, first 8 hours postburn = (Total Volume /2) /(8h - elapsed time in hours since burn).

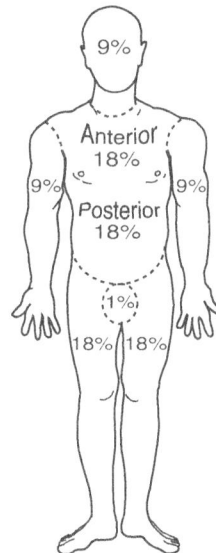

Fig. 28-2. Rule of nines, showing distribution of body surface area by anatomical part in the adult.

> Assume: 40% burn, 70-kg person, time of injury 1 h ago,
> (no fluids received yet).
> Fluid Requirements for First 24 h = 2 x 40 x 70 = 5600 ml
> One half of this to be given over first 8 h = 5600/2 = 2800 ml
> But one hour has elapsed, therefore hourly rate =
> 2800 ml/7 h = 400 ml/h

- **These calculations are only an initial estimate.** Patients with inhalation injury, predominantly full-thickness burns, and delay in resuscitation will have higher fluid requirements. The rate of infusion of LR must be adjusted every 1–2 hours, based on physiologic response (see below). Despite the formula, no abrupt change is made at the 8-hour mark.
- If LR is not available, use other crystalloids such as normal saline. If crystalloid supplies are severely limited, consider starting colloid at the 12-hour mark, at the rate recommended for the second 24 hours (see below).
- Children (< 30 kg) have a greater surface-to-weight ratio, and their fluid requirements are greater. The formula for children is based on 3 cc/kg/% burn.
  - o In addition, children must be given a standard maintenance infusion of D5 $\frac{1}{2}$NS concurrently.

Monitoring the Burn Patient
- Two intravenous catheters (IVs), a Foley catheter, continuous ECG, pulse oximeter, core thermometer, and nasogastric (NG) tube are needed for ICU care of a patient with burns of 20% TBSA or greater.
- Vital signs and fluid input/output are recorded every hour on a flow sheet.
- NG decompression is essential for all patients with burns over 20% TBSA, due to potential gastric ileus.

Secondary Survey
- Perform a thorough head-to-toe secondary survey, looking for nonthermal injuries, to include corneal abrasion, tympanic membrane rupture, fractures, or dislocations.
- If there is a question of intra-abdominal injury, diagnostic peritoneal lavage, through burned skin if necessary, is appropriate.

Resuscitation Management, First 24 Hours

> On an hourly basis, reassess the patient's urine output, which is the single most important indicator of the adequacy of resuscitation.

- Seek a urine output of 30–50 mL/h in adults or 1 mL/kg/h in children. If the urine output is less than the target for 1–2 consecutive hours, increase the LR infusion rate by about 25%. If it is greater than the target, decrease it by about 25%.
- Avoid over-resuscitation, which may lead to edema-related complications (eg, compartment syndromes and pulmonary edema).
- Other indices of adequate resuscitation include a decreasing base deficit, a moderate tachycardia (typically a pulse of 100 to 130 is normal in adult burn patients), and an acceptable mental status.
- Diuretics are never indicated in the treatment of burn shock, except when gross pigmenturia is present (see below).
- Glycosuria is common following severe thermal injury and may cause hypovolemia secondary to osmotic diuresis. Check the urine for glucose and treat hyperglycemia with IV insulin as needed.

Resuscitation Management, Second 24 Hours

> At the end of the first 24 hours postburn, discontinue the LR. For the second 24 hours, use 5% albumin in normal saline.

- The 24–hour albumin volume is as follows:

5% albumin volume = (* mL) • (% TBSA burned) • (preburn wt, kg)

% TBSA burn	30–49	50–69	70+
* mL	0.3	0.4	0.5

For example, in a burn of approximately 40% in a 70-kg patient:
Albumin volume = (* ml) • (40%) • (70kg) = (0.3) • (2,800) =
840 mL/24 h = **35 mL/h**

- Burns < 30% TBSA do not require colloid infusion.
- It is rarely necessary to adjust the colloid infusion rate.
- If albumin is not available, fresh frozen plasma or synthetic colloid can be used at the same dose. If none of these is available, continue the LR until the 48th hour postburn, monitoring urine output, and so forth.
- At 24 hours, start D5W at half the last hourly rate of LR.
- Follow serum sodium closely. Resuscitation is usually complete by the 48th hour postburn. Continued evaporative water loss replacement is needed thereafter—**beware of hypo- or hypernatremia!**

Burn Wound Care
- The burn wound is not an early management priority, but must be attended to by 24 hours postburn.

> **Initial burn wound care includes adequate IV pain management, removal of foreign bodies, debridement, cleansing with surgical soap (use only saline around the face), unroofing of all blisters, and application of a topical antimicrobial.**

- Adequate wound care requires adequate pain control. Small, intermittent boluses of IV morphine or fentanyl are effective for background pain control. Ketamine (Bristol-Myers Squibb, NY), 1 mg/kg IV, is generally effective for painful wound care.
- Apply a topical antimicrobial cream twice daily after thorough cleansing with a surgical detergent such as chlorhexidine gluconate (Hibiclens, Zeneca Pharmaceuticals, Wilmington, DE).
- One-percent silver sulfadiazine (Silvadene, Monarch Pharmaceuticals, Bristol, TN) and/or 11.1% mafenide acetate (Sulfamylon, Bertek Pharmaceuticals, Morgantown, WV) burn creams should be used. They are applied as a thick (1/16- to 1/8-in. thick) layer—not as a lotion.
- Following burn cream application, burns may be treated open or closed (wrapped in gauze).

o Extremity wounds can be wrapped in a thick layer of roller gauze that is changed twice daily.

o During the period of active wound exudation, it is helpful to place bulky dressings beneath the burned parts to absorb the exudate.

o Burn cream should be reapplied to open burns as often as needed to keep them covered.

Burn victims must be adequately immunized against tetanus and (if arrival at the burn center will take longer than 24 hours) should be treated with a 5-day course of penicillin or similar antibiotic (intravenously for large burns, orally for small ones).

- Definitive burn surgery in the combat zone is generally not recommended.
- Prevent thermal (cold) stress by keeping the environment as warm as possible (> 85°F).
- Corneal abrasions in burn patients can lead to full-thickness ulceration and blindness, and require aggressive treatment with antibiotic ointments, preferably gentamicin or a quinolone every 4 hours, alternating with erythromycin every 4 hours.
- It is common for patients to develop a sterile, chemical cellulitis, manifested by an erythematous rim of normal tissue extending 1–2 cm around the wound margin. **Erythema extending beyond this margin, with other clinical evidence of infection, likely represents beta-hemolytic streptococcal cellulitis.** Consider vancomycin if penicillin has already been given. Treat with appropriate IV antibiotics.
- Invasive gram-negative burn-wound infection is heralded by striking changes in the color of the burn wound and a clinical course consistent with sepsis.
  - o Initiate an aminoglycoside and a semi-synthetic anti-pseudomonal penicillin; apply Sulfamylon (Bertek Pharmaceuticals, Morgantown, WV) cream bid if available; and plan urgent evacuation.
  - o Consider subeschar clysis (injection via a spinal needle) with the daily dose of an antipseudomonal penicillin

(ticarcillin, piperacillin) in a suitable volume of crystalloid solution (eg, 500 mL). This is done at time of diagnosis, and then immediately prior to excision to fascia.

Daily inspection of the burn wound by a surgeon is essential to identify early infection complications.

Extremity Care
- Carefully monitor the extremities throughout the resuscitation period. The management of the burned extremity can be summarized as follows:
  o Elevate;
  o Exercise burned extremities hourly;
  o Evaluate pulses and neurologic status hourly; and
  o Perform escharotomy as indicated.
- **In extremities with full thickness, circumferential burns, edema formation beneath the inelastic eschar may gradually constrict the venous outflow and, ultimately, arterial inflow.** Adequate perfusion must be assessed hourly during resuscitation.

Progressive diminution of audible arterial flow by Doppler flowmetry is the primary indication for escharotomy. Doppler pulses should be sought in the palmar arch, not the wrist.

- Pulses may be difficult to palpate in edematous, burned extremities. However, **in the absence of a Doppler flowmeter, and in the appropriate clinical setting, loss of palpable pulses may indicate a need for escharotomy.**
- Patients requiring escharotomy often present with a tight and edematous extremity. They may have progressive neurologic dysfunction such as unrelenting deep tissue pain or paresthesias, and/or distal cyanosis.
- Prior to prolonged transport, strongly consider prophylactic escharotomy.
- Note that loss of the palmar arch Doppler signal, in the presence of adequate radial and ulnar pulses, is an indication for dorsal hand escharotomies. These are performed over the dorsal interossei. Digital escharotomies may be useful in some cases.

- **Following escharotomy, document restoration of normal pulses and continue to monitor the patient.** If one incision fails to restore pulses, make a second incision on the other side of the limb.
- After escharotomy, cover wounds, including the escharotomy incisions, in burn cream.
- The patient may still develop a true intramuscular, subfascial compartment syndrome requiring fasciotomy.
- Fractures associated with thermal injury are best treated by skeletal traction or by external fixation to permit exposure of the burns and their treatment with topical antimicrobials. Plaster, if used, should be bivalved immediately to permit access for wound care and to accommodate edema of the burned limb.

Other Considerations

- Burn patients manifest a hypermetabolic state, with hyperthermia, tachycardia, and hypercatabolism, which may be difficult to distinguish from early sepsis.
- Stress ulcer prophylaxis is critical (see Chapter 19, ICU Care).
- Early enteral nutrition—once hemodynamically stable, generally at 24 hours.
- Respiratory care.
  - o About one week after injury, patients with subglottic inhalation injury may develop obstructing bloody casts. Inhaled heparin sodium, at a dose of 10,000 units, may be given by nebulization every 4 hours in order to prevent the formation of these casts.
  - o **Subglottic inhalation injury may persist longer than clinically evident. Extubation must be performed with caution after adequate airway assessment.**
- Patients with large burns are at risk for abdominal compartment syndrome.

Electrical Injury

- High-voltage electrical injury (>1,000 volts) causes muscular damage that often is much greater in extent than the overlying cutaneous injury.
- Examine the extremities for compartment syndrome and perform urgent fasciotomy as needed.

- Gross pigmenturia (myoglobinuria) may result, and fluid resuscitation must be modified to protect against renal injury.
  - o Pigmenturia is diagnosed by reddish-brownish urine, with a dipstick test which is positive for blood, but with insignificant numbers of red blood cells on microscopy.
  - o Increase the hourly LR rate until a urine output of 100 ml/h is achieved.
  - o If this fails to cause a progressive clearing of the urinary pigmenturia over 3 to 4 hours, add 12.5 g mannitol to each liter of LR infused and consider invasive monitoring.
  - o Infusion of sodium bicarbonate in water (150 mEq/L) in order to alkalinize the urine may be useful.
- Hyperkalemia may occur as a result of rhabdomyolysis, and must be carefully assessed and treated, with calcium gluconate infusion, insulin, and glucose.
- Surgical debridement of nonviable muscle is the definitive treatment of myoglobinuria.

> **High-voltage electric injury requires consideration of deep muscle injury, with resultant rhabdomyolysis, hyperkalemia, acute renal failure, and compartment syndrome. Cardiac monitoring, aggressive fluid and electrolyte management, fasciotomy, and debridement are often required.**

- Patients with electrical injuries are also at high risk for spinal fractures.

Chemical Burns
- Initial treatment requires immediate removal of the offending agent.
  - o Brush any dry materials off the skin surface before copious water lavage.
  - o In the case of alkali burns, lavage may need to be continued for several hours.
  - o Resuscitate and manage just as a thermal burn.

White Phosphorus Burn
- Most of the cutaneous injury resulting from phosphorus burns is due to the ignition of clothing, and is treated as a conventional burn.

- Fragments of this metal, which ignite upon contact with the air, may be driven into the soft tissues.
- First aid treatment of casualties with imbedded phosphorus particles includes **copious water irrigation, and placement of a saline-soaked dressing that must be kept continuously wet.**
- Profound hypocalcemia, and hyperphosphatemia, have been described as effects of white phosphorus injury. Treat with IV calcium.
- Rapid surgical removal of the identifiable particles is often required. UV light can be used to help locate them.
  - o A dilute (1%) freshly mixed solution of copper sulfate has been used to help identify white phosphorus particles. However, this is no longer recommended because if the solution is absorbed, it can cause fatal hemolysis. If it is used, immediately wash it off with copious saline irrigation. Never apply it as a wet dressing.
- Liberally apply topical antimicrobial burn creams postoperatively.

"How I Do It": Excision and Grafting

Definitive burn care, including surgery and rehabilitation, is manpower and resource intensive; therefore it is generally inadvisable to perform excision and grafting of burns in a theater of operations. However, under certain circumstances, this may be unavoidable.

Patient Selection

Do not attempt to autograft patients with grossly colonized or infected wounds. Such patients are best treated with deep tangential excision or primary excision to fascia, followed by immediate placement of a biologic dressing such as gamma-irradiated allograft (Gammagraft, Promethean LifeSciences, Inc., Pittsburgh, PA). Many second-degree (partial thickness) wounds are likely to heal in 14–21 days with acceptable cosmetic and functional outcomes. Partial-thickness wounds which take longer to heal, are likely to heal with fragile or hypertrophic scar, and should be considered for grafting. Likewise, full-thickness burns will only heal by contracture and should be considered for grafting.

Preparation

When performing burn surgery in a theater of operations, it is preferable to perform several limited procedures (eg, 10% TBSA or less at each operation) in order to limit the physiologic stress of the operation. Plans for the operation must be discussed and rehearsed with all personnel involved, and the availability of OR equipment and postoperative dressings and splints must be ascertained. At least 4 units of PRBCs should be available for a patient undergoing a 10% TBSA excision. A single dose of prophylactic intravenous antibiotic, such as a first-generation cephalosporin, should be administered. (However, antibiotics effective against *Pseudomonas* and other gram-negative wound pathogens should be considered for patients with heavily colonized wounds.) Total IV general anesthesia (TIVA), based on ketamine, is very effective in burn patients. Select the donor sites to be used. Often, the anterior thighs are available and easy to harvest. However, any area of clean unburned skin can be harvested. Hair is removed from the donor site, and both the area to be excised and the donor site are prepped.

Tangential vs Fascial Excision

Many surgeons recommend that extensive burn wound excision of the extremities be performed after exsanguination and pneumatic tourniquet application to limit blood loss. Using a Weck knife for small areas, or a Blair knife (or similar) for large areas, the burn is tangentially excised to the level of viable tissue. When an area has been exsanguinated, absence of hemosiderin staining of the dermis or fat is the usual endpoint for tangential excision. When an area has not been exsanguinated, the usual endpoint is diffuse punctuate bleeding (in the dermis) or viable-appearing fat. When the surgeon believes that all nonviable tissue in the surgical field has been excised, gauze soaked in a 1:100,000 solution of epinephrine in lactated Ringer's can be applied, followed by a tight ace wrap. The tourniquet is released and the wound is reassessed after 5–10 minutes. Hemostasis in the bed is then achieved by electrocautery. If available, topical hemostatic agents such as spray thrombin and fibrin sealant can be applied before letting the tourniquet down.

Alternatively, if the burn extends into fat and/or demonstrates evidence of invasive burn wound infection, the burn wound can be excised to the level of the investing muscle fascia, using electrocautery.

Donor Site Harvesting

The subcutaneous space of the selected donor site is clysed with a saline solution containing a 1:1,000,000 dilution of epinephrine. This technique reduces bleeding and can be used to round out irregular contours of the donor site when skin must be harvested from bony or irregularly shaped areas. It is particularly important to do this prior to harvesting the scalp to control bleeding. It is optional for most other locations. A pneumatic or electric dermatome is loaded with a wide blade and the thickness of the skin to be harvested is adjusted to a depth between 8/1,000 and 15/1,000 inch. It would be appropriate to use 10/1,000 for grafting of most sites. Many surgeons use skin harvested at a depth of 12/1,000 to 15/1,000 inch for the hands. If a powered dermatome is not available, skin grafts can be harvested using a manual dermatome or a Weck knife. Hemostasis of the donor site is achieved with the application of warm gauze packs, soaked in a 1:100,000 solution of epinephrine.

At the end of the procedure, the packs are removed and the donor site is dressed with a single sheet of rolled, fine-mesh gauze or xeroform (petrolatum and 3% bismuth tribromophenate) gauze. Donor sites can alternatively be dressed in a biosynthetic membrane material such as Biobrane (Bertek Pharmaceuticals Inc., Morgantown, WV). When the donor site is small, another alternative is to apply an occlusive transparent film dressing such as a large OpSite (Smith & Nephew, Largo, FL) to the donor wound.

Application and Securing of the Graft

The harvested split-thickness skin may be meshed. It would be appropriate in this case to use 1.5:1 or 2:1 for the arms; but unmeshed skin, or skin meshed 1:1 or 1.5:1, is preferred for the hands. If a mesher is not available, the graft can be pie-crusted using a scalpel. The graft is applied to the prepared bed and stapled in place. Over the hands, the graft is minimally expanded. Bridal veil (or another product to prevent shear, such as fine-mesh gauze) is applied over the grafted areas, followed by a moist gauze dressing. Dressings should be kept slightly moist, for example, by application of normal saline or aqueous 5% Sulfamylon solution (Bertek Pharmaceuticals Inc., Morgantown, WV) every 6–8 hours. Another option, when the grafted area is surrounded by normal skin, is the use of a vacuum-assisted closure device (V.A.C., Kinetic Concepts, Inc., San Antonio, TX).

Following dressings, the extremities are splinted, with the axilla at 90° horizontal with bedside troughs or in an airplane splint, elbow fully extended. Hands and wrist are splinted in the "beer can" position: wrist slightly extended (10°), metatarsophalangeal joints of the fingers flexed, interphalangeal joints fully extended, and thumb in 40°–50° of abduction with interphalangeal joint extended.

Postoperative Care

Donor sites dressed with fine-mesh gauze are treated open, with a heat lamp applied until the gauze is dry. Grafted extremities are immobilized for 4–5 days. Grafted sites are inspected 4–5 days after surgery. They should be inspected sooner in case of fever, malodor, or other evidence of infection. Moist dressings are continued until the interstices of the grafted area have entirely closed.

Physical and occupational therapy are begun as soon as graft take is sufficient to discontinue immobilization, usually 5 days after surgery. Extremities are splinted in the position of function at night. The dried gauze on the donor site is allowed to separate spontaneously, at which time the donor site can be recropped as necessary for further grafting. After all wounds are closed, the patient is fitted for custom compression garments. If garments are not available, compression can be achieved with ace bandages.

Chapter 29

Environmental Injuries

Introduction
The successful prevention and control of cold, heat, and altitude injuries depend on vigorous command interest, the provision of adequate clothing, and a number of individual and group measures. The medical officer must ensure that he or she understands how military duties impact the occurrence and severity of environmental conditions and advise the commander on preventive measures.

Cold Injuries
Trench foot and frostbite together have accounted for over 1 million US casualties in WW I, WW II, and the Korean War. Influencing factors include previous cold injury; fatigue; concomitant injury resulting in significant blood loss or shock; geographic origin; nutrition; tobacco use; activity; drugs and medication; alcohol; duration and exposure; dehydration; environment (temperature, humidity, precipitation, and wind); and clothing.

Non–Freezing Cold Injury
- Chilblain.
  - o Results from intermittent exposure to temperatures above freezing, usually accompanied by high humidity and moisture; 1 to 6 hours of exposure.
  - o Swelling, tingling pain, and numbness with pink-to-red flushing of skin (especially the fingers).
  - o Extremities will be pruritic as they warm up.
  - o Symptoms usually subside overnight; some superficial scaling may occur.
  - o Mild joint stiffness may occur acutely but subsides in a few hours.
  - o No permanent damage occurs.

- Pernio.
  - o Continuum of events from chilblain.
  - o Exposure for > 12 hours to cold and/or wet conditions.
  - o Tight-fitting footwear can shorten exposure time and increase severity of injury.
  - o Swelling is more severe; pain is more persistent than with chilblain.
  - o Thin, partial-skin thickness, and necrotic patches (from dorsum of the hands or feet).
  - o Plaques may slough without scarring but may be particularly painful for months or years.
- Trench foot.
  - o Epidemiology/clinical appearance.
    - ◆ Occurs from prolonged exposure to cold, wet conditions or prolonged immersion of feet at temperatures as high as 17°C for > 12 hours. Shorter duration at or near 0°C results in the same injury.
    - ◆ Occurs in nonfreezing temperatures 0°C–12°C.
    - ◆ Can occur at higher temperatures from prolonged water immersion.
    - ◆ Blunt trauma of marching can produce more serious injury.
    - ◆ First symptom often is the feet becoming cold, mildly painful, and numb.
    - ◆ Tight footwear increases risk of trench foot.
    - ◆ Common symptoms are "cold and numb" or "walking on wood."
    - ◆ Foot may appear swollen, with the skin mildly blue, red, or black.
    - ◆ Limb is hot and often hyperhidrotic.
    - ◆ On rewarming, pain is excruciating and does not respond to pain medication, including morphine.
    - ◆ As time progresses, liquefaction necrosis occurs distally, but more proximal tissue may also be compromised.
    - ◆ No sharp line of demarcation of dead from viable tissue.
    - ◆ Nerve, muscle, and endothelial cells are most susceptible to this long-term cooling.
    - ◆ Microvascular vasospasm with tissue ischemia is the apparent etiology of trench foot.

- ◆ Postinjury sequelae include pain, numbness, loss of proprioception, and cold feet. Hyperhidrosis with subsequent paronychial fungal infections are common.
- ◆ Life-long, life-changing injury.
- o **Treatment.**
  - ◆ Prevent further cold exposure.
  - ◆ Do not massage.
  - ◆ Dry extremity, warm torso, and allow slow passive rewarming of feet. **Never immerse feet in warm or hot water.**
  - ◆ Elevate feet.
  - ◆ Rehydrate.
  - ◆ If **vesicles** develop do not debride.
  - ◆ Pain medication. The only effective approach is amitriptyline 50–150 mg at bedtime. Other analgesics are either completely ineffective, or (as with narcotics) do not actually relieve pain.
  - ◆ Blisters should be left intact; ruptured blisters require meticulous antisepsis after unroofing.
  - ◆ Systemic antibiotics and tetanus prophylaxis are indicated when there are nonviable tissues, as with any other contaminated wound, or when there is evidence of infection.
  - ◆ Debridement of necrotic tissue may be required in trench foot.
  - ◆ Macerated or damaged skin requires topical antibacterial precautions.
  - ◆ Avoid trauma.
  - ◆ Early mobilization is vital to prevent long-term immobility.
  - ◆ Recovery is protracted and may require evacuation because trench foot may lead to weeks-to-months of pain and disability.
  - ◆ Long-term sequelae are very common and include sensitivity to the cold (secondary Raynaud's phenomenon), chronic pain, neurological impairment, and hyperhydrosis.

- Frostnip.
  - o Exposed skin appears red or minimally swollen.
  - o Tissue is not actually damaged.
  - o Not true frostbite; freezing is limited to skin surface only.
  - o Signals imminent likelihood of frostbite developing.
  - o Resolves quickly with warming.
- Frostbite.
  - o Results from crystallization of water in the skin and adjacent tissues exposed to temperatures below freezing.
  - o Depth and severity of injury is a function of temperature and duration—the lower the temperature, the shorter the time required to produce injury.
  - o At low temperatures in the presence of wind, exposed skin can freeze within a few seconds—starts distally and progresses up the finger or toe.
  - o Freeze-front (line where the ice is formed in the tissues) is where liquefaction and necrosis occur. Tissues immediately proximal to this line may also die, but therapeutic modalities are directed at improving their survival.
  - o Clinical appearance.
    - ◆ Skin initially becomes numb and feels stiff or woody.
    - ◆ Mottled, bluish, yellowish, "waxy," or "frozen."
    - ◆ Depth of involvement may be difficult to determine until demarcation occurs, which may take an extended period.
  - o Frostbite grading.
    - ◆ Classification into degrees is primarily a retrospective evaluation and has little treatment value.
    - ◆ A more clinically useful grading typically divides injuries into superficial or deep.
    - ◆ Superficial frostbite.
      - ◊ Involves only the skin with swelling, mild pain, and minor joint stiffness.
      - ◊ No blisters form.
      - ◊ Nonmedical personnel can manage simply by rewarming.
    - ◆ Deep frostbite.
      - ◊ Involves deeper tissues to include bone.
      - ◊ White-hard, anesthetic, blanched, and inflexible.

◊ Skin will not move over joints.

◊ On rewarming, there is great pain and a blue-gray-to-burgundy color change.

◊ Blisters form and are clear, fluid-filled, or hemorrhagic (the latter indicates a more severe, deeper injury). They should be left in place; will slough in 7–10 days without consequence.

◊ Failure to form vesicles in an obviously deep-frozen extremity is a grave sign.

◊ Postinjury sequelae include Raynaud's phenomenon; pain; paraesthesias; hyperhidrosis; loss of proprioception; cold, discolored feet; and gait modification.

- Field treatment (first aid).
  o Superficial (blanched cheeks, nose, ears, fingertips).
    ♦ Warm with palm of hand or warm, wet cloth; warm fingers in armpits.
    ♦ Emollients may help prevent skin from drying or cracking.
    ♦ Do not massage, rub with snow, or warm part by an open fire or high-heat source.
    ♦ Meticulous skin care is required.
  o Deep frostbite.
    ♦ Prevent further cooling of body part as well as the patient as a whole.
    ♦ Apply dry, sterile bandage and elevate involved extremity.
    ♦ Protect from refreezing during evacuation.
    ♦ Evacuate promptly to definitive medical care.

Avoid thawing and refreezing; this leads to the greatest damage to tissue and the poorest outcome.

- MTF treatment.
  o **The outcome of a frozen extremity is not directly related to length of time frozen, but more importantly to the method of rewarming and any subsequent refreezing.**
    ♦ If the soldier will again be at risk for refreezing, no attempt at rewarming should be initiated; the soldier

should ambulate on the frozen extremities until he reaches definitive care.

♦ For transport, the patient's extremity should be splinted, and padded with dry dressings and protected from heat sources that would slowly rewarm the extremity.

o **Rapid rewarming (without the possibility of refreezing) is the treatment of choice.**

♦ Immerse in gently circulating water (whirlpool bath) at 40°C (104°F) for at least 30 minutes longer than could be needed to defrost all affected tissues. If deep freezing of the leg or arm has taken place, thorough surgical fasciotomy is mandatory prior to rewarming, to prevent lethal increase in deep tissue pressures as ice melts. Extremities are rewarmed until pliable and erythematous at the most distal areas.

♦ Twice daily whirlpool baths at 40°C with topical antibacterial added to the water, together with oral ethanol. The alcohol reduces the need for analgesia and may improve outcome. Other drug regimens remain unproven.

♦ After rewarming, edema will appear within a few hours and vesicles form within the next 6–24 hours.

♦ Intensive mobilization is essential to avoid long-term immobility.

o Vesicles.

♦ Frostbite vesicles are typically left intact.

♦ Debridement is not recommended. Early surgery is only indicated in severely infected cases. Normally surgery should be delayed for at least 6 months.

o General considerations.

♦ Ibuprofen or ketorolac should be given as systemic thromboxane/prostaglandin inhibitors.

♦ Systemic antibiotics and tetanus prophylaxis are indicated when there are dead tissues, as with any other contaminated wound, or when there is evidence of infection.

♦ Dry, loose dressings may be applied.

♦ Cigarette smoking and/or nicotine use is contraindicated during treatment due to its effect on the microvasculature.

♦ Daily hydrotherapy is recommended. Pain control with NSAIDs and narcotics will be needed.
♦ Sequelae include contractures, cold sensitivity, chronic ulceration, arthritis, and hyperhidrosis.
♦ Frostbite cases will require prolonged hospital care (9 d on average); therefore, all but those with the most trivial injuries should be evacuated to more definitive care as soon as possible.
♦ Early surgery is indicated only in the most severe freeze-thaw-refreeze cases, where massive tissue destruction has taken place, and in some more severely infected cases. Normally, surgery should be delayed for at least 6 months ("Freeze in January, operate in July").

Due to the inability to reliably predict the outcome in the postthaw period, there is no role for debridement/ amputation of necrotic or potentially necrotic tissue in the initial treatment of frostbite.

Hypothermia

Hypothermia is classically defined as whole-body cooling below 35°C. Degree of hypothermia is further defined according to the body's core temperature and the clinical effects seen in a given temperature range.

● Causative factors and prevention.
  o Water immersion.
  o Rain and wind.
  o Prolonged exposure to severe weather without adequate clothing. The insulation effect of clothing is markedly decreased with wetness, which increases the conductive heat loss.
  o Stay dry and avoid windy exposure.
  o Shivering can provide five times the normal metabolic heat production. Exhaustion and glycogen depletion decrease the time of shivering. Compromise of shivering due to inadequate food intake (skipping meals), exhaustion, heavy exercise, alcohol, and drugs increases threat of hypothermia.

- Mild hypothermia > 33°C (> 91°F).
  - o Shivering, hyperreflexia.
  - o Amnesia, dysarthria, poor judgment, ataxia, apathy.
  - o Cold diuresis.
- Moderate hypothermia 28°C–33°C (82°F–91°F).
  - o Standard hospital thermometers, mercury as well as digital, cannot measure temperatures below 34°C (93°F).
  - o Stupor, loss of shivering.
  - o Onset of atrial fibrillation and other arrhythmias.
  - o Progressive decrease in level of consciousness, respiration, and pupillary reaction, eventual pupil dilation.
- Severe hypothermia < 28°C (< 82°F).
  - o Increased incidence of ventricular fibrillation, which often occurs spontaneously.
  - o Loss of motion and reflexes, areflexic at approximately 23°C (72°F).
  - o Marked hypotension/bradycardia.
- Profound hypothermia < 20°C (< 68°F).
  - o Asystole.
  - o Lowest known adult survival from accidental hypothermia is 13.7°C (56°F).

Treatment
- Prehospital (field) treatment.
  - o Awake patients.
    - ♦ Remove wet clothing; dry and insulate the patient.
    - ♦ Give oral sugar solutions to hydrate.
    - ♦ Walk out or transport to MTF. (This should be attempted if it is the only alternative because it is likely to worsen the condition.)
    - ♦ Although walking may deepen hypothermia due to the return of peripheral colder blood to the core, adequate prehydration decreases the postexposure cooling.
  - o Comatose patients.
    - ♦ Patient should remain horizontal and be handled gently to avoid inducing arrhythmias; do not massage.
    - ♦ IV fluids, warmed to 40°C–42°C, if possible.
    - ♦ Do not use lactated Ringer's solution because the cold liver cannot metabolize lactate; warm (40°C–42°C

[104°F–107.5°F]), D5NS is the fluid of choice.

♦ Remove wet clothes, dry, insulate, and add an outer vapor barrier. Wrap patient in multiple layers of insulation.

♦ Limit active rewarming principally to the body's center/ core only.

◊ Heated (40°C–45°C), humidified air/O_2 is the method of choice.

◊ Norwegian personal heater pack (charcoal heater), with warming tube placed into insulation wrap.

◊ Forced air (Bair Hugger) with rigid chest frame.

◊ Hot water bottles in groin/axilla.

♦ Intubation and heated ventilation may be performed.

♦ If apneic and asystolic, consider CPR, because the brain may survive longer.

Remember: The patient is not dead until he is warm and dead. Continue resuscitation, if possible, until patient has been rewarmed.

● Medical treatment.

o Ventilate; apply CPR if asystolic or in ventricular fibrillation.

o As the body cools, the peripheral vasculature constricts, causing pooling of cold acidotic blood.

o Rewarming the periphery of the body rather than the core causes an inrush of this cold acidotic blood into the core, further dropping the core temperature (afterdrop), and worsening cardiac instability.

o Core rewarming—peritoneal dialysis, thoracic lavage, heated and humidified oxygen, external warm blankets, and warm-water torso immersion.

o For ventricular fibrillation.

♦ Bretylium tosylate, 10 mg/kg. Bretylium is the only known effective antidefibrillation drug for hypothermia. It remains functional in a cold heart. Other medications have not proven effective.

♦ Warmed IV (lactate and potassium-free).

♦ Monitor core temperature via esophageal (preferred) or rectal probes.
♦ Careful correction of acid/base balance.
♦ Rewarm core to 32°C (90°F) and attempt cardioversion (360 J). Continue rewarming and repeat. Defibrillate after every 1°C rise in temperature.
♦ Monitor potassium, glucose, temperature, and pH.
♦ Major causes of failure to resuscitate include elevating central venous pressure too fast or too early; attempting defibrillation when core temperature is below 32°C, or continuing to rewarm past 33°C when potassium levels are high and pH is low. If serum potassium levels are high, consider the use of intravenous glucose and insulin.
♦ Avoid other antiarrhythmics and other medications.
♦ Patients with core temperature (rectal) above 30°C can generally be rewarmed externally in a variety of methods including warm blankets, warm-water torso immersion. Patients below 30°C rectal should be considered more fragile and will often require internal methods of rewarming (ie, warm gastric, colonic, and/or bladder lavage; warm peritoneal lavage dialysis; warm thoracic lavage; and arteriovenous (blood rewarming). Lavage fluids should be warmed to 40°C–42°C (104°F–107.5°F).
♦ Core temperature will continue to drop after the patient is removed from the cold exposure. Continued temperature drop can have grave prognostic implication and increases the likelihood of fibrillation. Post-rewarming collapse of an apparently functional heart often leads to a nonresuscitable heart and death.

● Cardiopulmonary resuscitation.
  o If cardiac monitor shows any electrical complexes, check carefully for apical and carotid pulses before initiating CPR. If any pulse—however thready—is present, **do NOT initiate CPR.**

> **Trauma patients should be considered to have hypothermia more profound than the core temperature indicates and be warmed more aggressively.**

- Treatment of mild stable hypothermia.
  - o Insulation.
  - o Heat lamps.
  - o Warmed IV fluids.
  - o Warmed forced air (Bair Hugger). Hair dryers have been jury-rigged for this purpose.
  - o Consider arteriovenous anastomoses (AVA) warming.
    - ♦ Immerse hand, forearms, feet, calves in water heated to 44°C–45°C (111°F–113°F).
    - ♦ Opens AVAs in the digits causing increased flow of warmed venous blood to the heart and decreases afterdrop.
- **Treatment of severe hypothermia with hemodynamic instability**.
  - o Cardiopulmonary bypass with rewarming, when available, is the ideal technique in this circumstance because it provides core rewarming while ensuring circulatory stability.

Heat Injury

In the military setting, heat illness occurs in otherwise healthy individuals, and ranges from mild (heat cramps) to life threatening (heatstroke). Individuals typically present with exertional heat illness and are hot and sweaty, not hot and dry as seen in classic heatstroke.

> **Lack of sweating is not a criterion for heatstroke. Some military casualties of heatstroke have profuse sweating; especially with rapid onset of heatstroke.**

Minor heat illnesses include heat cramps and heat exhaustion. Major heat injuries include exertional heat injury (EHI), exertional rhabdomyolysis, and heat stroke. The diagnostic categories of heat exhaustion, EHI, and heat stroke have overlapping features and should be thought of as different regions on the continuum rather than discrete disorders, each with its own distinct pathogenesis.

- Heat injury prevention.
  - o Easier to prevent than treat.
  - o Occurs most commonly in unacclimatized individuals.
    - ◆ Acclimatization to heat requires 7–10 days.
    - ◆ Predeployment training in artificially warm environments does aid heat acclimatization.
    - ◆ One hour of progressively more difficult exercise sufficient to induce moderate sweating each day will maximize acclimatization. (Regular strenuous exercise sufficient to stimulate sweating and increase body temperature will result in a significant degree of heat acclimation.) Aerobic fitness provides cardiovascular reserve to maintain the extra cardiac output required to sustain thermoregulation, muscular work, and vital organs in the face of heat stress.
  - o Utilize published work–rest cycle guides (eg, FM 21-10/ MCRP 4-11.1D) or work–rest cycles tailored to the individual's physical capacity by direct medical oversight.
  - o **Water restriction/discipline leads to increased heat injury and is contraindicated.**
    - ◆ Acclimatization does not reduce, and may actually increase, water requirements.
    - ◆ Service members will on average not feel thirsty until 1.5 L (1%–2%) dehydrated.
    - ◆ Fluid intake should be monitored to ensure urine appears dilute. Additionally, soldiers should be monitored for body weight changes and orthostatic blood pressure changes due to hydration.
    - ◆ The GI tract can absorb only 1–1.5 L/h.
    - ◆ Daily rehydration should not exceed 12 L/d orally. **Too much hydration can also be dangerous and lead to water intoxication!**
    - ◆ Leaders must reinforce hydration by planning for all aspects of adequate hydration—elimination as well as consumption. (Soldiers may not drink at night to avoid awakening and having to dress to urinate, or soldiers may not drink prior to a convoy because no rest stops are planned.)

o MOPP gear will increase fluid losses and the incidence of heat injuries.
o In the first few days of acclimatization, sweat–salt conservation will not be fully developed. Salt depletion is a risk if soldiers are exposed during this time to sufficient heat or work stress to induce high sweating rates (> several liters per day), particularly if ration consumption is reduced. Salt depletion can be avoided by providing a salt supplement in the form of salted water (0.05%–0.1%). Acclimation should eventually eliminate the need for salt supplementation
o Salt supplements are not routinely required and are only recommended in rare instances where adequate rations are not consumed.
o Coincidental illnesses increase heat casualty risk through fever and dehydration. Fever reduces thermoregulatory capacity leading to increased risk, even after clinical evidence of illness has disappeared. Requires increased command supervision and moderate work schedule.
o Sunburn and other skin diseases of hot environments reduce the ability of the skin to thermoregulate. Sunburn must be prevented by adequate clothing, shade, and sunscreen. Skin diseases are best prevented by adequate hygiene.
o Medications that effect thermoregulatory adaptations and increase risk of heat injury include anticholinergics, antihistamines, diuretics, tricyclic antidepressants, major tranquilizers, stimulants, and beta blockers.

Despite preventive measures, service members may suffer from heat illness. One case of heat illness is a warning sign that many others are imminent. The most life-threatening condition is heatstroke. Severity of heat illness depends on the maximum core temperature and duration.

● Heatstroke.
Heat stroke is distinguished from heat exhaustion by the presence of clinically significant tissue injury and/or altered mental status. Degree of injury appears to relate to both the degree of temperature elevation and duration of exposure.

o Clinical presentation.

♦ Heat stroke is a true emergency. Involves five organ systems: brain, hemostatic, liver, kidneys, and muscles.

♦ Encephalopathy ranges from syncope and confusion to seizures or coma with decerebrate rigidity. Profound neuropsychiatric impairments present early and universally in casualties of advanced exertional heat stroke.

♦ Coagulopathy: thermal damage to endothelium, rhabdomyolysis, and direct thermal platelet activation causes intravascular microthrombi. Fibrinolysis is secondarily activated. Hepatic dysfunction and thermal injury to megakaryocytes slow the repletion of clotting factors. Hepatic injury is common. Transaminase enzyme elevation (values 100 or more times the upper normal limit), clotting factor deficiencies, and jaundice (within 24–36 h of onset). Transaminase levels may be transient and reversible, but if they persist 48 hours, it is indicative of more severe injury. Hypoglycemia is a frequent complication of exertional heat stroke.

♦ Renal failure: myoglobinuria from rhabdomyolysis in exertional heat stroke, acute tubular necrosis due to hypoperfusion, glomerulopathy due to disseminated intravascular coagulation (DIC), direct thermal injury, and hyperuricemia.

♦ Muscles are often rigid and contracted: Rhabdomyolysis is a frequent acute complication of exertional heat stroke. Acute muscular necrosis releases large quantities of potassium, myoglobin, phosphate, uric acid, and creatine, and sequesters calcium in exposed contractile proteins.

If heat stroke is suspected and temperature is elevated, cooling should not be delayed to accomplish a diagnostic evaluation. Cooling and evaluation should proceed simultaneously.

The patient with heat stroke requires immediate evacuation to medical facilities with intensive care capabilities. Active cooling should be started immediately and continued during evacuation.

- ◆ Prodromal symptoms include headache, dizziness (lightheadedness), restlessness, weakness, ataxia, confusion, disorientation, drowsiness, irrational or aggressive behavior, syncope, seizures, or coma.
- ◆ Collapse is a universal feature of heat stroke.
- ◆ An individual with a core temperature of ≥ 40°C (104°F) and CNS dysfunction that results in delirium, convulsions, or coma has heat stroke.
- o Casualties who are **unconscious** and have a core temperature of ≥ 39°C (102.2°F) have heatstroke.
  - ◆ Core temperature is often lower on arrival at a treatment area.
  - ◆ Seizures.
    - ◊ Occur frequently (> 50% of cases) with heatstroke.
    - ◊ Hinder cooling efforts.
    - ◊ Treat with diazepam 5–10 mg.
- o Treatment.
  - ◆ Rapid cooling can reduce heat stroke mortality anywhere from 50% down to 5%. Cooling by spraying cool water over the body and vigorous fanning can be effective though not as effective as ice water immersion. Any effective means of cooling is acceptable.
  - ◆ A variety of techniques have been used, and, while evaporative cooling is less effective, the ice immersion method may prevent safe cardiac monitoring or rapid resuscitation.
  - ◆ Cool water immersion (20°C) with skin massage is the classic technique. It provides rapid cooling. Closely monitor patient for, and prevent, shivering.
  - ◆ Cooling with cool-water–soaked sheets or ice chips and vigorous fanning is highly effective.
  - ◆ Do not use alcohol in the cooling solution because freezing of the skin can occur.

The goal of treatment is to effect a rapid lowering of the core temperature to 38°C (101°F), without inducing shivering.

♦ Rectal temperature should be closely monitored during cooling. Discontinue cooling efforts when core temperature reaches 38.3°C (101°F) to avoid hypothermia.

♦ Aspirin and acetaminophen should **NOT** be given to casualties of heatstroke.

♦ Aggressive fluid resuscitation is not required. Fluid requirements of 1 L in the first 30 minutes, with an additional 2 L or more in the next 2 hours may be sufficient. Because heat stroke patients are frequently hypoglycemic, the initial fluid should include dextrose (chilled IV fluid is of limited benefit).

◊ Base further hydration on fluid status/urinary output (Foley required).

◊ Overhydration can lead to congestive heart failure, cerebral edema, and pulmonary edema in the heat-stressed lung.

♦ If shivering develops, treat with diazepam (5–10 mg IV) or chlorpromazine (50 mg IV).

♦ Patients are frequently agitated, combative, or seizing. Diazepam is effective for control and can be administered IV, endotracheally, or rectally, but should be used with caution.

♦ Airway control is essential. Vomiting is common and endotracheal intubation should be used in any patient with a reduced level of consciousness, or otherwise unable to protect the airway. Supplemental oxygen should be provided when available.

♦ Hypotensive patients who do not respond to saline should receive inotropic support. Careful titrated use of dopamine or dobutamine is reasonable and has the potential added advantage of improving renal perfusion.

♦ Pulmonary artery wedge pressure monitoring should be used in patients with persistent hemodynamic instability.

♦ Management of encephalopathy is supportive in nature and is directed at minimizing cerebral edema by avoiding fluid overreplacement and by assuring hemodynamic, thermal, and metabolic stability. IV mannitol has been used to treat life-threatening cerebral edema, but is questionable unless renal function is adequate and the patient is fully hydrated. The efficacy of dexamethasone for treating heat-stroke–induced cerebral edema is not known.

o Complications.

♦ Rhabdomyolysis and secondary renal failure due to myoglobinuria and hyperuricemia; hyperkalemia; hypocalcemia; and compartment syndromes due to muscle swelling.

◊ Elevated creatine phosphokinase (CPK) (in the thousands).

◊ Administer IV fluid and possibly furosemide to maintain urinary output > 50 cc/h. (Assurance of adequate renal perfusion and urine flow will moderate the nephrotoxic effects of myoglobin and uric acid.)

◊ Hyperkalemia can be managed by K/Na ion exchange resin (Kayexalate) given orally or rectally as an enema. If available, dialysis may occasionally be indicated.

◊ Hypocalcemia does not usually require treatment.

◊ Increasing tenderness or tension in a muscle compartment may represent increasing intracompartmental pressures. Direct measurement of intramuscular pressure or fasciotomy should be considered. Pain and paresthesia from a compartment syndrome may not be present until after permanent damage has occurred.

♦ Alkalinize urine with sodium bicarbonate IV (2 amps NaHCO$_3$/L D5W). Management of acute renal failure requires exquisite attention to fluid and electrolyte balance. Uremic metabolic acidosis and hyperkalemia require dialysis for control.

♦ Coagulopathy due to hepatic injury.

◊ Hepatic injury is common, resulting in transaminase enzyme elevation, clotting factor deficiencies, and jaundice. Transaminase levels may be transient and reversible, but if they persist 48 hours, then it is indicative of more severe injury.

◊ Worst prothrombin time occurs at 48–72 hours postinjury.

◊ Thrombocytopenia and disseminated intravascular coagulation (DIC) peak at 18–36 hours postinjury.

◊ Beware of the coagulopathy timeframe when planning evacuation.

◊ Subclinical coagulopathy does not require active management. Clinically significant bleeding is an ominous sign. Treatment is directed at reducing the rate of coagulation and replacement of depleted clotting factors. Intravascular coagulation can be slowed by cautious heparin infusion (5–7 U/kg/h), followed in 2–3 hours by FFP and platelets. Successful management leads to a decline in indices of fibrinolysis (eg, fibrin split products). Heparin is tapered gradually over 2–3 days as directed by laboratory evidence of control.

◊ Monitor for hypo- or hyperglycemia.

♦ Prognosis is worse in patients with more severe degrees of encephalopathy. Permanent neurologic sequelae can develop after heat stroke, including cerebellar ataxia, paresis, seizure disorder, and cognitive dysfunction.

♦ Neurologic deterioration after initial recovery may represent intracranial hemorrhage related to diffuse intravascular coagulation or hematoma related to trauma unrecognized at the time of initial presentation.

♦ Other complications include gastrointestinal bleeding, jaundice, aspiration pneumonia, noncardiogenic pulmonary edema, and myocardial infarction. Immune incompetence and infection are late complications, particularly in patients with severe renal failure.

♦ Hyperkalemia is the most life-threatening early clinical problem. Measurement of serum potassium is an early priority.

● Heat cramps.

o Clinical presentation.

♦ Brief, intermittent, recurring, and often excruciating tonic muscle contractions that last 2–3 minutes. Preceded by palpable or visible fasciculations.

- ♦ Typically involve muscles of the abdomen, legs, and arms (voluntary muscles of the trunk and extremities). Smooth muscle, cardiac muscle, the diaphragm, and bulbar muscles are not involved.
- ♦ Occur often with heat exhaustion. (Despite the salt depletion associated with heat cramps, frank signs and symptoms of heat exhaustion are unusual.)
- ♦ There are no systemic manifestations except those attributable to pain.
- ♦ Occur in healthy individuals who exercise for prolonged periods in warm environments.
- ♦ Occur in salt-depleted patients, generally during a period of recovery after a period of work in the heat.
- ♦ Differential diagnosis: tetany due to alkalosis (hyperventilation, severe gastroenteritis, cholera), hypocalcemia, strychnine poisoning, black widow spider envenomation, and abdominal colic.
  - o Treatment.
    - ♦ Mild cases can be treated with oral 0.1%–0.2% salt solutions. Salt tablets should not used as an oral salt source.
    - ♦ Most "sports drinks" (diluted 1:1 with water) effective for mild cases.
    - ♦ IV NS provides rapid relief in more severe cases
    - ♦ Patients with heat cramps usually have substantial salt deficits (15–30 g over 2–3 days, usual dietary intake). These individuals should be allowed 2–3 days to replenish salt and water deficits before returning to work in the heat.
- ● Heat exhaustion.
  - o Clinical presentation.
    - ♦ Thirst, headache, dyspnea, lightheadedness (orthostatic dizziness), profound physical fatigue, anorexia, confusion, anxiety, agitation, mood change, chills, piloerection, nausea, and vomiting. There is no combination of presenting symptoms and signs that is pathognomonic.
    - ♦ Often accompanied by heat cramps.
    - ♦ Oliguria, clinical dehydration, ataxia, tachycardia, and

tachypnea resulting in symptomatic hyperventilation with acroparesthesia and carpopedal spasm.

♦ Syncope may occur.

♦ Core temperature is < 39°C (102.2°F), even at time of collapse.

o Treatment.

♦ Oral rehydration (if patient is not vomiting).

♦ Parenteral fluids produce more rapid recovery: no more than 250 mL NS bolus without laboratory surveillance; after 2.5 L of plain saline, add dextrose as a source of energy (D2.5^1/$_2$NaCl); subsequent fluid replacement should be D5^1/$_2$NS or D5^1/$_4$NS. Individuals with significant salt depletion have coincident potassium depletion, often amounting to 300–400 mEq of KCl. To begin restoration of potassium deficit, inclusion of potassium in parenteral fluids after volume resuscitation is appropriate if there is no evidence of renal insufficiency or rhabdomyolysis.

♦ Does not require active cooling; however, because symptoms are difficult to distinguish from heat stroke, the **safest course** is to provide active cooling for all casualties who are at risk for heat stroke.

♦ Removal from hot environment.

♦ Stop exercising, move out of the sun.

• Minor heat illnesses.

o Miliaria rubra, miliaria profunda, and anhidrotic heat exhaustion.

♦ Subacute (miliaria rubra) pruritic inflamed papulovesicular skin eruption that appears in actively sweating skin exposed to high humidity. Becomes generalized and prolonged (miliaria profunda); lesions are truncal, noninflamed papular, with less evidence of vesiculation than the lesions of miliaria rubra.

♦ Each miliarial papulovesicle represents an eccrine sweat gland whose duct is occluded at the level of the epidermal stratum granulosum by inspissated organic debris.

♦ Eccrine secretions accumulate in the glandular portion of the gland and infiltrate into the surrounding dermis.

- ◆ Pruritus is increased with increased sweating.
- ◆ Miliarial skin cannot fully participate in thermoregulatory sweating, therefore the risk of heat illness increases in proportion to the amount of skin surface involved. Sweat does not appear on the surface of affected skin.
- ◆ Sleeplessness due to pruritus and secondary infection of occluded glands has systemic effects that further degrade optimal thermoregulation.
- ◆ Miliaria is treated by cooling and drying affected skin, avoiding conditions that induce sweating, controlling infection, and relieving pruritus. Eccrine gland function recovers with desquamation of the affected epidermis, which takes 7–10 days.
- ◆ Miliaria profunda causes an uncommon but disabling disorder: anhidrotic heat exhaustion (or tropical anhidrotic asthenia). Miliaria profunda causes a marked inhibition of thermoregulatory sweating and heat intolerance similar to that of ectodermal dysplasia. That individual is more at risk for heat exhaustion and at high risk of heat stroke in conditions tolerated by others.
- ◆ Evacuation to a cooler environment until restoration of normal eccrine gland function.
- o Heat-induced syncope.
  - ◆ Due to a reduced effective blood volume. (Thermal stress increases risk of classic neurally mediated [vasovagal] syncope by aggravating peripheral pooling of blood in dilated cutaneous vessels.)
  - ◆ Symptoms range from light-headedess to loss of consciousness.
  - ◆ Typically someone standing in a hot environment.
  - ◆ Greatest risk on first day of heat exposure, subsequent risk decreases daily.
  - ◆ Risk almost zero after 1 week of heat exposure; however, syncope occurring during or after work in the heat, or after more than 5 days of heat exposure, should be considered evidence of heat exhaustion.
  - ◆ Core temperature is not elevated or only very minimally so.
  - ◆ Patient regains consciousness immediately after syncope.

- ◆ Clinical evaluation and management should be directed toward the syncopal episode, not potential heat illness. Treatment is oral hydration and continued acclimatization.
- o Heat edema.
  - ◆ Seen early in heat exposure.
  - ◆ Plasma volume expanding to compensate for the increased need for thermoregulatory blood flow.
  - ◆ In absence of other disease, condition is of no clinical significance.
  - ◆ Will resolve spontaneously.
  - ◆ Diuretic therapy is not appropriate and may increase risk of heat illness.
- o Sunburn.
  - ◆ Reduces thermoregulatory capacity of skin.
  - ◆ Systemic effect: hyperthermia.
  - ◆ Preventable.
  - ◆ Affected soldiers should be kept from significant heat strain until the burn has healed.
- o Heat tetany.
  - ◆ Rare; occurs in individuals acutely exposed to overwhelming heat stress.
  - ◆ Extremely severe heat stress induces hyperventilation.
  - ◆ Manifestations include respiratory alkalosis, carpopedal spasm, and syncope.
  - ◆ Treatment: removal from heat source and control of hyperventilation (rebreathing into paper bag to reverse respiratory alkalosis).
  - ◆ Dehydration and salt depletion are not prominent features.

Altitude Illness
Exposure of troops to the hypobaric hypoxia of altitude results in a decrement of performance, as well as the possible development of altitude illness. Altitude illness spans a spectrum from high-altitude bronchitis, to acute mountain sickness (AMS), to death from high-altitude pulmonary edema (HAPE) and high-altitude cerebral edema (HACE).

- Altitude basics.

The occurrence of altitude illness is based on altitude and rapidity of ascent. Contributory factors include level of exertion, physiologic susceptibility, age, and coexisting medical conditions.

- o Physiologic changes due to altitude begin to occur at just over 1,500 m (4,900 ft).
- o These changes are the body's attempt to acclimatize to altitude.
- o Symptoms occurring below 2,250 m (7,400 ft) are rarely due to altitude illness.
  - ◆ Rapid ascent to high altitudes results in a high incidence of altitude illness.
  - ◆ Climbing Mt. Rainier brings one from sea level to 14,500 ft (4,400 m) in 36 hours and results in a 70% incidence of altitude illness. An ascent to a similar height over the course of 5 days would only result in a 5% incidence of altitude illness.
  - ◆ 10%–20% of soldiers who ascend rapidly (< 24 h) to altitudes between 1,829–2,446 m (6,000–8,000 ft) experience some mild symptoms
  - ◆ Rapid ascent to elevations of 3,670–4,300 m (12,000–14,000 ft) results in moderate symptoms in over 50% of the soldiers, and 12%–18% may have severe symptoms.
  - ◆ Rapid ascent to 5,333 m (17,500 ft) causes severe, incapacitating symptoms in almost all individuals.
- Descent basics.
  - o Almost everything improves with prompt descent.
  - o For illness requiring descent, one should try to descend at least 1,000 m (3,300 ft) if not more.
  - o A Gamow bag (USA) (portable fabric hyperbaric chamber) or Certec SA (Europe) can temporize a patient if evacuation /descent is not possible.
  - o Symptoms typically resolve quickly with descent, but may linger for several days.
  - o Victims of HACE and HAPE should not reascend until 72 hours after symptoms abate, and then must ascend much slower than previously.

o Victims of HACE or HAPE should descend at the earliest sign, before they become moribund and incapable of aiding in their own descent.

o **There are no reliable predictors of susceptibility to AMS except prior experience at altitude.**

Incidence and severity of symptoms vary with initial altitude, rate of ascent, level of exertion, and individual susceptibility.

---

o Vigorous physical activity during ascent or within 24 hours after ascent will increase both the incidence and severity of symptoms.

♦ If a soldier became ill previously at a given altitude he or she will likely become ill at the same altitude unless the ascent is slower to allow for better acclimatization.

♦ Physical fitness level has **no effect** on susceptibility to altitude illness.

♦ Oral sildenafil (Viagra) 50 mg qd increases exercise tolerance in healthy volunteers at altitude (5,200 m [17,000 ft]), although it has not been approved for this purpose. The role of this drug in the treatment and/or prophylaxis of AMS and HAPE has not been established.

♦ If a rapid ascent to altitude must be made, use prophylaxis against AMS.

● Acute mountain sickness.

o AMS is the most common form of altitude illness.

o Onset is shortly after arrival at high altitude. Onset occurs 3–24 hours after ascent. Symptoms reach peak severity in 24–72 hours and usually subside over the course of 3–7 days.

o Further ascent without an acclimation period usually exacerbates symptoms and can result in increased incidence of HAPE and HACE. The majority of AMS cases do not progress to more serious altitude illness without continued ascent.

o Symptoms.

♦ Headache: Symmetric, global in location, and throbbing in character. Most intense during night and shortly after arising in the morning, attributed to increased hypoxemia caused by altitude-induced sleep apnea.

♦ Anorexia.
♦ Nausea.
♦ Fatigue (weakness).
♦ General malaise.
♦ Decreased coordination.
♦ Dizziness or light-headedness.
♦ Oliguria.
♦ Emesis (vomiting).
♦ Lassitude.
♦ Insomnia: Sleep disturbances with periodic breathing with recurrent apneic periods during sleep are usually present, but are not necessarily a component of AMS.

o Diagnosis.

♦ Occurrence of a headache and at least one other sign/symptom in an individual who ascended from low (1,524 m or < 5,000 ft) to high altitude, or high altitude to higher altitude in the previous 24–48 hours.
♦ Differential diagnosis includes viral gastroenteritis, hangover, exhaustion, dehydration, carbon monoxide poisoning, and HACE.
♦ Presence of neurologic symptoms such as incoordination, ataxia, and excessive lethargy or cognitive dysfunction is indicative of progression to HACE, which requires immediate therapeutic intervention.

o Prophylaxis for AMS.

♦ Gradual acclimation.

◊ Staged ascent: Soldiers ascend to intermediate altitudes and remain there for 3 or more days before ascending further.
◊ Graded ascent: Limits daily altitude gain to allow partial acclimation. Sleep altitude is most important. Have soldiers spend 2 nights at 2,743 m (9,000 ft) and limit the sleeping altitude to no more than 305 m (1,000 ft) per day above previous night's sleep altitude.
◊ Combination of both staged and graded ascent is the safest and most effective prevention method.

♦ Diet: High carbohydrate diet (< 70% of total energy intake as carbohydrates) (stimulation of ventilation through increased carbon dioxide produced from metabolism of carbohydrates).

♦ Acetazolamide, 250 mg qid or 500 mg bid po, starting 48 hours before ascent, continuing for 48 hours after ascent. Side effects include peripheral paresthesias, fatigue, increased urination (polyuria), and altered taste imparted to carbonated beverages. It prevents AMS in 50%–75% of soldiers and reduces symptoms in most others. Short-term use when changing altitude significantly (400 m). **Contraindicated in sulfa allergy**.

♦ Dexamethasone, 4 mg qid po is the prophylaxis of choice in sulfa-allergic individuals. Dexamethasone does not aid acclimatization and effects are gone when it is stopped. Dexamethasone +/– acetazolamide is also prophylaxis of choice for missions of a rapid, high (over 4,000 m [13,000 ft]), short-duration profile (raids, rescues).

♦ Cyanosis: Oxygen 2–6 L/min. Do not delay descent.

o **Treatment.**

♦ AMS alone does NOT mandate descent.

♦ Remain at the same elevation; do **not** ascend until symptoms abate.

♦ Acetazolamide, 125 mg qid to 500 mg, tid, po—do not use in patients with sulfa allergies. (If already receiving a preventive dose of acetazolamide (1,000 mg/d) and still symptomatic, 500 mg can be added with caution.

♦ Dexamethasone in doses of 2–4 mg q6h (has the same potentially serious side effects as when used as a prophylaxis). Symptoms may recur when medication stopped.

♦ Oxygen by nasal cannula 2–6 L/min (severe headache).

♦ Do NOT advance sleeping altitude.

♦ Symptomatic treatment with ASA, acetaminophen, prochlorperazine for nausea and vomiting 5–10 mg tid–qid, po or IM, or 25 mg bid prn also stimulates respiration; ibuprofen for headache.

♦ Minimize utilization of sleeping agents at altitude; they

can worsen illness. Acetazolamide for sleep disorders, 250 mg qid or tid po. Temazepam for insomnia 30 mg qhs po; triazolam for insomnia 0.125–0.25 mg qhs po. Short-term use only. Possible short-term memory loss.

- High-altitude pharyngitis and bronchitis.
  - o Common condition occurring after 2–3 weeks at altitude.
  - o Common at altitudes over 5,486 m (18,000 ft).
  - o Sore throat, chronic cough, and severe cough spasms (severe enough to cause rib fractures).
  - o Environmental, from breathing cold dry air.
  - o Altitude-induced tachypnea aggravates the problem.
  - o Cold-induced vasomotor rhinitis, especially at night, stimulates mouth breathing and also aggravates problem.
  - o Usually not caused by infection, although infection can occur.
  - o Patient will **not** have dyspnea at rest.
  - o Symptomatic treatment with lozenges, mild cough suppressant, and decongestant nasal sprays. Personnel can use a mask or a porous, breathable silk balaclava as a mouth covering to reduce respiratory heat and moisture loss.
  - o Maintain hydration.
- High-altitude peripheral edema.
  - o Altitude-related edema of hands and face.
  - o Hypoxia-induced retention of sodium and water.
  - o Not considered related to AMS/HACE edema-spectrum or HAPE.
  - o Decreased urine output and weight gain of 2.7–5.4 kg (6–12 lb) over several days; most evident upon awakening.
  - o Diagnosis based on association of characteristic peripheral edema with ascent to high altitude; recurs consistently with repeat ascents; more common in females.
  - o Differential diagnosis includes cardiogenic edema, allergic reactions, and edema of the upper extremities caused by pack straps or binding by tight clothes.
  - o Prophylaxis includes salt restriction. The acetazolamide regimen used to prevent AMS is often successful in preventing peripheral edema.

- o Treatment with diuretics (one 20–40 mg dose of furosemide, or 250 mg of acetazolamide every 8 h for 3 doses) and salt restriction.
- High-altitude retinal hemorrhage (HARH).
  - o Bleeding from retinal vessels during altitude exposure. One of the manifestations of hypoxia-induced retinopathy.
  - o Caused by BP "surges" within the distended vessels.
  - o Usually asymptomatic; normally does not adversely affect military operations; however, can affect an individual soldier's vision.
  - o Hemorrhages are self-limiting and resolve in 1–2 weeks after descent.
- Thromboembolic events.
  - o Increased possibility of thromboembolic event with ascent to high altitude: thrombophlebitis, deep venous thrombosis, pulmonary embolus, transient ischemic attacks (TIAs), and stroke.
  - o Probably result from hypoxia-induced polycythemia and clotting abnormalities but also may result from environmental and mission factors such as dehydration, cold, and venous stasis caused by prolonged periods of inactivity during inclement weather or by constriction of tight-fitting clothing and equipment.
  - o Unusual below 4,267 m (14,000 ft). At very high and extreme altitudes (> 4,200 m [13,700 ft]) these events are not uncommon, and thrombophlebitis appears to be relatively common.
  - o Clinical manifestations are similar to manifestations of thromboembolic events at low altitude, except for their occurrence in young and otherwise healthy personnel.
  - o Prevention relies on reducing the risk factors by maintaining adequate hydration and warmth and by avoiding conditions that might cause venous stasis.
  - o Evacuation to lower altitude is required. Treatment follows standard treatment guidelines, including appropriate anticoagulation. In the field setting, fractionated heparin (one dose of 250 IU/d) can be used prior to and during evacuation.
- Subacute mountain sickness.

o Prolonged deployment (weeks to months) to elevations above 3,658 m (12,000 ft).

o Common manifestations include sleep disturbances, anorexia, weight loss, fatigue, daytime somnolence, and subnormal mentation.

o Caused by failure to acclimatize adequately.

o Some relief of symptoms obtained from low-flow oxygen and from acetazolamide.

o Evacuate to lower altitude as soon as practical.

o Some degree of immune suppression and poor wound healing occurs in personnel at very high and extreme altitudes. Injuries resulting from burns, ballistics, and physical trauma should be considered more clinically significant at high altitude.

- High-altitude pulmonary edema.
  o Potentially fatal, **non**cardiogenic pulmonary edema.
  o Occurs in < 10% of personnel ascending above 3,700 m (12,000 ft).
  o Onset 2–4 days after rapid ascent to altitudes greater than 2,438 m (8,000 ft).
  o Repeated ascents and descents above 3,700 m (12,000 ft) increase susceptibility.
  o Risk factors.
    ♦ Moderate to severe exertion.
    ♦ Cold exposure.
    ♦ Anxiety.
    ♦ Young age.
    ♦ Male sex.
    ♦ Obesity (possibly).
  o Early symptoms (pulmonary edema).
    ♦ Nonproductive cough.
    ♦ Rales (few).
    ♦ Dyspnea on exertion.
    ♦ Fatigue.
    ♦ Weakness with decreased tolerance for physical activity and increased time for recovery after physical exertion.
    ♦ Resting tachycardia and tachypnea greater than induced by altitude alone.

♦ Once symptoms appear, HAPE can progress very rapidly (< 12 hours) to coma and death.
♦ Nail beds and lips may be more cyanotic than other unit members.

o Progressing pulmonary edema.
♦ Productive cough of frothy and sometimes pink or bloodstained sputum.
♦ Rales more numerous and widespread.
♦ Wheezing may develop.
♦ Lung sounds become audible even without stethoscope, especially when individual is supine.
♦ Orthopnea may occur (< 20%).
♦ Progressive hypoxemia causes dyspnea and cyanosis.
♦ Arterial blood gas (if available) documents hypoxemia, hypocapnia, and slight increase in pH.
♦ Mental status deteriorates with progressive confusion and sometimes vivid hallucinations.
♦ Obtundation, coma, and death occur without treatment.
♦ Subfebrile temperature < 38°C (100.5°F) and a mild increase in white blood cell count may be present
♦ Dyspnea at rest.
♦ Marked hypoxia by oximetry.
♦ **Dyspnea at rest and cough should be considered to be the onset of HAPE.**

DELAY IN TREATMENT OF PROGRESSIVE PULMONARY EDEMA AT ALTITUDE USUALLY RESULTS IN **DEATH.**

---

o Treatment.
♦ Depends on severity.
♦ Immediate descent is mandatory! Descent of even a few hundred meters (300–1,000 m) can be helpful or even lifesaving in severe cases.
♦ Mortality can approach 50% if descent cannot be accomplished rapidly.
♦ Oxygen by cannula 2–6 L/min (mild), or by mask 4–6 L/min (moderate and severe). DO NOT DELAY DESCENT!

- ◆ Portable fabric hyperbaric chamber may be lifesaving— Gamow bag/Certec SA.
- ◆ Nifedipine, 10 mg tid sublingually, or 20 mg po. A second 10-mg, sublingual dose can be administered in 15–20 minutes if no improvement in symptoms is apparent, followed by 30 mg qid.

Nifedipine should not be used in lieu of descent, supplemental oxygen, or treatment in a hyperbaric bag. It may be used in conjunction with other therapies.

- ◆ Immediate descent to lower elevation; if symptoms resolve, wait at least 72 hours before attempted return to previous elevation.

Neither furosemide nor morphine sulfate should be used in the treatment of HAPE unless other more effective treatment options are not available.

- ◆ Treatment after descent, at an MTF, is directed toward ensuring adequate oxygenation and reducing pulmonary artery pressure; includes bed rest, supplemental oxygen, and nifedipine.
- ◆ Invasive diagnostic procedures such as bronchoscopy or pulmonary artery catheterization are **NOT** indicated unless clinical course deteriorates and the diagnosis is in doubt. Endotracheal intubation is seldom necessary.
- o HAPE Prophylaxis.
  - ◆ Nifedipine, 20 mg tid, po, 24 hours before ascent, continuing 72 hours after ascent.
- ● High-altitude cerebral edema.
  - o Onset following ascent is highly variable and occurs later than either AMS or HAPE. Mean duration of onset 5 days with a range of 1–13 days.
  - o Incidence lower than AMS or HAPE (< 1% of individuals making rapid ascent).
  - o Potentially fatal, uncommon (< 2% above 3,700 m). Can occur as low as 2,430 m (8,000 ft) but vast majority of cases

above 3,600 m (12,000 ft). Untreated HACE can progress to death over 1–3 days or become more fulminant with death occurring in < 12 hours.

o Exacerbation of unresolved, severe AMS.

o **Most often occurs in people who have AMS symptoms and continue to ascend.**

o Signs and symptoms.

♦ Most signs and symptoms are a manifestation of progressive cerebral edema.

♦ **Early signs resemble AMS (these symptoms are not invariably present).**

♦ Severe headache

♦ Nausea

♦ Vomiting.

♦ Extreme lassitude.

o Progressing **signs.**

♦ Mental status changes: Confusion, disorientation, drowsiness, and impaired mentation.

♦ Truncal ataxia (swaying of upper body, especially when walking). As the edema progresses, soldier may also exhibit an ataxic gait in addition to the truncal ataxia.

♦ Soldier appears withdrawn, and behavior is mistakenly attributed to fatigue or anxiety.

♦ Cyanosis and general pallor are common.

♦ Symptoms of HAPE.

o Untreated HACE.

♦ Variety of focal and generalized neurologic abnormalities may develop: visual changes, anesthesias, paresthesias, clonus, pathological reflexes, hyperreflexia, bladder and bowel dysfunction, hallucinations, and seizures.

♦ Papilledema may be present in up to 50% of the soldiers, but is **NOT** universal.

o Coma.

Ataxia at altitude is HACE.

o Prophylaxis.

No definitive evidence; however, due to similarity with AMS, prophylactic measures for HACE include use of staged or graded ascent, high carbohydrate diet, and use of acetazolamide.

o Treatment.

♦ Immediate descent is mandatory. Definitive treatment of HACE is immediate descent. In general, the greater the descent the better the outcome. Descent of more than 300 m (1,000 ft) may be required for clinical improvement, and descents to altitudes of less than 2,500 m (8,000 ft) is optimal.

♦ If descent is delayed, treatment with a portable cloth hyperbaric chamber may be lifesaving. May require at least 6 hours of pressurization in chamber.

♦ Oxygen by mask or cannula 2–6 L/m; should not be used as a substitute for descent.

♦ Dexamethasone, 4–8 mg initially and then 4 mg qid, po, IV, or IM. DO NOT DELAY DESCENT! Few side effects if used only 3–4 days.

♦ Loop diuretics and osmotic diuretic agents, such as mannitol, urea, and glycerol, have been suggested, but there is little experience with them in this role. Careful attention is required before diuretics are used. Individual may have altitude-induced decrease in intravascular volume concomitant with cerebral edema.

♦ Hospital management consists of supplemental oxygen (if needed to maintain arterial oxygen levels), supportive care, and possibly diuretics. Comatose patients may require intubation and bladder catheterization.

HACE and HAPE often coexist. Individuals with HACE will often have HAPE; however, most individuals with HAPE do not have concomitant HACE.

Chapter 30

Radiological Injuries

> The reader is strongly advised to supplement material in this chapter with the following two references:
> 1. *Medical Management of Radiological Casualties Handbook*, 2003, Armed Forces Radiobiology Research Institute, Bethesda, MD.
> 2. *Medical Management of the Acute Radiation Syndrome: Recommendations of the Strategic National Stockpile.* Radiation Working Group, Strategic National Stockpile (*Annals of Internal Medicine*, 15 June 2004).

Introduction

Radiological casualties on the battlefield may occur with improvised or conventional nuclear devices or radiological dispersal devices ("dirty bombs") (Table 30-1).

- Conventional nuclear weapons.
  - o The relative casualty-causing potential depends primarily on four factors:
    - ◆ Yield of the weapon.
    - ◆ Height of burst.
    - ◆ Environmental conditions in which the detonation occurs.
    - ◆ Distribution and shielding of troops in the target area.
  - o A nuclear detonation generally causes injuries with the following distribution:
    - ◆ Blast injury: 50%.
    - ◆ Thermal injury: 35%.
    - ◆ Ionizing radiation injury.
      - ◊ Initial: 5%.
      - ◊ Residual: 10%.

- A radiological dispersal device (RDD) is any device, including any weapon or equipment, other than a nuclear explosive device, specifically designed to spread radiation.
  - o RDDs contaminate conventional casualties with radionuclides, complicating medical evacuation.
  - o RDDs are ideal weapons for terrorism and are used to intimidate and deny access to an area by spreading radioactive material.

Table 30-1. Radiological casualties.

Weapon Effect	Weapon Yield (Kiloton)/Distance (Meters)			
	1 kt	10 kt	100 kt	1,000 kt
Blast (50% casualties)	140 m	360 m	860 m	3,100 m
Thermal radiation (50% deep burns)	370 m	1,100 m	3,190 m	8,020 m
Ionizing radiation (50% immediate transient ineffectiveness)	600 m	950 m	1,400 m	2,900 m
Ionizing radiation (50% lethality)	800 m	1,100 m	1,600 m	3,200 m

Triage

- Different from conventionally injured patients, because survivable radiation injury is not manifested until days to weeks after exposure.
  - o **Based primarily on conventional injuries**, then modified by radiation injury level.
  - o Make a preliminary diagnosis of radiation injury only for those with exposure symptoms, such as nausea, vomiting, diarrhea, fever, ataxia, seizures, prostration, hypotension.
  - o Radiation patient triage classifications.
    - ◆ **Delayed:** casualties with only radiation injury, without gross neurological symptoms (ataxia, seizures, impaired cognition). For trauma combined with radiation injury, all surgical procedures must be completed within 36–48 hours of radiation exposure, or delayed until at least 2 months after the injury.

♦ **Immediate:** those requiring immediate lifesaving intervention. Pure radiation injury is not acutely life-threatening unless the irradiation is massive. If a massive dose has been received, the patient is classified as Expectant.

♦ **Minimal:** buddy care is particularly useful here. Casualties with radiological injury should have all wounds and lacerations meticulously cleaned and then closed.

♦ **Expectant:** receive appropriate supportive treatment compatible with resources; large doses of analgesics as needed.

● Table 30-2 provides medical aspects of radiation injuries.

Table 30-2. Medical aspects of radiation injuries.

Probability/degree of exposure		Signs and Symptoms						
		Nausea	Vomiting	Diarrhea	Hyperthermia	Erythema	Hypotension	CNS dysfunction
	Unlikely	–	–	–	–	–	–	–
	Probable	++	+	+/–	+/–	–	–	–
	Severe	+++	+++	+/+++	+/+++	–/++	+/++	–/++

The lethal dose of radiation, which will kill 50% of a population within 60 days of exposure, is called $LD_{50/60}$. The $LD_{50/60}$ is approximately 3–4 Gray (Gy) for a population with radiation injury alone and with no significant medical care. The $LD_{50/60}$ for a population with radiation injury alone and the best available medical care (including antiemetics, antivirals, antibiotics, hematopoietic cytokines, and transfusion) may be 6 Gy or more. Combined injuries with radiation and trauma and/or burns will markedly lower the LD_{50}.

Significant medical care may be required at 3–5 weeks for 10%–50% of personnel. Anticipated problems should include infection, bleeding, fever, vomiting, and diarrhea. Wounding or burns will markedly increase morbidity and mortality.

- Treatment.
  - o Fluid and electrolytes for GI losses.
  - o Cytokines for immunocompromised patients (follow granulocyte counts).
  - o Restricted duty. No further radiation exposure, elective surgery, or wounding. May require delayed evacuation from theater during nuclear war IAW command guidance.
  - o If there are more than $1.7 \bullet 10^9$ lymphocytes per liter, 48 hours after exposure, it is unlikely that an individual has received a fatal dose.

Patients with low (300–500) or decreasing lymphocyte counts, or low granulocyte counts, should be considered for cytokine therapy and biological dosimetry using metaphase analysis where available.

- Asymptomatic patients with lethal radiation dose may perform usual duties until symptomatic.

Potential Injuries
- **Thermal/flash burns** or thermal pulse burns are caused directly by infrared radiation. Close to the fireball, the thermal output is often so great that everything is incinerated, and even at great distances, thermal/flash burns will occur (see Chapter 28, Burns, for management).
  - o Burn mortality rates associated with radiation exposure are significantly higher due to bone marrow suppression and infection (a 50% TBSA burn associated with radiation exposure has a mortality of 90%).
- **Blast injuries** associated with a nuclear detonation include:
  - o Direct blast wave overpressure forces measured in terms of atmosphere overpressure.
  - o Indirect blast wind drag forces, measured in terms of wind velocity, which may displace large objects such as vehicles or cause the collapse of buildings.

- **Radiation injuries** are due to ionizing radiation released both at the time of the nuclear detonation and for a considerable time afterward. The two types of radiation released are electromagnetic (gamma) radiation and particulate (alpha, beta, and neutron) radiation.
  - o Alpha particles can be shielded against by clothing.
  - o Beta particles shielding requires solid materials, like a wall.
  - o Gamma and neutron radiation are the most biologically active, and require lead equivalent shielding for protection.
  - o Fission products are the major radiation hazard in fallout, because a large number emit penetrating gamma radiation. This can result in injuries, even at great distances.
  - o Fallout causes whole body irradiation from gamma-emitting isotopes, because they do not actually have to be on a person's skin to cause damage.
- **Flash blindness** may occur as the result of a sudden peripheral visual observation of a brilliant flash of intense light energy. **Retinal burns** may also occur and result in scarring and permanent altered visual acuity.

Treatment of Combined Injuries
- Following the detonation of a nuclear device, the majority of resulting casualties will have sustained a combination of blast, thermal, and radiological injuries.
- The usual methods of treatment for blast injuries must be modified in those casualties simultaneously exposed to ionizing radiation.

Traditionally, combat wounds are left open. However, wounds left open to heal by secondary intention in the irradiated patient will serve as a nidus of infection. <u>Wounds exposed to ionizing radiation should be debrided and closed at a second-look operation within 36–48 hours.</u>

- Hypotension should always be assumed to be hypovolemia and not due to radiologic injury.
- Hyperthermia is common.
- Radiological injuries increase the morbidity and mortality of injuries due to compromise of the normal hematopoietic and

immune responses to injury. Surgical procedures may need to be delayed during bone marrow suppression if at all possible.

- Potassium iodide may be used for prevention of thyroid uptake of radioisotopes after nuclear reactor accidents.
- Chelating agents may be used to eliminate metals from the bloodstream before they reach target organs.
- Mobilizing agents are used to increase the excretion of internal contaminants.
- Prussian blue is used to remove radionuclides from the capillary bed surrounding the intestine and prevents their reabsorption. Delay until patient is stable. Treat ABCs first.

Decontamination

- No healthcare provider has ever been injured with radiation while performing ABCs on a radiation victim.
- Removal of the casualty's clothing can remove as much as 90% of the radiological contamination.
- The first priority of surface decontamination should be to open wounds, then other areas.
  - o To prevent rapid incorporation of radioactive particles, wounds should be copiously irrigated with normal saline for several minutes.
  - o The eyes, ears, nose, mouth, areas adjacent to uncontaminated wounds, hair, and remaining skin surface should be decontaminated with soap and water.
  - o Personnel providing decontamination must protect themselves from ionizing radiation exposure with:
    - ♦ Protective outer clothing.
    - ♦ Aprons, gloves, and masks.
- Amputation should be seriously considered when the contamination burden is great and severe radionecrosis is likely.

Logistics of Casualty Management

- **If nuclear weapons are employed within the theater, the entire medical evacuation and treatment system will be severely overburdened** and some system of classification and sorting of casualties must be added to the normal procedures of evacuation and hospitalization.

- Patients entering a medical treatment facility should be routinely decontaminated if monitoring for radiation is not available.
- These two requirements, the sorting of casualties and the holding of the excess numbers, must be planned for and drilled as part of the normal organization and operation of the health service support system in a theater of operations where radiation exposure potential is high.

Chapter 31

Biological Warfare Agents

Introduction
Biological warfare (BW) agents infect the body via the same portals of entry as infectious organisms that occur naturally. These include inhalation into the respiratory tract, ingestion into the GI tract, and absorption through mucous membranes, eyes, skin, or wounds. Most BW agents will enter the body through inhalation. Usually, the disease produced by a BW agent will mimic the naturally occurring disease, but the clinical presentation can be different if delivery of an agent occurs through a portal that differs from the natural portal.

Detection
- Compressed epidemiology with record numbers of sick and dying in a short time.
- High attack rates (60%–90%).
- High incidence of pulmonary involvement when usual form of infection is not (eg, anthrax).
- Incidence of a particular disease in an unlikely location.
- Increased deaths of animals of all species.
- Near simultaneous outbreaks of several different epidemics at the same site.
- Biological Identification Detection System or standoff BW detectors alarming.
- Direct evidence of an attack such as contaminated or unexploded munitions.

Diagnosis

> The first indication of an attack may be when large numbers of patients present with the same constellation of signs and symptoms, especially for a disease that is not endemic to the area of operations.

Rapid diagnostic tests may be available in forward areas to assist clinicians in early diagnosis:

- Isolation of the etiologic agent can occur within 1–2 days for some agents.
- Enzyme-linked immunosorbent assays (ELISA).
- Genome detection by polymerase chain reaction (PCR).
- Antibody detection.

Prevention and Protection

- Immunizations: Anthrax, and in specific scenarios, smallpox and plague.
  - o Pre- or postexposure chemoprophylaxis—anthrax, plague, Q fever, and tularemia. Chemoprophylaxis for anthrax is presently FDA-approved for postexposure only.
    - ♦ Investigational new drugs exist for the treatment of Argentine hemorrhagic fever, botulinum toxin, Q fever, Rift Valley fever, Venezuelan Equine Encephalitis (VEE), and tularemia.
- Protective clothing and mask.

Decontamination —Personnel, Equipment, and Clothing

- **Mechanical** decontamination removes, but not necessarily neutralizes, the BW agent.
  - o Brushing to ensure loosening of the BW agent from the surface.
  - o Filtration and chlorination of drinking water to remove organisms.
- **Chemical** decontamination renders BW agents harmless through the use of disinfectants.
  - o Soap and water followed with copious rinsing with water is often sufficient.
  - o For patients requiring urgent decontamination, biologic agents are neutralized within 5 minutes when contaminated areas are washed with a 0.5 % hypochlorite solution (1 part household bleach mixed with 9 parts water).
  - o **Do not use hypochlorite in the eyes, abdominal cavity, or on nerve tissue**.
  - o A 5% hypochlorite solution (ie, household bleach) may be used to decontaminate clothing or equipment.

- **Physical** decontamination such as heat and solar ultraviolet (UV) radiation.
  - o Dry heat for 2 hours at 160°C.
  - o Autoclaving at 120°C under 1 atm of overpressure for 20 minutes.
  - o UV radiation difficult to standardize.
- Dry biological agents can be a hazard through secondary aerosolization; but adequate liquid decontamination will prevent this hazard. There is no vapor hazard, and special protective masks are generally not required for surgical personnel.

Infection Control

Infection control procedures should be reinforced for situations involving BW agents. Standard precautions are appropriate for BW agents once they have been identified. For an undifferentiated febrile illness following a BW agent attack:

- Place patients together in an isolated setting such as a designated tent or other structure.
- Surgical masks may be placed on patients when isolation is not possible.
- Employ respiratory droplet precautions along with standard precautions until diseases transmissible by droplet (such as plague and smallpox) have been excluded.

Medical Evacuation

- If plague, smallpox, and the hemorrhagic fevers can be **excluded**, patients may be evacuated using standard precautions and the disease-specific precautions.

> **Plague and smallpox are internationally quarantinable diseases (IQDs). Do not evacuate patient across international borders unless authorized by the theater surgeon.**

- Isolation precautions should be added to standard precautions.
- Immediately upon diagnosing patients with smallpox, the line and medical chain of command must be notified.
- Observe strict quarantine.

o Standard and respiratory droplet isolation precautions.
- ◆ **Standard precautions**.
  - ◊ Hand washing after patient contact.
  - ◊ Use of gloves when touching blood, body fluids, secretions, excretions, and contaminated items.
  - ◊ Use of mask, eye protection, and gown during procedures likely to generate sprays of blood, body fluids, secretions, or excretions.
  - ◊ Handle contaminated patient-care equipment and linen in a manner that precludes transfer of micro-organisms to individuals or equipment.
  - ◊ Practice care when handling sharps and use pocket mask or other ventilation device when ventilating the patient.
  - ◊ Place patient in private room when possible. Limit the movement or transfer of patient.
- ◆ **Droplet precautions**.
  - ◊ Standard precautions plus:
    - ▪ Place patient in private room or with someone with the same infection. If not feasible, maintain at least 1 m distance between patients.
    - ▪ Use of a mask when working within 1 m of patient.
    - ▪ Mask the patient if he/she needs to be moved.

o All contacts should be vaccinated within 7 days of exposure and quarantined together for at least 17 days following the most recent exposure.

Hemorrhagic fevers—Hanta, Ebola, Lassa, Rift Valley, HFRS
- Except for yellow fever, quarantine is not mandatory; however, person-to-person transmission is possible, therefore, universal precautions are recommended.
- Medical evacuation may result in increased morbidity and mortality, thus treatment at local MTFs is preferred.
- When necessary, patients may be evacuated using universal and respiratory droplet isolation precautions.

Biological Agents

There are two biological toxins that are potential BW agents: botulinum and ricin (see Table 31-1).

Table 31-1

Biological Toxin	Signs/Symptoms	Medical Management
Botulinum	Cranial nerve palsies Paralysis Respiratory failure	Antitoxin/supportive care
Ricin	Fever, cough, SOB Arthralgias, pulmonary edema	Nonspecific/Supportive care

Bacterial Agents

The bacteria or rickettsia most often considered to be potential BW threat agents include *Bacillus anthracis* (anthrax), *Brucella* sp. (brucellosis), *Vibrio cholerae* (cholera) *Burkholderia mallei* (glanders), *Yersinia pestis* (plague), *Francisella tularensis* (tularemia), and *Coxiella burnetii* (Q Fever) (see Table 31-2).

Table 31-2

Bacterial	Signs/Symptoms	Medical Management
Anthrax	Fever, malaise, cough, SOB, cyanosis	Ciprofloxacin
Plague	High fever, chills, headache, cough, SOB, cyanosis	Streptomycin
Brucellosis	Fever, headache, myalgias, sweats, chills	Doxycycline
Cholera	Massive watery diarrhea	Fluid therapy and antibiotics (tetracycline, doxycycline or ciprofloxacin)
Tularemia	Local ulcer, lymphadenopathy, fever, chills, headache, and malaise	Streptomycin
Q-fever	Fever, cough, and pleuritic chest pain	Tetracycline

Viral Agents

A number of viruses are BW agents, including smallpox, the viral hemorrhagic fevers (VHF), and the alpha virus that causes VEE (see Table 31-3).

Table 31-3

Viral	Signs/Symptoms	Medical Management
VEE	Fever and encephalitis	Nonspecific/supportive care
Smallpox	Malaise, fever, rigors, vomiting, headache followed by pustular vesicles	Antiviral under investigation
VHF	Flushing of the face, petechiae, bleeding, fever, myalgias, vomiting, and diarrhea	Nonspecific/supportive care

Chapter 32

Chemical Injuries

The reader is strongly advised to supplement material in this chapter with the *Medical Management Of Chemical Casualties Handbook*, 3rd ed., 2000, USAMRICD, Aberdeen Proving Ground, MD.

Personal Protection
- Prevention!
  - o Avoid becoming a casualty.
  - o Protect yourself and instruct your personnel to do the same.
- Prevent further injury of the casualty by instructing him/her to put on the protective mask and mission-oriented protective posture (MOPP) ensemble, and administer self-aid. If contaminated, tell the individual to remove clothing and decontaminate potentially exposed body surfaces.
- Provide buddy aid by masking the individual, administering antidotes, and spot decontaminating exposed body areas.
- Ensure completeness of decontamination process to the greatest extent possible at the collocated patient decontamination station.
  - o Potential for vapor exposure from an off-gassing residual agent or inadvertent contact with undetected liquid is a hazard for medical personnel.
  - o Avoid contamination of the medical treatment facility (MTF).

Initial Treatment Priorities
- There is no single "best" way to prioritize emergency treatment for chemical or mixed casualties, although respiratory insufficiency and circulatory shock should be treated first. One workable sequence is shown below.

1. Treat respiratory insufficiency (airway management) and control massive hemorrhage.
2. Administer chemical agent antidotes.
3. Decontaminate the face (and protective mask if donned).
4. Remove contaminated clothing and decontaminate potentially contaminated skin.
5. Render emergency care for shock, wounds, and open fractures.
6. Administer supportive medical care as resources permit.
7. Transport the stabilized patient to a contamination-free (ie, clean) area.

Specific Chemical Warfare (CW) Agents and Treatment Considerations

Nerve Agents (GA, GB, GD, GF and VX)

- **General:** Nerve agents are among the most toxic of the known chemical agents. They pose a hazard in both vapor and liquid states, and can cause death in minutes by respiratory obstruction and cardiac failure.
- **Mechanism of action:** Nerve agents are organophosphates that bind with available acetylcholinesterase, permitting a paralyzing accumulation of acetylcholine at the myoneural junction.
- **Signs/symptoms:** Miosis, rhinorrhea, difficulty breathing, loss of consciousness, apnea, seizures, paralysis, and copious secretions.
- **Treatment:** Each deployed US service member has three MARK I kits or Antidote Treatment-Nerve Agent Autoinjectors (ATNAAs) for IM self-injection in a pocket of the protective mask carrier; each kit delivers 2 mg injections of atropine sulfate and 600 mg pralidoxime chloride (2-PAMCl). Each US service member also carries a 10 mg diazepam autoinjector to be administered by a buddy.
  - o Immediate IM or IV injection with
    - ♦ Atropine to block muscarinic cholinergic receptors (may require multiple doses in much greater amounts than recommended by Advanced Cardiac Life Support [ACLS] doses).

♦ 2-PAM (if given soon after exposure) to reactivate cholinesterase.

- Pretreatment: Military personnel may have also received pretreatment prior to nerve agent exposure. In the late 1990s, the US military fielded pyridostigmine bromide (PB tablets) as a pretreatment for nerve agent exposure (this **reversibly** binds to the enzyme acetyl cholinesterase, enhancing the efficacy of atropine against Soman).

Vesicants (HD, H, HN, L, and CX)

- **General:** The vesicants (blister agents) are cytotoxic alkylating compounds, exemplified by the mixture of compounds collectively known as "mustard." Sulphur mustard is designated "HD" or "H"; nitrogen mustard is designated as "HN"; Lewisite is designated as "L"; and phosgene oxime is designated as "CX".
- **Mechanism of action:** Mustard is an alkylating agent that denatures DNA, producing a radiomimetic effect, produces liquefaction necrosis of the epidermis, severe conjunctivitis, and if inhaled, injures the laryngeal and tracheobronchial mucosa.
- **Signs/symptoms:** Skin blisters, moderate-to-severe airway injury (presentation can be delayed), conjunctivitis of varying severity that causes the casualty to believe he has been blinded, and mucus membrane burns. No delay with Lewisite: immediate burning of the skin and eyes.
- **Treatment:** Preventive and supportive. Immediate decontamination of the casualty has top priority. Agent droplets should be removed as expeditiously as possible by blotting with the M-291 kit, or flushing with water or 0.5% hypochlorite. The M-291 kit is extremely effective at inactivating mustard. Most military forces carry a decontamination powder or liquid that should be used immediately to remove the vesicant. Because mustard tends to be an oily solution, water may spread the agent. Dimecaprol is used by some nations in the treatment of Lewisite. Dimecaprol must be used with caution because the drug itself may be toxic.

Lung Damaging (Choking) Agents (Phosgene [CG], Diphosgene [DP], Chloropicrin [PS], and Chlorine)

- **General:** Lung damaging or choking agents produce pronounced irritation of the upper and the lower respiratory tracts. Phosgene smells like freshly mowed hay or grass.
- **Mechanism of action:** Phosgene is absorbed almost exclusively by inhalation. Most of the agent is not systemically distributed but rather is consumed by reactions occurring at the alveolar-capillary membrane.
- **Signs/symptoms:** Phosgene exposure results in pulmonary edema following a clinically latent period that varies, depending on the intensity of exposure. Immediate eye, nose, and throat irritations may be the first symptoms evident after exposure (choking, coughing, tightness in the chest, and lacrimation). Over the next 2–24 hours the patient may develop noncardiogenic fatal pulmonary edema.
- **Treatment:**
  - o Terminate exposure, force rest, manage airway secretions, O_2, consider steroids.
  - o **Triage considerations** for patients seen within 12 hours after exposure.
    - ♦ Immediate care in ICU if available for patients in pulmonary edema.
    - ♦ Delayed: dyspnea without objective signs of pulmonary edema, reassess hourly.
    - ♦ Minimal: asymptomatic patient with known exposure.
    - ♦ Expectant: patient presents with cyanosis, pulmonary edema, and hypotension. Patients presenting with these symptoms within 6 hours of exposure will not likely survive.

The Cyanogens (Blood Agents AC and CK)

- **General:** Hydrogen cyanide (AC) and cyanogen chloride (CK) form highly stable complexes with metalloporphyrins such as cytochrome oxidase. The term "blood agent" is an antiquated term used at a time when it was not understood that the effect occurs mostly outside the bloodstream.
- **Mechanism of action:** Cyanide acts by combining with cytochrome oxidase, blocking the electron transport system. As a result, aerobic cellular metabolism comes to a halt.

- **Signs/symptoms:** Seizures, cardiac arrest, and respiratory arrest.
- **Treatment:**
  o Immediate removal of casualties from contaminated atmosphere prevents further inhalation.
  o 100% oxygen.
  o If cyanide was ingested, perform GI lavage and administer activated charcoal. Administer sodium nitrite (10 mL of 3% solution IV) over a period of 3 minutes, followed by sodium thiosulfate (50 mL of 25% solution IV) over a 10-minute period. The sodium nitrite produces methemoglobin that attracts the cyanide; the sodium thiosulfate solution combines with the cyanide to form thiocyanate, which is excreted.

Incapacitation Agents (BZ and Indoles)

- **General:** Heterogeneous group of chemical agents related to atropine, scopolamine, and hyoscyamine that produces temporary disabling conditions with potent CNS effects that seriously impair normal function, but do not endanger life or cause permanent tissue damage.
- **Signs/symptoms:** Mydriasis, dry mouth, dry skin, increased reflexes, hallucinations, and impaired memory.
- **Treatment:**
  o Immediate removal of firearms and other weapons to ensure safety.
  o Close observation.
  o Physostigmine, 2–3 mg IM every 15 minutes to 1 hour until desired level is attained; maintain with 2–4 mg IV every 1–2 hours for severe cases.

Thickened Agents

- Thickened agents are chemical agents that have been mixed with another substance to increase their **persistency** (persistent agents may remain in the environment over 24 h).
- Casualties with thickened nerve agents in wounds are unlikely to survive to reach surgery.
- Thickened mustard has delayed systemic toxicity and can persist in wounds, even when large fragments of cloth have been removed.

Surgical Treatment of Chemical Casualties
● **Wound decontamination.**
The initial management of a casualty contaminated by chemical agents will require removal of MOPP gear as well as initial skin and wound decontamination with 0.5% hypochlorite before treatment.
  o Bandages are removed, wounds are flushed, and bandages replaced.
  o Tourniquets are replaced with clean tourniquets after decontamination.
  o Splints are thoroughly decontaminated.
Only the vesicants and nerve agents present a hazard from wound contamination. Cyanogens are so volatile that it is extremely unlikely they would remain in a wound.

Off-Gassing
● The risk of vapor off-gassing from chemically contaminated fragments and cloth in wounds is very low and insignificant.

> Off-gassing from a wound during surgical exploration will be negligible or zero.

Use of Hypochlorite Solution
● Household bleach is 5% sodium hypochlorite, hence, mix 1 part bleach with 9 parts water to create ~ 0.5% solution.
● Dilute hypochlorite (0.5%) is an effective skin decontaminant, but the solution is **contraindicated** for use in or on a number of anatomical areas:
  o Eye: may cause corneal injuries.
  o Brain and spinal cord injuries.
  o Peritoneal cavity: may lead to adhesions.
  o Thoracic cavity: hazard is still unknown although it may be less of a problem.
● Full strength 5% hypochlorite is used to decontaminate instruments, clothing, sheets, and other inanimate objects.

Wound Exploration and Debridement
Surgeons and assistants should wear well-fitting, thin, butyl rubber gloves or double latex surgical gloves. **Gloves should**

be changed often while ascertaining that there are no foreign bodies or thickened agents remaining in the wound.

Wound excision and debridement should be conducted using a no-touch technique. Removed fragments of tissue should be dumped into a container of 5% hypochlorite solution. Superficial wounds should be wiped thoroughly with a 0.5% hypochlorite and then irrigated with copious amounts of normal saline.

Following the Surgical Procedure

- Surgical and other instruments that come into contact with possible contamination should be placed in 5% hypochlorite for 10 minutes prior to normal cleansing and sterilization.
- Reusable linen should be checked with the chemical agent monitor (CAM), M8 paper, or M9 tape for contamination. Soak contaminated linen in 5% hypochlorite.

Chapter 33

Pediatric Care

Introduction
The military surgeon needs to be familiar with the unique challenges the pediatric population presents, not only in war, but also in military-operations-other-than-war scenarios. This includes proper diagnostic evaluation and resuscitation, and the necessary equipment to ensure success. For US Army medical units, the humanitarian augmentation medical equipment set (MES), requested by the hospital commander through command channels, provides medical supplies and equipment for a population of 10,000 people. Additionally, the special care augmentation team can be requested for this mission.

Anatomic and Physiologic Considerations
- Fluid, electrolyte, and nutrition.
  - o Normal fluid requirements in children are estimated via a weight-based method (Table 33-1).

Table 33-1

Weight (kg)	Volume
0–10	120 mL/kg/d (after the first week of life)
11–20	1,000 mL + 50 mL/kg over 10 kg
over 20	1,500 mL + 20 mL/kg over 20 kg

  - o Maintenance IV fluid replacement is $D_5 1/2NS + 20$ mEq/dL KCl for children over 3 months or $D_{10} 1/2NS + 20$ mEq/dl KCl for children under 3 months.
  - o Fluid resuscitation is best performed with isotonic fluids at 20 cc/kg boluses. (See Evaluation and Diagnosis below.)
  - o Total fluid requirement should be adjusted for a goal urine output of 1–2 cc/kg/h.

- o Daily sodium requirements are 2–3 mEq/kg/d and daily potassium requirements are 1–2 mEq/kg/d.
- o Daily caloric and protein requirements are estimated by weight and age as follows (Table 33-2):

Table 33-2

Age (y)	kcal/kg body weight	Protein (g/kg body weight)
0–1	90–120	2.0–3.5
1–7	75–90	2.0–2.5
7–12	60–75	2.0
12–18	30–60	1.5
> 18	25–30	1.0

- o Breast milk is always the first choice when initiating oral intake in infants. Alternatively, infant formulas contain 20 kcal/oz. An estimate of the amount of formula needed to provide 120 kcal/kg/d is

Infant's wt (kg) • 22 = Amt (in cc) of formula needed q 4 h.

- **Pulmonary.**
  - o Newborns tend to be obligate nasal breathers, thus nasal airways should be avoided if possible.
  - o The child's larynx is positioned more anterior in the neck, thus making it more difficult to visualize during intubation, and necessitating a more forward position of the head.
  - o The acceptable range of PaO_2 (60–90 mm Hg) correlates to oxygen saturations of 92%–97%. A premature infant's oxygenation saturation should never exceed 94% to avoid retinopathy of the premature.
  - o Infants breathe mostly with their diaphragm, thus increases in intraabdominal pressure or other problems that limit diaphragmatic movement can significantly inhibit respiration.
- **Cardiovascular.**
  - o Vital signs by age group (Table 33-3).

Table 33-3

Age	Weight (kg)	Resp. Rate	Pulse	BP (systolic)
Premie	< 3	40–60	130–150	42+10
Term	3	40	120–140	60+10
1–5 yr	~10–20	20–30	100–130	95+30
6 –10 yr	20–32	12–25	75–100	100+15
Adolescent	50	12–18	70	120+20

o Cardiac stroke volume in children is relatively fixed. Therefore, bradycardia or relative bradycardia can significantly decrease cardiac output. Stimulation and oxygen therapy are corrective for over 90% of significant bradycardias in infants.

> Limit peripheral IV access attempts to 2 within 60 seconds for the child in shock, then immediately proceed to saphenous vein cutdown or intraosseous (IO) infusion (see Chapter 8, Vascular Access).

- Burns.
  o An infant or child's head tends to encompass more of the BSA, with the lower extremities being a smaller percentage. The palm of the child's hand can be used to estimate 1% of total BSA for burn calculations (Fig. 33-1).
- Gastrointestinal.
  o Reflux is a common finding, especially in the newborn period. This predisposes some children to difficulty with digestion and frequent emesis.
  o Children are predisposed to hypoglycemia due to low glycogen storage capacity of their liver. Full-term infants will tolerate NPO status for approximately 5 days (with an appropriate D_{10} solution). Premature infants will tolerate only 3 days of NPO status prior to the initiation of TPN.

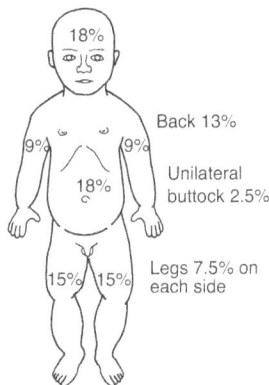

18%

Back 13%

Unilateral buttock 2.5%

18% c

Legs 7.5% on each side

9% 9%

15% 15%

Fig. 33-1. BSA percentages for infants and children.

o A child's GI tract is very sensitive to most insults, including electrolyte abnormalities and systemic illnesses. This can result in an ileus and manifest as feeding intolerance, and may precipitate necrotizing enterocolitis (NEC).

- Hematology and blood volume.
  o Infants have a physiologic anemia during the first 3–5 months with a hematocrit of 30%–33%.
  o Estimates of blood volume are as follows:

Age	Volume (cc/kg)
Premature	85–100
Term	~80
1–3 mo	75–80
> 3 mo	~70

- Renal.
  o Infants and young children have a limited ability to concentrate urine (max 400–600 mOsm/L) and a fixed ability to excrete sodium, causing an inability to handle excess sodium, resulting in hypernatremia if they receive too much sodium. Premature infants are salt wasters and full-term infants are salt retainers. It takes 6 years to achieve normal tubular concentrating ability.
  o Infants can excrete water just like an adult. At 2 weeks of age the glomerular filtration rate (GFR) is 75% of the eventual adult rate and reaches maximum capacity at 2 years.
  o Total body water is 80% at 32 weeks, 75% at term, 60% beyond 1 year.

- Thermoregulation.
  o Infants and young children are predisposed to heat loss and they poorly compensate for wide fluctuations in ambient temperatures.
  o Reduce exposure and keep infants and children in a regulated warm environment.

- Immune system.
  o Premature infants have incomplete development of their immune system, causing a 60-fold increased risk of sepsis. All elective surgery in infants under 30 days of age requires 48 hours of prophylactic antibiotics (with anaerobic coverage added when appropriate) after the first week of life.

o Early signs of sepsis can include lethargy, intolerance to feedings, fever, hypothermia, tachycardia, and irritability before a rise in the white blood cell count.

Evaluation and Diagnosis
- History.
    - o Duration/location of pain is important in injury diagnosis. Over one third of pediatric patients evaluated for abdominal pain lasting more than a few hours will have an underlying pathologic condition.
    - o Any bilious emesis, especially in the newborn period, may be a sign of intestinal obstruction, and mandates further workup.
    - o GI bleeding requires immediate attention. The character (bright red vs melena), quantity, and associated stool history (ie, diarrhea with infectious source or currant-jelly–like with intussusception) may provide clues as to the underlying disorder.
- Physical examination.
    - o Basic ATLS guidelines should direct the initial assessment and evaluation for all children involved in traumas. It is essential to keep the patient warm because children are much more prone to heat loss than adults.
        - ♦ Modified GCS for children < 4 years old:

Verbal Response	V-Score
Appropriate words/social smile/fixes/follows	5
Cries, but consolable	4
Persistently irritable	3
Restless, agitated	2
None	1

- Radiological studies.
    - o All bilious vomiting in infants and children should be evaluated with contrast radiographic imaging. As a general rule contrast enemas are safer as an initial approach.
        - ♦ Ultrasound is an excellent screening test for the identification of free abdominal fluid and is also used

in cases of abdominal pain to evaluate appendicitis (noncompressible appendix with fecolith) and intussusception (target sign), and others.

◆ Constipation is a common complaint in children that can be readily diagnosed with plain radiographs and by history.

Treatment

● The treatment algorithm shown below provides the proper sequence for the rapid sequence intubation (RSI) of the pediatric patient (Fig. 33-2).

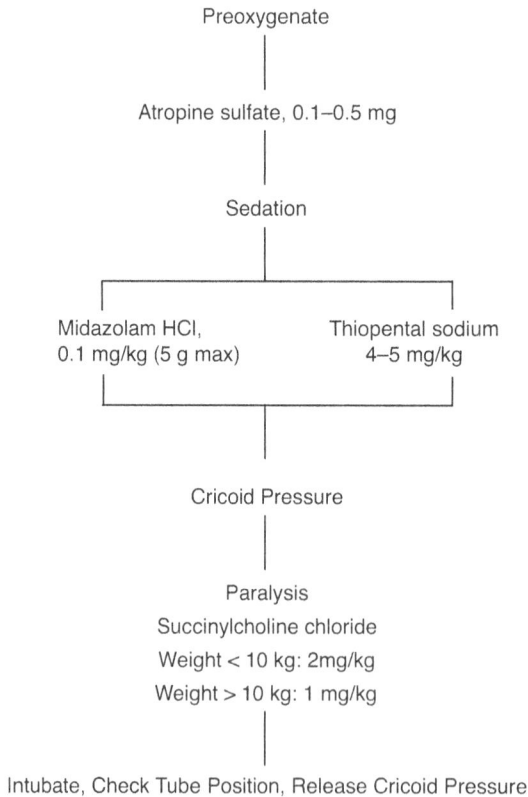

Preoxygenate

Atropine sulfate, 0.1–0.5 mg

Sedation

| Midazolam HCl, 0.1 mg/kg (5 g max) | Thiopental sodium 4–5 mg/kg |

Cricoid Pressure

Paralysis
Succinylcholine chloride
Weight < 10 kg: 2mg/kg
Weight > 10 kg: 1 mg/kg

Intubate, Check Tube Position, Release Cricoid Pressure

Fig. 33-2. Rapid sequence intubation for the pediatric patient.

Equipment and Supplies

- Accessory pediatric medical/surgical equipment arranged according to age and weight (Table 33-4).

Table 33-4

AGE, WEIGHT (kg)	AIRWAY/BREATHING							CIRCULATION		SUPPLEMENTAL EQUIPMENT				
	O₂ Mask	Oral Airway	Bag-valve	Laryngo-scope	ET Tube	Stylet	Suction	BP Cuff	IV Cath	NG Tube	Chest Tube	Urinary Cath	C-collar
Premie 3 kg	Premie Newborn	Infant	Infant	0 Straight	2.5–3.0 No Cuff	6 F	6–8 F	Premie Newborn	24-gauge	12 F	10–14 F	5 F Feeding	—
0–6 mo 3.5 kg	Newborn	Infant Small	Infant	1 Straight	3.0–3.5 No Cuff	6 F	8 F	Newborn Infant	22-gauge	12 F	12–18 F	5–8 F Feeding	—
6–12 mo 7 kg	Pediatric	Small	Pediatric	1 Straight	3.5–4.0 No Cuff	6 F	8–10 F	Infant Child	22-gauge	12 F	14–20 F	8 F	Small
1–3 y 10–12 kg	Pediatric	Small	Pediatric	1 Straight	4.0–4.5 No Cuff	6 F	10 F	Child	20–22 gauge	12 F	14–24 F	10 F	Small
4–7 y 16–18 kg	Pediatric	Medium	Pediatric	2 Straight or Curved	5.0–5.5 No Cuff	14 F	14 F	Child	20-gauge	12 F	20–32 F	10–12 F	Small
8–10 y 24–30 kg	Adult	Medium Large	Pediatric Adult	2–3 Straight or Curved	5.5–6.5 Cuffed	14 F	14 F	Child Adult	18–20-gauge	12 F	28–38 F	12F	Medium

- Surgical instruments.
  - o If a pediatric surgical set is not immediately available, a peripheral vascular set will usually contain instruments delicate enough to accomplish most tasks in newborns.

Commonly Used Drugs and Dosages

- Phenobarbital 2–3 mg/kg IV.
- Diazepam 0.25 mg/kg IV
- Midazolam HCl 0.1 mg/kg IV (max 5 mg).
- Atropine 0.1–0.5 mg IV.
- Phenytoin 15–20 mg/kg, administered at 0.5 to 1.5 ml/kg/min as a loading dose, then 4–7 mg/kg/d for maintenance.
- Mannitol 0.5–1.0 g/kg IV.
- Succinylcholine chloride 2 mg/kg IV for < 10 kg, and 1 mg/kg IV for > 10 kg.
- Ampicillin 25–50 mg/kg IV q8h (q12–18h in newborns).
- Gentamicin 2.5 mg/kg IV q8h (q12–18h in newborns).
- Metronidazole 10 mg/kg IV.
- Acetaminophen 15 mg/kg po.

33.7

Surgical Management

- Basics.
  - o As a general guideline, transverse incisions should be used in infants. This minimizes the risk of postoperative dehiscence, while still allowing adequate exposure.
  - o Absorbable suture such as Vicryl or PDS (2-0) should be used to close the rectus fascia, regardless of the incision. The skin can then be closed using staples or absorbable monofilament suture (eg, Monocryl 4-0).
  - o When placing retention sutures for severe malnutrition, permanent sutures such as Prolene or nylon can be used as a full thickness through the rectus muscle and skin. Care should be taken to avoid the epigastric vessels. The sutures can be passed through small pieces of a 14F red rubber catheter prior to tying to avoid excess pressure on the skin.
  - o Personnel: Remember that if obstetrics is part of the mission, pediatric support will be required!

Chapter 34

Care of Enemy
Prisoners of War/Internees

Introduction

Healthcare personnel of the Armed Forces of the United States have a responsibility to protect and treat, in the context of a professional treatment relationship and universal principles of medical ethics, all detainees in the custody of the Armed Forces. This includes enemy prisoners of war, retained personnel, civilian internees, and other detainees. For the purposes of this chapter, all such personnel are referred to as **internees**.

It is the policy of the Department of Defense that healthcare personnel of the Armed Forces and the Department of Defense should make every effort to comply with "Principles of Medical Ethics Relevant to the Role of Health Personnel, Particularly Physicians, in the Protection of Prisoners and Detainees Against Torture and Other Cruel, Inhuman or Degrading Treatment or Punishment," adopted by United Nations General Assembly Resolution 37/194 of 18 December 1982 (and provided as Appendix 1 to this book). This is in addition to compliance with all applicable DoD issuances.

The Geneva Conventions

- Define medical personnel as those individuals "exclusively engaged in the search for, or the collection, transport, or treatment of the wounded or sick, or in the prevention of disease; and staff exclusively engaged in the administration of medical units and establishments" (Geneva Convention for the Amelioration of the Wounded and Sick in Armed Forces in the Field [GWS]).

- Medical personnel of enemy forces are not considered internees, but are classified as "retained" in order to treat other EPWs. Internees are also entitled to the protections afforded under the provisions of the Geneva Convention Relative to the Treatment of Prisoners of War (GPW). Detained persons who are not protected under GWS and GPW, may be protected under the provisions of the Geneva Convention Relative to the Protection of Civilian Persons in Time of War (GC).

The GWS states that belligerents must care for the sick and wounded without any adverse distinction founded on sex, race, nationality, religion, political opinions, or any other similar criteria. *Only* medical urgency can justify priority in the order of treatment.

EPW/Retained/Detained Medical Care (Internees)

Workload

The number of internees and retained/detained personnel requiring medical in-processing and/or medical care can be staggering. The US captured approximately 425,000 prisoners in WW II and 105,000 in the Korean conflict. Coalition forces captured over 62,000 internees during Operation Desert Storm. During the 1-week ground war, 308 internees were treated by US military medical treatment facilities (MTFs). From the end of the ground war (28 February 1991) until the end of March 1991, 8,979 internees were treated.

- Fragment wounds accounted for 44% of the surgical admissions during the ground war.
- 23% of surgical admissions required treatment for fractures.
- Surgical intervention was required in 28% of Iraqi casualties admitted.
- Most common operative procedures included
  - Wound debridement.
  - Open reduction and internal fixation of fractures.
  - Exploratory laparotomies.
  - Incision and drainage of abscesses.

- The most common internee medical condition reported during Operation Desert Storm was dental disease (24%) such as periodontal infections, fractures, and extensive caries. Other common medical illnesses were unexplained fever, nephrolithiasis, peptic ulcer disease, and malaria.

> **Wounds in internees may be different than those seen in friendly forces due to differences in personal protective gear, preexisting diseases, malnutrition, and neglect.**

Medical Care of Internees

- What healthcare providers **should** do.
  - o No matter the setting, healthcare providers have a responsibility to report information, the consequences of which constitute a clear and imminent threat to the lives and welfare of others. Information gained from patients who are internees should be treated no differently.
  - o As given below, healthcare providers have specific responsibilities for the care and treatment of internees. The overarching principle of this guideline, however, is that internees of any status should whenever possible receive medical care equal to that of our own troops.
    - ♦ As one would expect for our own troops, physicians should report any suspected abuse or maltreatment of a detainee or prisoner.
    - ♦ Just as one would write a profile or duty limitation for one of his own service members, physicians have a responsibility to inform the detention facility chain of command of internees' activity limitations. This includes "clearing the prisoner for interrogation," with the expectation that interrogation will conform to the standards of AR 190-8. Medical recommendations concerning internee activities are exactly that—recommendations. Decisions concerning internee activities are made by the chain of command.
  - o Healthcare providers should be trained in the tenets of the Geneva Conventions of 1949 and other documents and principles of internee care. They should also be trained to

recognize the symptoms and signs of internee maltreatment or abuse.

- What healthcare providers **should not** do.
  - o Healthcare professionals charged with any form of assistance with the interrogation process, to include interpretation of medical records and information, should not be involved in any aspect of internee healthcare.
  - o Healthcare providers charged with the care of internees should not engage in any activities that jeopardize their protected status under the Geneva Conventions.
  - o Healthcare providers charged with the care of internees should not be actively involved in interrogation, advise interrogators how to conduct interrogations, or interpret individual medical records/medical data for the purposes of interrogation or intelligence gathering.
- Recusal. Healthcare providers who are asked to perform duties they feel are unethical should ask to be recused. Requests for recusal should first go to the healthcare provider's commander and chain of command. If the chain of command is unable to resolve the situation, providers should engage the technical chain by contacting the Command Surgeon. If these avenues are unfruitful, healthcare providers may contact their specialty consultants or the Inspector General.
- Specific medical requirements. Medical requirements for internee care are provided in AR 190-8/OPNAVINST 3461.6/AFJI 31-40/MCO 3461.1. Internees are entitled to medical treatment. Each must have an examination on arrival at the detention facility, as well as a chest radiograph (tuberculin skin test for children up to age 14 years). Sick call must be available daily, and each internee must be weighed at least once a month. Sanitation and hygiene must be maintained at all times (AR 190-8, para 3-4 i.).
- Medical records.
  - o Internee medical records, like the medical records of all Service members, retirees, and their dependents are property of the US Government. Internees are entitled to copies of their medical records upon their release. The original records; however, remain the property of the

United States. Entries should be made into internee medical records as they would for any other patients.

o The Health Insurance Portability and Accountability Act does not apply to the medical records of internees (DoD 6025 C5.1, C7.10, C7.11). However, the handling, disposition, and release of all types of medical records is governed by regulation. Commanders and other officials who have an official need to know can access information contained in internee medical records by following the procedures given in AR 40-66, Chapter 2 using DA Form 4254. Patient consent is not required. Receiving MTFs file and maintain all DA Form 4254s. The MTF commander or commander's designee, usually the patient administrator, determines what information is appropriate for release. Only that specific medical information or medical record required to satisfy the terms of a legitimate request will be authorized for disclosure. Healthcare providers should expect that released medical information will be used by the chain of command, to include interrogators, in accordance with Medical Information, which follows.

- Medical information.
  o Because the chain of command is ultimately responsible for the care and treatment of internees, the detention facility chain of command requires some medical information. For example, patients suspected of having infectious diseases such as tuberculosis should be separated from other internees. Guards and other personnel who come into contact with such patients should be informed about their health risks and how to mitigate those risks.
  o Releasable medical information on internees includes that which is necessary to supervise the general state of health, nutrition, and cleanliness of internees, and to detect contagious diseases. Such information should be used to provide healthcare; to ensure health and safety of internees, soldiers, employees, or others at the facility; to ensure law enforcement on the premises; and ensure the administration and maintenance of the safety, security, and good order of the facility. Under these provisions,

34.5

healthcare providers can confirm that an internee is healthy enough to work or perform camp duties.

- Reporting.
  - o The chain of command is the first and foremost channel for information and reporting. Healthcare providers should report routine medical information, clear and imminent threats, suspicions of abuse or maltreatment, and any other relevant information to their commanders or their commanders' designees. If the healthcare provider is not assigned to the detention facility, mechanisms must be in place to also inform the detention facility chain of command.
  - o Alternative means of reporting exist for healthcare providers who are unable to resolve issues through the chain of command. The technical chain is the first alternative, and begins with the Command Surgeon responsible for medical oversight of the provider's activities. Other alternatives include the provider's specialty consultant, the Inspector General, and Criminal Investigations.

Setup/Planning
- Develop plans for prisoners on a hunger strike or who refuse treatment.
- Prisoners from separate armies should be housed apart—this is the responsibility of the internment camp commander.
- Care should be exercised in the selection of medical personnel to serve in internee facilities.
- Enemy forces may do little or no medical screening prior to conscription. Chronic medical problems will be more likely in these forces. Enemy forces may have preexisting diseases that are not present in the AO or US forces. Planning for appropriate medications may be required.
- Maintain medical records for internees in the same manner as for friendly forces.
- Ensure that any internee/retained/detained person evacuated to the MTF for treatment is escorted by an armed guard as designated by the nonmedical (echelon) commander. The guard must remain with the patient while in the medical

evacuation and treatment chain. To the greatest extent possible, keep all internees segregated from friendly forces' patients; but treat all enemy patients with the same level of care as provided to friendly forces' patients.

- An internee identification number must be secured for any internee evacuated through medical channels. This is accomplished by reporting the patient to the theater Prisoner of War Information System (PWIS). Medical personnel **do not** search, guard, or interrogate internees while in medical channels; this is the responsibility of the echelon commander.
- Internees are housed in internment facilities that are established, maintained, and guarded by forces designated by the echelon commander. Medical personnel **are not** involved in the daily operations of these facilities. However, these facilities normally have a medical staff embedded in the organization to accomplish medical examinations and to conduct routine sick call and preventive medicine activities. Control procedures (guards, physical layout, and precautionary procedures) are regulated by the facility commander. If a patient must be transferred to an established MTF for specialized care, transfer procedures and guards are governed by the facility commander.
- In a mature theater (such as during WW II and the Gulf War of 1991 [Desert Storm]), there are often sufficient internee patients to warrant the designation of a specific hospital for their exclusive care. In this case, coordination between the senior command and control headquarters, and the senior medical command and control headquarters is required to provide security, establish prisoner-control procedures, and regulate other nonmedical matters involved in establishing and administering a medical facility specifically for internees. The standard of care for this facility is required to be the same standard of care as practiced in other deployed hospitals.

It is critical that medical personnel not enter the general EPW holding area, but have patients brought out to them for sick call and any medical treatment.

Interpreters—Always a Shortage
- Internees may not know any other language but their own.
- NATO STANAG 2131, Multinational Phrase Book for Use by the NATO Medical Services - AMedP-5(B) provides basic medical questions in a number of NATO languages, published as DA Pam 40-3/NAVMED P-5104/AFP 160-28.
- Use other retained persons/internees (especially medical personnel) as translators.
- Simulation of mental illness by EPWs is a potential technique for evading interrogation, especially if combined with a captured interpreter.

Screening
- Ensure internees are screened for hidden weapons and other potentially dangerous materials. **This is not a medical function**; it should be accomplished by the guards. **Medical personnel, however, must remain vigilant of these threats and mentally prepared should a threat or attack occur.**
- Each prisoner who comes into the facility must receive a complete physical examination including a dental examination. Vital statistics are recorded for each internee treated. Essential care should be given at this point. Other follow-up evaluations are dependent on the baseline health of the combatant population.
- During internment, routine sick call is provided on a daily basis; this includes medication dispensing, wound care, and indicated minor procedures.
- During transfer, release, and/or repatriation, another medical examination should be performed. Final documentation of any ongoing medical, surgical, or wound care problem is completed and forwarded to the gaining facility or to the appropriate medical records repository.

Supply
- The internment facility must enforce field hygiene and sanitation principles.
- Plan for personal hygiene requirements and protective measures (insect netting, insect repellent, sunscreen).

- Coordinate with the supporting medical HQ for additional Preventive Medicine support (pest management, potable water, dining facility sanitation, and waste disposal) and Veterinary Services support for food safety as required.
- For medicolegal purposes, **a high-quality camera is important**.

Medical Staffing

- Dictated by the organizational structure of the facility. The same standard of care as that provided to US forces must be maintained.
- Retained medical personnel should be utilized for care of their compatriots in conformity with the Geneva Conventions.

Legal

- If possible, signed permission should be obtained for all surgical or invasive procedures.
- In contrast to civilian medical photography, the patient's identity should be absolutely clear in each photograph. This is invaluable should there be a claim of unnecessary surgery or amputation. With clearly identifiable photographs, the state of the wound for that patient can be demonstrated.

> **Any patient who requires amputation or major debridement of tissue should be photographed (face as well as wound images).**

Internee Advocate

- The military physician is the commander's advisor for medical ethics. The physician should be alert for potential and actual ethical conflicts, and exert all efforts to remedy any perceived conflicts. As the patient's advocate (in this case, the captured enemy soldier), the military physician and all military healthcare providers must maintain the patient's health. They must also strive to maintain a "moral distance" from participating in any proceeding potentially adverse to the patient's interest.

Security

- There is **always** an element of danger to the medical staff in treating internees.
- Physical security will be provided by nonmedical personnel as designated by the appropriate leadership.
- The security routine must be maintained at all times. Security personnel must accompany all internees whenever they are in a treatment area or holding area. In forward areas, it may not be possible to have separate and secure medical treatment/holding areas for internees. The limited size and compact layout of Level I and II MTFs and the forward surgical team normally necessitate that internees are treated and held in close proximity. To the extent possible, internees should be segregated from allied, coalition, and US forces.
- If possible, medical equipment should not be taken into the patient wards for security reasons—ie, bring the patient to the equipment.
- If an EPW is to be discharged back to the general EPW population, the physician should alert internment medical personnel of any special needs the internee may have.

> **Personal safety should <u>never</u> be taken for granted by the medical team, regardless of familiarity with internees and surroundings.**

Envoi

I would say that two contrary laws seem to be wrestling with each other nowadays: The one, a law of blood and death, ever imagining new means of destruction and forcing nations to be constantly ready for the battlefield— the other a law of peace, work, and health ever evolving new means of delivering man from the scourges which beset him. Which of these two laws will ultimately prevail God alone knows.

—Louis Pasteur

Principles of Medical Ethics relevant to the role of health personnel, particularly physicians, in the protection of prisoners and detainees against torture* and other cruel, inhuman or degrading treatment or punishment

Adopted by United Nations General Assembly Resolution 37/194 of 18 December 1982

Principle 1
Health personnel, particularly physicians, charged with the medical care of prisoners and detainees have a duty to provide them with protection of their physical and mental health and treatment of disease of the same quality and standard as is afforded to those who are not imprisoned or detained.

Principle 2
It is a gross contravention of medical ethics, as well as an offence under applicable international instruments, for health personnel, particularly physicians, to engage, actively or passively, in acts which constitute participation in, complicity in, incitement to or attempts to commit torture or other cruel, inhuman or degrading treatment or punishment.

Principle 3
It is a contravention of medical ethics for health personnel, particularly physicians, to be involved in any professional

relationship with prisoners or detainees the purpose of which is not solely to evaluate, protect or improve their physical and mental health.

Principle 4

It is a contravention of medical ethics for health personnel, particularly physicians:

(a) To apply their knowledge and skills in order to assist in the interrogation of prisoners and detainees in a manner that may adversely affect the physical or mental health or condition of such prisoners or detainees and which is not in accordance with the relevant international instruments;

(b) To certify, or to participate in the certification of, the fitness of prisoners or detainees for any form of treatment or punishment that may adversely affect their physical or mental health and which is not in accordance with the relevant international instruments, or to participate in any way in the infliction of any such treatment or punishment which is not in accordance with the relevant international instruments.

Principle 5

It is a contravention of medical ethics for health personnel, particularly physicians, to participate in any procedure for restraining a prisoner or detainee unless such a procedure is determined in accordance with purely medical criteria as being necessary for the protection of the physical or mental health or the safety of the prisoner or detainee himself, of his fellow prisoners or detainees, or of his guardians, and presents no hazard to his physical or mental health.

Principle 6

There may be no derogation from the foregoing principles on any ground whatsoever, including public emergency.

----

*1. For the purpose of this Declaration, torture means any act by which severe pain or suffering, whether physical or mental, is intentionally inflicted by or at the instigation of a public official on a person for such purposes as obtaining from him or a third person information or confession, punishing him for an act he has committed or is suspected of having committed, or intimidating him or other persons. It does not include pain or suffering arising only from, inherent in or incidental to, lawful sanctions to the extent consistent with the Standard Minimum Rules for the Treatment of Prisoners.

2. Torture constitutes an aggravated and deliberate form of cruel, inhuman or degrading treatment or punishment.

Article 7 of the Declaration states:

"Each State shall ensure that all acts of torture as defined in article 1 are offences under its criminal law. The same shall apply in regard to acts which constitute participation in, complicity in, incitement to or an attempt to commit torture."

Glasgow Coma Scale

GLASGOW COMA SCALE

Component	Response	Score
Motor Response (best extremity)	Obeys verbal command	6
	Localizes pain	5
	Flexion-withdrawal	4
	Flexion (decortication)	3
	Extension (decerebration)	2
	No response (flaccid)	1
	Subtotal	**(1–6)**
Eye Opening	Spontaneously	4
	To verbal command	3
	To pain	2
	None	1
	Subtotal	**(1–4)**
Best Verbal Response	Oriented and converses	5
	Disoriented and converses	4
	Inappropriate words	3
	Incomprehensible sounds	2
	No verbal response	1
	Subtotal	**(1–5)**
	Total	**(3–15)**

Appendix 3

Theater Joint Trauma Record

General

Evidence-based medicine has become the goal of all specialties. Unfortunately, because of the realities of Combat Trauma, timely and accurate data collection and interpretation of results are difficult. Quality information on casualties for combatant commanders is essential because it facilitates optimal placement, utilization, and resupply of scarce medical resources, and rapid identification of new trends in wounding and treatment. Accurate, aggregated theater information is necessary to shorten quality improvement cycles in deployed treatment facilities.

Furthermore, these data placed on a website could provide rapid feedback to the sending physicians, allowing individual follow-up on their patients. These concepts are not new: they are routinely employed in the > 1,000 verified trauma centers in the US. Application of these principles to the battlefield, using a limited set of jointly approved data elements is described below. This data collection effort is not designed to be an extra step. The proposed form can be used as the trauma chart (both battle and nonbattle injury) and sent to the next evacuation Level with the casualty.

Situational Awareness

The revolution in warfighting which has digitized the battlefield to display friendly positions, intelligence, and engagements electronically has not been equally applied to the casualty side of the equation. This places demands on medical organizations to provide online and continuously updated status and location information on killed, wounded, ill, and psychologically impaired combatants and noncombatants; which includes both the casualty loss to the unit and the return to duty patient. This need will only escalate, as medical situational awareness plays an increasing role in the tactical risk assessment process. At a minimum, commanders should be able to assess Killed In Action (KIA, died before reaching medical care/force wounded) and Died Of Wounds (DOW, die after reaching medical care/force wounded) in order to measure risk associated with operations and the capability of the medical force to control mortality.

$$\text{Percentage KIA} = \frac{\text{No. killed before reaching a BAS}}{\text{No. of casualties (killed + admitted)}} \bullet 100$$

$$\text{Percentage DOW} = \frac{\text{No. died after reaching a BAS}}{\text{No. of admitted}} \bullet 100$$

Where admitted is defined as any casualty that stays at a Level II facility or above. These definitions do not include the carded for record category in the denominator

A breakdown of casualties by type of injury and the major body regions (ie, face, head and neck, chest, abdomen and pelvis, upper and lower extremities, and skin) will enable an analysis of injury patterns that can be utilized to design interventions resulting in a decrease in morbidity and mortality.

Other Uses
Data on types of wounds, their causes, and appropriate procedures have potential value in constructing predictive models for medical force development and placement, logistical delivery systems, and research on improved medical interventions. The history of improvements in medicine and surgery are grounded on the battlefield, and dissemination should not be limited to the isolated innovator with a personal spreadsheet for documentation. Individual providers at individual medical treatment facilities (MTFs) have long recorded clinical data and observations. This Joint Theater Trauma Record effort is an extension of their efforts.

Minimum Essential Data

In addition to recording the standard contents of the postprocedure note (ie, who did what, on whom, why, and a plan), the standard data components of a trauma registry are especially helpful (eg, demographics, circumstance and mechanism of injury, pre-hospital monitoring and care, hospital monitoring and care, outcome, participants, direct assessment against standards). Figure A-1 (see next four pages) is a sample form that can serve as both the trauma chart and the data entry source. These minimum essential elements have been agreed on by the US Army, Air Force and Navy. Data will be collated and placed on a website at the first Level IV facility in the evacuation chain.

Recommended Methods and Technology

The process to document emergency trauma care can be employed on either the immature or mature battlefield. This would entail utilizing paper or computer-assisted electronic technology, respectively. In the ideal environment, this would be a single step process. Reality is much different. It is important to recognize that documentation should occur at all Levels, while aggregation of data should occur at the first Level that can support such activity. At a minimum, paper documentation should be used for each casualty and the chart should accompany the patient to the rear as evacuation occurs. When electronic records are available, this process will be simplified.

Trauma Record
DISCHARGE SUMMARY

MEDICATIONS:

LABS

XRAYS:

PMH:

Alergies

REGION	DIAGNOSIS, PROCEDURES and COMPLICATONS
Face	
Head & Neck (incl C-spine)	
Chest (incl T-spine)	
Abdomen (incl L-spine)	
Pelvis	

A3.4

Theatre Joint Trauma Record

UPPER /LOWER Extremities

Skin

DISPOSTION ☐ EVAC to

DTG: ☐ RTD ☐ DECEASED (see below)

Evacuation Priority
☐ ROUTINE
☐ PRIORITY
☐ URGENT

Damage Control Procedures? Y / N   Hypothermic (< 34°C)? Y / N   Coagulopathy? Y / N

Cause of Death at _____

ANATOMIC:
Airway Head Neck Chest Abdomen Pelvis Extremity (Upper/Lower)
Other

PHYSIOLOGIC:
Breathing CNS Hemorrhage Total Body Disruption Sepsis Multi-organ failure

COMMENTS:

SURGEON: _____ (printedName)

A3.5

Trauma Record

For use of this form, see DoD Memo. Subject Trauma Record, dtd 1 APR 04, the proponent agency is OTSG

AUTHORITY AR 40-66
PURPOSE To provide a standard means of documenting all trauma care at echelons 1-3
ROUTINE USES The "Blanket Routine Uses" set forth at the beginning of the Army compilation of systems of records notice apply
DISCLOSURE This is protected health information HIPAA laws apply

MTF DESIGNATION
Number

TYPE

CASUALTY NAME
FIRST
LAST

CASUALTY SSN

Arrive Date-Time Group (DTG):

Rank

Date of Birth

Gender
□ Male □ Female

Unit

ARRIVAL METHOD:
□ WALKED
□ CARRIED
□ Non-MED AIR
□ OTHER

□ Non-MED GND
□ SHIP EVAC
□ GND AMB
□ AIR AMB

Nation
□ US
□ Host Nation
□ Enemy(   )
□ Coalition(   )

Service
□ Civilian
□ Combatant
□ Contractor
□ USA

□ USN
□ USMC
□ USAF
□ SOF

□ NGO (   )
□ Other

Wound DTG:

PROTECTION:
□ UNK

	Not Worn	Worn	Struck	Penetrated
HELMET				
FLAK VEST				
CERAMIC PLATE				
EYE PROTECTION				
OTHER				

TRIAGE CATEGORY
□ IMMEDIATE □ MINIMAL
□ DELAYED □ EXPECTANT

GLASGOW COMA SCALE (circle one)
3   8   12   15
UNC   STUPOR   LETHARGY   ALERT

TIME	
Pulse	
Temp	
B/P	
Resp	
SpO₂	

WOUNDED BY:
□ US/COALITION(Nation   )
□ ENEMY   □ NonENEMY
□ CIVILIAN (Nation   )
□ TRAINING
□ SELF ACCIDENT
□ SELF NON-ACCIDENT
□ SPORTS-RECREATION
□ OTHER

MECHANISM OF INJURY:
□ GSW/BULLET
□ BLUNT TRAUMA
□ SINGLE FRAGMENT
□ MULTI FRAGMENT

□ KNIFE / EDGE
□ BLAST
□ CRASH(av, veh, pe)
□ Chem/Rad/Nucl
□ BURN (thermal, flash)

□ CRUSH
□ FALL
□ SMOKE Inhalation
□ HEAT
□ COLD

□ BITE / STING
□ OTHER

INJURY Description (Location, nature and size in cm)

R   L R   L   R   L   R

TX & PROCEDURES		
SEDATED		
CHEM PARALYZED		
INTUBATED		
CRIC		
NEEDLE DECOMP		
Chest Tube	L R	
IO line		autoboid
COLLOID		ml
CRYSTALLOID	L/R/NS/HTS ml	
TOURNIQUET	Time on / Time off	
Collar / C spine / Back board		
HEMOSTATIC DEVICE		
OXYGEN	Liters/min	
RBC		Units
FFP		Units
CRYO		Units
Plts		Packs
Fresh Whole Bld		Units
rFVIIa		mcg/kg
EXT Fixation		Extremity

AM Amputation   BL Bleeding   D Deformity   H Hematoma
AV Avulsion   B Burn   F Foreign Body L Laceration
P Puncture   X Fracture   S Stab Wnd   G Gunsh Wnd

Vent On / Off	ICU in / Out	SPECIALTY
OR Start / Stop		
PROVIDER		

Index